OTHER BOOKS ON COLONIAL AUSTRALIA BY THE AUTHOR

IN FOR THE LONG HAUL
The First Fleet Voyage and Colonial Australia:
The Convicts' Perspective

ANDREW THOMPSON
From Boy Convict to
Wealthiest Settler in Colonial Australia

www.annegrethall.com

DOCTOR REDFERN

*Mutineer, Convict,
Medical Pioneer, Rights Activist*

ANNEGRET HALL

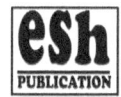

First published in 2023.

Copyright © Annegret Hall 2023
www.annegrethall.com

ESH Publication, Nedlands 6009, Australia.

All reasonable attempts have been made to communicate with copyright holders of the images reproduced in this book. Any corrections to information provided about these images should be communicated to the author.

This book is copyright. Apart from any fair dealing for the purpose of private study, research, criticism or review, as permitted under the *Copyright Act*, no part of this book may be reproduced by any process without written permission from the author.

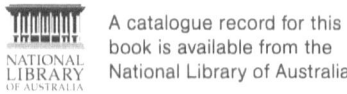 A catalogue record for this book is available from the National Library of Australia

ISBN: 978 0 9876292 4 1 (paperback)
ISBN: 978 0 9876292 5 8 (ebook)

Cover images:
Front – A portrait of William Redfern painted in 1832 by George Mather, courtesy of the State Library of New South Wales (PXA 2144/Box 86, 84. Pic.Acc.2406) reproduced with the permission of Damian Greenish.
Back – Part of an 1817 painting by Edward Close showing the harbour of Sydney Cove and the Macquarie Street hospital on the hill to the left, courtesy of the State Library of New South Wales (SAFE/PXA 1187).

Text set in Garamond typeface

Printed in Australia by Ingram Lightning Source

To

my parents

Margret & Friedel

Contents

Chapter 1	Surgeon's Mate	1
Chapter 2	Mutiny at the Nore	7
Chapter 3	Court Martial	17
Chapter 4	Banished to NSW	36
Chapter 5	Norfolk Island	47
Chapter 6	Norfolk Farmer & Trader	66
Chapter 7	Medical Qualifications	86
Chapter 8	Sydney Hospital Surgeon	97
Chapter 9	The Rum Hospital	109
Chapter 10	Miss Sarah Wills	123
Chapter 11	Medical Pioneer	135
Chapter 12	Mountain Crossing	153
Chapter 13	Bank Director	167
Chapter 14	Calm Before the Storm	181
Chapter 15	The Inquisitor	192
Chapter 16	The Slaughter House	206
Chapter 17	Rights Activist	222
Chapter 18	Angel of Discord	239
Chapter 19	A New Governor	254
Chapter 20	Fractious Times	269
Chapter 21	Edinburgh Finale	287
Epilogue		307
Maps & Illustrations		viii
Conversion Chart		x
Acknowledgements		313
Bibliography		314
Notes		320
Index		346

MAPS & ILLUSTRATIONS

Page

6   Surgical instrument set, London 1810-1812. (WL: zava88mp)

9   Etching of seamen complaining of their rations from *Cassell's Illustrated History of England*, Vol 6, 1865.

11 Etching of the mutiny at Portsmouth from Frederick Whymper, *The Sea: Its Stirring Story of Adventure, Perily & Heroism*, Vol 1, 1887.

28 Etching of the Coldbath Fields Prison, Clerkwell in 1798. (WL: 37714i)

30 A page from Redfern's notebook. (SLNSW: MAV/FM3/709)

33 Etching of the gate to the Coldbath Fields Prison in *The Criminal Prisons of London* by Henry Mayhew.

37 1829 etching of a prison hulk in Portsmouth by Edward Cooke. (NLA: nla.obj-135934086)

53 1798 etching of Sydney on Norfolk Island by Wilson Lowry. (NLA: nla.obj-135681919)

54 Record of sick, death and birth on Norfolk Island. (TNA: CO201/29)

56 Watercolour by John Eyre of Queenborough on Norfolk Island in 1804. (SLNSW: SV8/Norf I/2)

65 Excerpts from Redfern's notebook. (SLNSW: MAV/FM3/709)

69 Map of Norfolk Island showing settlement areas.

72 Silhouette of D'Arcy Wentworth in ca 1815. (SLNSW: PXA 2100/Box 38)

72 Miniature portrait of Captain John Piper in 1815. (SLNSW: MIN 75)

76 Portrait of Philip Gidley King in ca 1800-1805. (SLNSW ML: MIN 62)

76 Portrait of William Bligh painted by Alexander Huey in 1814. (NLA: nla.obj-136207002)

89 View of Sydney from the western side of the Cove painted by George Evans in 1803. (SLNSW: XV1/1803/1)

93 View of Sydney Cove painted by George Evans in 1802 and engraved in 1804 by F. Jukes. (SLNSW DX: DL Pf 121a)

99 View of Sydney from the western side of the Cove painted by John Eyre in 1806. (SLNSW DX: XV/201)

103 View of Sydney Cove painted by John Eyre in 1808. (SLNSW XV1/1808/9)

108 Miniature portrait of Elizabeth Macquarie in 1810. (SLNSW ML: MIN 70)

108 Portrait of Lachlan Macquarie painted by John Opie in ca 1805. (SLNSW ML: ML 37)

118 An 1811 drawing of the new General Hospital. (TNA: CO 201/57)

125 Miniature portrait of William Redfern painted in Edinburgh in August 1832 by George Marshall Mather, courtesy of Damian Greenish. (SLNSW ML: PXA 2144/Box 86, 84. Pic.Acc.2406)

125 Miniature portrait of Sarah Redfern in c. 1815 by unknown artist, courtesy of Damian Greenish. (SLNSW ML: PXA 2144/Box 86, 84. Pic.Acc.2406)

126 Watercolour of St Philip's Church by George Evans in 1809. (SLNSW ML: PXD 388)

127 Town plan of Sydney by James Meehan at Governor Bligh's request in 1807. (NLA: MAP F 105B)

140 Government House painted by George Evans in 1809. (SLNSW ML: PXD 388)

156 Painting of track across Blue Mountains by John Lewin in 1815. (SLNSW ML: PXE 888)

158 Bathurst Plains painting by John Lewin in 1815. (SLNSW ML: V*/Expl/2)

169 Painting of Sydney hospital seen from Darlinghurst by Joseph Lycett in 1818. (SLNSW: SAFE/PXE 1072)

172 Part of an 1840 map of Port Jackson by W. Meadows Brownrigg. (SLNSW: Z/M3 811.15/1840/2)

193 Portrait of Commissioner John Bigge painted by Thomas Uwins in 1819. (SLNSW: P2/290)

211 Lithograph of the new Sydney hospital by Frederick Terry in the late 1860s. (NLA: 2407 #S1997)

219 Part of an 1840 map of the Country of Cumberland by W. Wells showing Redfern's Campbellfield estate. (NLA: MAP F 263)

224 Pencil drawing of Campbellfield by Steve Roach in 1963, courtesy of Andrew Thomson.

241 Portrait of William Wentworth ca 1848. (SLNSW: PXA 2100/Box 38);

241 Portrait of William Wentworth by James Anderson in 1872. (SLNSW ML: ML 411)

246 Engraving of the University of Edinburgh in 1820 by J. & H. Storer, *Views in Edinburgh and its vicinity*.

253 View of Sydney by Joseph Lycett in 1825. (SLNSW: MRB/F980.1/L)

263 Portrait of Sir Thomas Brisbane engraved by Frederick Bromley from painting by Robert Frain in 1842. (SLNSW ML: P3/230)

263 Portrait of Ralph Darling painted by John Linnell in 1825. (NLA: nla.obj-134769948)

280 Engraving of buildings on George Street by John Carmichael in 1829. (SLNSW: PXB 359/no. 3)

294 Engraving of Moray Place in Edinburgh in 1829 by T. H. Shepherd, *Modern Athens, displayed in a series of views; or Edinburgh in the nineteenth century*.

298 Engraving of University of Edinburgh in 1829 by W. Lizars. (WL: 17093i)

299 Engraving of Surgeons' Square in Edinburgh in 1830 by T. Barber. (WL: 17457i)

312 Family trees of William and Sarah Redfern

CONVERSION CHART

For historical accuracy, imperial measurements have been retained in the text.

1 foot (ft)	30 centimetres
1 mile	1.6 kilometres
1 nautical mile (nm)	1.85 kilometres
1 acre	4047 square metres
1 gallon	4.5 litres
1 pint	0.57 litres
1 ton	1016 kilograms
1 pound (lb)	0.46 kilograms
1 bushel wheat	27.2 kilograms
1 bushel maize	25.4 kilograms
1 pound Sterling (£)	20 shillings Sterling
1 crown	5 shillings Sterling
1 shilling (s)	12 pence Sterling
1 penny (d)	1/240th of 1 pound Sterling

To preserve historical authenticity, quotations in the body of the text are given verbatim with original spelling and grammar. Occasional insertions have been made, bounded by square brackets, to assist comprehension.

Chapter 1

SURGEON'S MATE

The rank-and-file of medical practitioners throughout the country was not of high type. Anyone could set himself up as a general practitioner, and there was no control whatever over medical practice before the Apothecaries' Act of 1815. Medical training in the eighteenth century was almost entirely by apprenticeship to older practitioners, and unless a man wished to become a consultant, or to achieve promotion in one of the services, he rarely troubled to take a degree from one of the universities. John Comrie, 1935[1]

William Redfern sat staring at the glimmer of daylight piercing the narrow vent near the roof of his cell in the Coldbath Fields prison. He and his shipmates had spent the last three years in the cruellest gaol in England for the 1797 mutiny on Royal Navy ships at the Nore. So brutal was their confinement that many claimed the sailors dangling from the yardarm had got the better deal. The 25-year-old Redfern was bitter and dejected at his involvement in this affair. He had seen the protests on his ship HMS *Standard* as a plea by sailors for better food and pay, and it seemed inconceivable that the government had construed their demands as mutiny. In any case he was appalled at being drawn into the protests and, even worse, at being seen to encourage them. He was, after all, only a surgeon's mate, a non-commissioned officer of low rank, who had played no part in the issues being contested. But all such reasoning had little value now – the mutineers were being treated like vermin and surrounded by death; he believed his days were numbered.

The solitary confinement had seriously depressed Redfern and led him to question his very reason for being. He cursed his tendency to try and right the wrongs of the world, and for being at all involved in other peoples' problems. In the depths of his despair Redfern blamed his righteous upbringing, but his affection for his family quickly suppressed such thoughts. He had been raised to believe that equity and justice were fundamental rights, and that these rights were worth fighting for. Placed in the same situation again, he probably would have acted no differently. Not that this mattered; recrimination would not reverse the charge of mutiny or the life sentence of transportation *Beyond the Seas*. For now, he had to focus on surviving long enough to get out of this putrid prison.

Details of William Redfern's early life have largely been lost. Prior to 1785 there are no records of his family in England, Ireland or Canada.[2] This was an era when birth, marriage and death dates were not routinely kept, and few early immigration papers have survived. Much more is known about imprisoned felons than law-abiding commoners in 18th century Britain.

Based on the 1797 HMS *Standard* muster log, William Redfern was born in 1775 in Canada.[3] It seems that his parents Robert and Margaret Redfern left Ireland in the 1760s and migrated, along with many other Northern Irish and Scottish Protestants, to Nova Scotia Canada. Around 1785 Robert and Margaret with their sons Thomas aged 22, Robert 16, William 10 and Joseph 1, returned to Britain where they opened a saddlery in Trowbridge, Wiltshire. Here Robert Jr was apprenticed to his father, and Thomas studied to be a surgeon, opening an apothecary in 1789 with surgeon John Dodd. Fluent in French and Latin, 15-year-old William completed school in 1790 and began an apprenticeship in surgery with his brother Thomas.[4] An apprenticeship was the usual way to become a surgeon or physician because of the exorbitant cost of university studies. Apprentices and university students sat the same final examination before the Company of Surgeons and serving in the army or navy offered the same future job opportunities.

With sons Thomas and William securely employed, the Redfern parents moved back to Belfast accompanied by Robert Jr and Joseph. Soon after, Robert Redfern Sr bought James Martin's saddlery on Castle Street Belfast and specialised in leather accessories for horses, coaches and carts.[5] Two more Redfern children were born in 1792 and 1796, daughters Margaret and Eliza, respectively.

From early childhood William Redfern was a prolific reader and, in his lifetime, he would accumulate thousands of books on medical and classical literature.[6] One of his earliest acquisitions was *A Treatise on the Theory and Practise of Midwifery* by William Smellie, given to him by John McMullin in 1794. This book is today in the RACP (Royal Australasian College of Physicians) History of Medicine Library in Sydney. William continued his apprenticeship until 1796 when he moved to London to finish his studies.[7]

The earliest record of William Redfern's life is from the 25 May 1796 entry in his notebook; a book he would retain and treasure for the rest of his life. On that day, Redfern sailed on the schooner *Hibernia* from Dublin to Porto in Portugal, arriving on 16 June and the next day meeting for breakfast with the English Consul John Hitchcock. A week later he sailed back to London, arriving on 17 July 1796.[8] It seems likely William was an assistant to the surgeon on the *Hibernia* and had visited his family in Ireland before starting his career in the navy the following year. As his short erratic life in the navy unravelled, this may have been the last time he saw his mother and father.

On 19 January 1797, after seven year's training as a surgeon and physician, the 22-year-old Redfern sat before the examiners of the Company of Surgeons in London to get his accreditation.[9] Shortly after this he was accepted into the Royal Navy with qualifications to become either a physician on all rates of warships or a surgeon on warships of third-rate and below. First-rate warships carried up to 100 cannons and a crew of over 1000 men, whereas the smaller third-rate warships carried fewer guns and crew. On 23 January 1797 Redfern received a warrant from the Sick and Hurt Board to be a Surgeon's First Mate on HMS *Standard* in Yarmouth harbour, captained by Thomas Parr. HMS *Standard* was a third-rate full-rigged battleship of 64 guns, 159 feet (48.5 m) long, 44 feet (13.5 m) beam and a crew of 491 men – it was part of Admiral Duncan's North Sea Fleet. The newly qualified William Redfern boarded HMS *Standard* on 23 January where he was recorded in the ship's log as a 22-year-old surgeon's first mate, born in Canada.[10]

When Redfern joined the navy, Britain had been at war with the Spanish, French and Dutch for four years, and the inhabitants of the British Isles were burdened down by the constant threat of invasion. Rumours abounded that Austria, Britain's last ally, was seeking peace with France, and that the French intended joining the Spanish and the Dutch to invade Britain. Adding to external threats, clandestine networks of republicans in the country, encouraged by the French Revolution and inspired by Thomas Paine's 1791 publication the *Rights of Man*, wanted to overthrow the monarchy and the government. The Tory government of William Pitt the Younger was wary of seditious activities and carried out an active campaign of repression.

Two separate naval fleets guarded Britain against invasion. The Channel Fleet, commanded by Admiral Lord Bridport was anchored in Spithead outside Portsmouth on the south coast. The North Sea Fleet, commanded by Admiral Adam Duncan, comprised two groups: one anchored at the Yarmouth Roads just off Great Yarmouth in Norfolk, the other off the Nore sandbank in the Thames River Estuary. Duncan's responsibility was to deter Dutch warships from attacking Britain along the eastern coastline.

On HMS *Standard* in Yarmouth, William Redfern was first mate to the ship's surgeon Robert Kirkwood, and had a young assistant (a loblolly boy) to help him. Next to Kirkwood's cabin, Redfern occupied a small dispensary only large enough for a medicine chest and a small desk.[11] As a first mate, he slept in a hammock between cannons with the rest of the non-commissioned crew.

Medical practitioners at that time were generally addressed as surgeons, physicians or apothecaries. However, Royal Navy ship surgeons covered all three duties and were expected to treat every medical condition. Accompanied by the surgeon's mate, a surgeon saw patients at least twice a day and kept a journal on each patient. As well as treating injured sailors, he attended to the daily sick calls at the mainmast. During sea battles, the surgeon worked in the ship's cockpit, a protected area in the rear part of the orlop, the lowest deck on the ship. Here, a space near a hatchway was permanently partitioned off for wounded men to be lowered into the cockpit. This was a relatively safe place to treat the wounded but, being near the gun decks, the blasts of cannons made it a deafening hellhole. At other times the ship's sickbay was located on a higher deck where there was more air and light. In addition to treating the sick and wounded, surgeons were responsible for enforcing hygiene aboard the ship.[12]

The health of the ship's crew was especially important to the navy as common seamen were responsible for most duties on the warships and did the bulk of fighting during a naval action. Their ability to do hard physical labour was essential. Despite Admiralty regulations aimed at ensuring the crew's health, more Royal Navy sailors died from illness than from enemy action. Medical practices were under continual review and many naval surgeons published ways to improve health standards aboard warships.[13]

The most common health threat to sailors was scurvy (*scorbutus*) caused by a lack of vitamin C in the diet. This disease presented as sore joints, fever, ulcers, bleeding under the skin, rotting gums and slow wound healing, and, if left untreated, death soon followed. The non-perishable foods commonly provided to seamen were biscuits, salt beef, pork, cheese and salt fish. All lacked the vital ingredient of vitamin C, and, although the surgeon James Lind had advised the navy in the 1740s that citrus fruits reduced scurvy, no real attempt was made to improve ship diets until much later. The Admiralty did suggest antiscorbutic supplements such as essence of malt mixed with wine, sauerkraut and wort of malt though these only partly helped. Lind published his work in 1753 but it was not until Gilbert Blane advocated citrus fruits in 1795 that it was accepted.[14]

Another devastating maritime illness was 'ship fever' (*typhus*), transmitted through lice often present in unhygienic overcrowded conditions and dirty clothing. Although most surgeons encouraged personal hygiene through regular use of soap and clean clothing, the Admiralty regulations intended to minimise this disease were not routinely enforced. It was usually left to the discretion of the ship surgeon as to what preventive actions were needed to avoid the spread of typhus. Other ailments routinely reported to the ship's sickbay were dysentery, smallpox, venereal disease, stones (kidney and bladder), intoxication, tooth decay and the seasonal diseases of catarrh and rheumatism. Adding to the constant threat of disease, sailors faced many physical dangers on board a warship. When the red-hot cannons were not blasting away on multiple decks, the precarious task of rigging the enormous sails at great heights tested the fittest of men, even in calm weather. Shipboard injuries were a daily occurrence and the wounds inflicted during sea battles often led to limb amputations.

Many of the diseases encountered by ship surgeons had no known cure in the 18th century and, consequently, most medical treatments were palliative. The more dedicated ship surgeons sought ways to limit illness by increasing air circulation below decks, improving nutrition, promoting safe practices and ensuring adequate clothing.[15] Regular fumigation of ships was used to expel the foul odours of the bilge water and to destroy insect and rodent infestations. This involved the burning of gunpowder, brimstone (sulphur), tar oil, tobacco or vinegar between decks; fumigation practices were not without their own health hazards.[16]

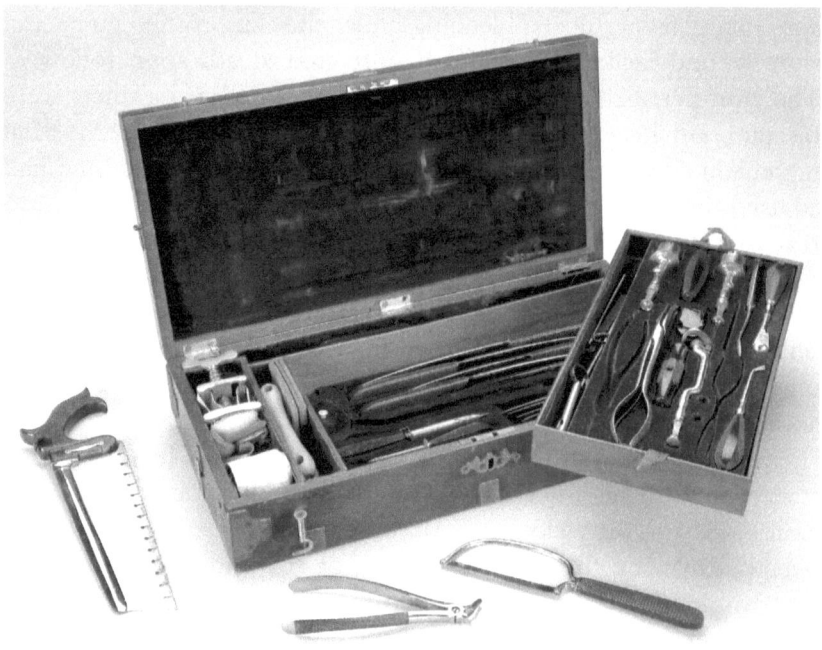

Surgical instruments used by British army surgeons in 1810. William Redfern would have used similar instruments.

First Mate William Redfern was now fully ensconced in this challenging maritime world and, although his life as a surgeon's mate on HMS *Standard* was to be brief, it gave him a short intense internship in practicing medicine on a Royal Navy warship. Later in life this would lead him to write influential guidelines for preventing diseases on ships transporting convicts.

Chapter 2

MUTINY AT THE NORE

At present we are all quiet in our Fleet; and, if Government hang some of the Nore Delegates, we shall remain so. I am entirely with the Seamen in their first Complaint. We are a neglected set, and, when peace comes, are shamefully treated; but, for the Nore scoundrels, I should be happy to command a Ship against them. Horatio Nelson, 30 June 1797[1]

Prior to commencing duties aboard HMS *Standard* in Yarmouth harbour in January 1797, First Mate William Redfern had little or no knowledge of the parlous state of common seamen in the Royal Navy. Discontent among sailors had become much more than the usual grievances voiced below decks where grumbles about harsh discipline aboard Royal Navy ships had existed for centuries and were an accepted part of naval life. The anger fermenting in 1797 was quite different and much more serious – it centred on the non-payment and unfairness of wages, an existential issue for the lives of seamen and their families. Many sailors in the British fleets had received no pay for over a year, and the wages of the lower ranks had not changed for over a century – nor had their pensions.

Pitiful pay was not the only issue. Recruitment of common seamen had become haphazard and brutal. Four years of war with continental enemies had depleted ships of sailors who had signed up voluntarily and they were replaced by men forcefully enlisted by press gangs that scoured ports and taverns. Even homeward-bound merchant ships were boarded to compel men to sail for the Crown. On some warships half of the lower ranks, many of them Irish, served against their will.[2] The surliness and incompetence of pressed crewmen was eroding the morale of the professional sailors in the Royal Navy and led to increased desertions.

To prevent further loss of crew some naval captains started to refuse shore leave, effectively imprisoning seamen on their own ships. Sailors protested that the navy treated them 'more like convicts than free-born Britons', complaining that shipboard punishments, which had always been harsh, were now tyrannical.³ Seamen were poorly fed, underpaid and received little medical care. Even trivial offences incurred flogging that was so excessive sailors preferred 'to throw themselves off the yards into the sea rather than face the skinning they were promised'. Others protested vehemently that they were being 'treated worse than the dregs of London Streets'.⁴

Reinforcing the ferment among lower ranks was a belief that the Admiralty was intentionally depriving the backbone of the navy of their basic rights and that the treatment of seamen had not improved since Samuel Pepys reorganised the Royal Navy in the 17th century. The aspirations of ordinary seamen now matched the rising expectations of the working class across Britain, and they no longer accepted the brutal naval discipline or that the orders of officers could not be challenged. Apart from the inadequacy and non-payment of wages, the abysmal food rations and medical care for ordinary seamen had to change. The inconsistent enforcement of navy regulations meant that the wellbeing of seamen hinged on the competence of their commanding officer. Since the capability and compassion of officers varied greatly, so did the conditions on ships. Often drinking water was so foul that the grog ration, served twice a day, was the only liquid drinkable, and this invariably led to drunkenness and accidents.

In February 1797, only a month after William Redfern had joined the Navy, the sailors on four ships in the Channel Fleet at Spithead sent a joint formally-worded petition to Admiral Lord Richard Howe, Chief of the Navy, asking that seamen's wages be paid and increased. When no response was received, further polite requests were made. The seamen took special care that no sign of disobedience existed on the four ships. Ironically, it was probably for this reason alone that Admiralty officials ignored the petitions arguing that these conditions had existed for generations, so why change it because of a few malcontents?⁵

Eleven carefully worded petitions to Howe went unanswered. This would soon have far-reaching consequences; the Admiralty had completely misjudged the determination of the seamen to resolve longstanding grievances. Sailors aboard some ships elected delegates to handle future negotiations but to avoid an overreaction, informed the Admiralty that the war readiness of ships would not be affected. The admirals, who had never negotiated with lower ranks before, were astonished at the insolence and immediately ordered the Channel Fleet at Spithead be put to sea. When the order was given to the Channel Fleet in April 1797 to weigh anchor, seamen aboard 16 ships refused, and the fleet remained at Spithead. A mortified Admiralty realised that this was far more than a petty grievance and, with Britain at war they had a potential mutiny on their hands! Indeed, the military's definition of 'mutiny' was any unlawful attempt to seize authority, an offence that carried the death penalty.

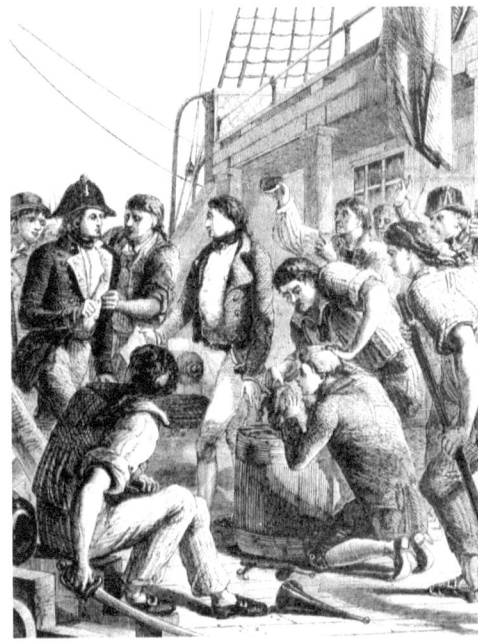

Etching of seamen on a Royal Navy warship protesting about their food and pay prior to the 1797 Nore mutiny.

Because of Britain's war footing, the Admiralty resisted sending armed Royal Marines to make widespread arrests; without crew replacements, this would have totally disabled the Channel Fleet. Instead, each ship captain was ordered to muster ordinary seamen and have them assign two delegates to compile a list of grievances. The non-payment of unfair wages headed these lists, followed by five other issues: food rations should be larger and better quality; flour must not be substituted for meat when in port; fresh vegetables be provided more often; the care of the sick must be improved; shore leave granted when in port; men wounded in action be paid until cured and discharged.[6]

On seeing the complaints, the senior physician of the Channel Fleet, Thomas Trotter, challenged delegates on their concerns about health care. He claimed that since 1795 he had insisted that fresh vegetables and meat be distributed to ships to reduce illness, and lemons be provided as a cure for scurvy. The delegates pointed out that his orders were repeatedly ignored, and many men still perished from diseases and avoidable accidents.[7] After a few weeks of discussions with the government, Admiral Lord Howe successfully steered a bill through the British Parliament for improving working conditions in the Royal Navy. On 15 May 1797 the Channel Fleet dispute was peacefully resolved after delegates agreed to a series of proposals: better pay and working conditions; that several unpopular officers be retired; and that a pardon be granted to seamen involved in the dispute.

While negotiations were taking place on the Channel Fleet ships at Spithead, Admiral Duncan and North Sea Fleet captains at Yarmouth ignored similar complaints from their crews. Duncan declared that his men were 'perfectly satisfied and orderly'.[8] The reality was quite different. The concerns of North Sea Fleet seamen were identical to those of the Channel Fleet, and their anger became white hot when their compatriots at Spithead were offered better conditions and they were not.

A key concern of the North Sea Fleet sailors was an urgent need for better health care. There had been a major outbreak of ship's fever aboard HMS *Sandwich*, the 90-gun flagship of the fleet with 1500 men, currently stationed near the Nore sandbank in the Thames Estuary. Typhus infections were so high that weeks earlier Captain Mosse of HMS *Sandwich* had sent Admiral Duncan a report from the ship's Surgeon John Snipe expressing alarm at the virulence among seamen who were dirty and 'bare of common necessaries'. Surgeon Snipe requested a reduction of men on the ship to prevent further contagion, stating that he had never been 'in a situation more replete with anxiety, than the present as Surgeon of the *Sandwich*'.[9]

On 12 May 1797, with typhus still rampant, seamen took control of HMS *Sandwich*. News of the seizure soon reached the other North Sea Fleet ships at Yarmouth, and several mutinied and sailed to the Nore to join the flagship on which sailors had elected delegates to present their demands to the Admiralty. Able Seaman

Richard Parker on HMS *Sandwich* was elected 'President of Delegates'. Requests to rectify grievances were first made to the ships' captains and any refusals were reported to the delegate committee. One such report stated that the captain of HMS *Director*, the 45-year-old William Bligh – who had previously been involved in the mutiny on the HMS *Bounty* and later would become Governor of New South Wales – refused to hand over the ship's arsenal, or to gaol three unpopular officers. He was removed from his ship on 19 May.[10]

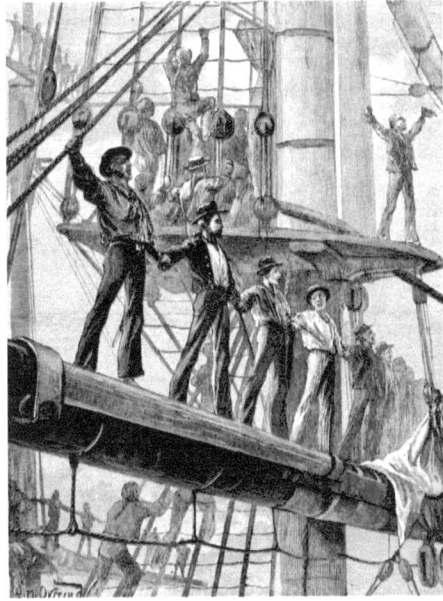

Etching of sailors protesting on the yard arm of a Royal Navy warship during the 1797 Nore mutiny.

Encouraged by the success of the Channel Fleet and newspaper articles hostile to the government, the seamen compiled a list of complaints.[11] The following day, their delegates met aboard HMS *Sandwich* and issued their demands to Admiral Charles Buckner, with a request for the same 'indulgences' granted to the Channel Fleet. These included pardons for all seamen, increased wages paid before departing for sea, shore leave when in port, and that no officer removed from the ships should return without consent of the crew. Additional demands were made that any seaman who had deserted his ship, and returned, should not be charged with desertion; that prize money from captured vessels be more fairly distributed among crew; and that the Articles of War be made more moderate.[12]

These demands went further than those of the Channel Fleet, and the Admiralty flatly refused to consider them. The situation worsened when two Navy frigates were fired upon when trying to leave their moorings at the Nore. *The London Chronicle* reported on 27 May that the mutineers had now begun to block the movement of ships in the Thames Estuary and refused a free passage of the river to private vessels.[13]

> The Seamen wanted Lord Howe to Negotiate with them, they wished for a procession of their delegates; and absolute refused to return to their duty till the same honours were paid them that had been shewn to the delegates at Portsmouth. The Admiralty endeavoured to pass over this conduct without notice, but the forbearance of Government only irritated the mutineers. They fired on two frigates that were putting to sea, compelling the crews to join them, and at last they actually blocked up the Thames, refusing a free passage up and down the River to London trade. They thought this a certain way of extorting compliance from the Admiralty, and they have succeeded.[14]

Londoners, who had previously backed the protesting seamen, became increasingly nervous and their support vanished entirely when the blockade threatened the city's economy. Newspaper editors took different sides – some supported the seamen and blamed their conduct on the government. The parliamentary Whig party sympathised with the seamen's efforts to improve conditions and blamed the Tory government for the disruption.[15] But this did not help and increasingly newspapers favoured the government.

With William Redfern still aboard HMS *Standard* stationed at Yarmouth, *The Hampshire Chronicle* wrote on 27 May that there had been 'enough concessions' to the mutineers and 'the refractory seamen must be brought back to their duty by other than lenient and palliative measures'.[16] The public mood was changing.

In late May 1797 the Admiralty closed the naval hospital at Sheerness on the Thames after renegade delegates visited seamen recovering there. When the patients accused two surgeons with maltreatment, the delegates threatened them to such an extent that one ran away and the other committed suicide.[17]

Captain Bligh, whose views on crew behaviour were listened to by the Admiralty, was appointed as an intermediary in the dispute. He boarded the North Sea Fleet warships remaining in Yarmouth and discussed with seamen if they would follow orders to attack the protesting ships at the Nore. Having talked with seamen on several ships, Bligh reported to the Admiralty that it would be unwise to expect sailors of the same fleet to fire upon each other.[18]

By mid-May 1797 eight ships of the North Sea Fleet remained at Yarmouth, but few were under Admiral Duncan's direct control. When the Admiralty instructed Duncan that these ships might be required to attack ships anchored at the Nore, he advised against it. However, he informed the Admiralty that he would not hesitate to take drastic action if the problem could not be solved in another way. He suggested HMS *Sandwich* might be 'cut adrift in the night and let her go on the sands, that the scoundrels may drown; for until some example is made they will not stop'.[19] On 26 May, Duncan was instructed to prepare the Yarmouth ships for action against the mutineers at the Nore. News of this order was leaked to the Yarmouth crews – they were outraged. But fate intervened.

With England still at war, Duncan was informed that the Dutch fleet was preparing to leave its sheltered harbour and the North Sea Fleet must blockade the Dutch coast. Most Yarmouth sailors considered Duncan's order for the blockade to be a ploy. They imprisoned their officers and prepared to sail for the Nore, leaving Duncan with two ships. Fortunately, the Dutch never attacked.[20]

On 29 May, HMS *Standard*, anchored at Yarmouth, hoisted a red flag to show that protesting seamen had taken control of the ship. Several officers were sent ashore but First Mate William Redfern remained on board.[21] With a red flag flying above the mainsail HMS *Standard* sailed for the Nore to join the other North Sea Fleet ships stationed there.[22] The decision to take control of HMS *Standard* was not unanimous among the seamen but most understood that unity was crucial if their cause was to succeed. This had become an *all or nothing* dispute.

HMS *Standard* docked at the Nore on 31 May, the same day King George III issued 'A Proclamation for the Suppression of the mutinous and treasonable Proceedings of the Crew of certain ships at the Nore'.[23] All communication between the mutineer ships and the shore then ceased and soldiers were stationed along the Thames shoreline to prevent any landings.[24] By now, 26 ships had joined the mutiny. Realising that this dispute would not end peacefully, Redfern submitted a written request to Captain Parr for his discharge from the Navy. Parr refused to accept it.

From his short time aboard HMS *Standard* Redfern had come to appreciate the deep-seated distrust ordinary seamen had for officers and surgeons. In fact there was an almost irreconcilable barrier between sailors and the higher ranks. Throughout their life most of the men had been discriminated against by the upper classes, and though some officers had achieved their commission through merit, most had purchased them. The majority of officers expected common seamen to show the same subservience they received from servants ashore and, despite some attempts at reform, the Admiralty allowed this attitude to flourish in the navy. There were many recent occurrences of discrimination and incompetence. Seamen on HMS *Minotaur* accused their surgeon of mistreating the sick and wounded, not being qualified, ignoring patients for months and being drunk. They complained that men had died because the surgeon failed to provide the sick with adequate rations – some men who had sought his medical help had been told that 'a flogging would do them most good'.[25]

Such incidents were not isolated. The surgeon on HMS *Marlborough* was accused of cruelty and of withholding provisions intended for the sick. He had a sick 'living skeleton' flogged and had ordered an ill sailor to set maintop sails. The same surgeon had insisted a swelling on the sailor's head was due to an excess of oatmeal porridge and molasses. The seaman died the following day. Another surgeon had been tarred and feathered at the Nore for drinking heavily and being totally incapable of doing his duty.[26]

Because of a general distrust of medical care on naval ships anchored at the Nore, some surgeons were put in the brig or sent ashore. Invariably surgeons' mates were required to take over their duties. A week after the HMS *Standard* arrived at the Nore, William Redfern was ordered by the ship's committee to replace Surgeon Kirkwood. Redfern promptly requested, for the second time, to be discharged and offered a sum of money for permission to leave the ship.[27] But Captain Parr refused again, and Redfern was ordered to assume the duties of the ship's surgeon. He was now certain that his life was at risk.

With all shipping on the Thames at a standstill, the outcome of the dispute took a more serious turn. Most Londoners and newspaper editors now saw the disruptions in their revered navy as a catastrophe that would imperil the country, and support for the North Sea Fleet protesters vanished. Moreover, the Admiralty decided they had been far too lenient with the Channel Fleet seamen and were determined not to repeat the mistake. Supplies of fresh water and food to the mutineer ships were cut off and all shore contact was stopped. The government expected that famine and disease would soon force mutineers to cooperate. But the Nore protesters were not finished yet. They forced the blockaded ships on the Thames to provide them with essential supplies thus impeding hundreds of vessels and affecting thousands of London merchants and inhabitants.[28]

On 3 Jun 1797 Prime Minister Pitt brought on a bill intended to suppress the Nore mutiny and to outlaw the mutineers.[29] The government sought cross-party support for the bill claiming that the mutiny was revolutionary sedition instigated by societies such as the United Irishmen. This society aimed to unite all religions in Ireland and introduce parliamentary reforms similar to those in America or France. In April 1797 eleven United Irishmen had been arrested in Belfast and charged with 'Treasonable Practises' and imprisoned in Dublin's Kilmainham Gaol. Among them was William Redfern's 28-year-old brother Robert.[30] It is unknown if William knew of his brother's arrest while on HMS *Standard*, or whether the navy had made any connection between the Redfern brothers. If it had, it would prejudice William's future.

With the passing of a bill outlawing the Nore mutineers, Prime Minister Pitt mobilised the army and threatened to storm the ships unless the seamen abandon their cause and leaders. Disagreements among the seamen's delegates soon arose, and the crews on some ships began to surrender unconditionally, others were fired upon. The crew of HMS *Director* imprisoned the leading mutineers on their vessel on 30 May, and this encouraged similar actions on other ships. HMS *Gorgon* Captain John Dixon even proposed to the Admiralty that he assassinate the President of Delegates, Richard Parker, 'the monster he considered as the head and fount of all the disgraceful trouble'. However, the offer of 'so very desperate a measure' was refused.[31]

The noose was tightening around the necks of the mutineers. In a desperate attempt at reconciliation, delegates sought a general amnesty. Admiral Buckner agreed to give pardons to all seamen except the delegates and activists – the government was well aware that punishing all protesters was impossible since it would disable the North Sea Fleet and leave Britain undefended. Delegates on some ships suggested sailing to France but all crews refused; support for the protest delegates among seamen was rapidly collapsing. The level of public outrage at the mutiny became apparent on 9 June 1797 when the Marine Society of merchants and shipowners in London offered a reward of £100 to any person who would bring to public justice anyone involved.[32]

By 12 Jun 1797, only seven warships at the Nore flew the mutineer's red flag. This was the day that the crew of HMS *Standard* was persuaded by her first lieutenant to surrender and to escape up the Thames flying the blue flag of peace. The mutineer delegate on HMS *Standard*, William Wallace, shot himself the next day. First Mate William Redfern was discharged at Gravesend on 14 June 1797 and, because of an accusation that he had supported the mutiny, he was put in prison. The mutiny ended the next day when all ships at the Nore surrendered.[33] Despite previous assurances of a general amnesty for non-delegates, hundreds of ordinary seamen were accused of treason and gaoled.

William Redfern's premonition of how the protest would end had been correct, and he considered his life to be in jeopardy. Because he continued to perform surgeon duties aboard HMS *Standard* at the Nore, the decision whether he was an active participant in the mutiny would depend on the views of fellow crewmembers. They would need to vouch that he had been forced to continue as a surgeon and to cooperate with the mutineers. He also hoped that his two attempts to resign as surgeon's mate on HMS *Standard* would be accepted as evidence that he tried to disengage from the rebellious conduct on the ship.

Chapter 3

COURT MARTIAL

The Mutiny commenced without my knowledge and was carried to an enormous height without my concurrence. William Redfern, 23 Aug 1797[1]

Over 10,000 seamen on 26 warships anchored at the Nore had been involved in the month-long mutiny from May to June 1797. At its closure, 560 of the most prominent protesters, especially the elected delegates and committee members, were arrested and incarcerated in London prisons and hulk gaols on the Thames. Of these men, 412 were court martialed and sentenced to either death by hanging, prison or flogging, or given a pardon. Some death sentences were later commuted to imprisonment or transportation. The courts also tried to identify those belonging to the Republican underground – none were uncovered; no mutineer was found to have endorsed a revolution or any ideology unpatriotic to Britain.[2]

Captain William Bligh resumed command of HMS *Director* on 16 June 1797 before the court martial trials began. Although his seamen were the last to surrender, he persuaded the Admiralty to pardon most of his crew. The twelve sailors who did appear before a martial court were released. Bligh showed the same compassion to his sailors that he later exhibited as Governor of New South Wales to small settlers struggling with flood debts in 1806. James Dugan wrote in his book *The Great Mutiny*, 'William Bligh knew the value of a good foreman hanging from the yard-arm as an example to others, as contrasted with a good foreman with a bit of mutiny on his record, pacing round the forecastle inspiring them'.[3] Other captains followed Bligh's example and all subsequent court martial proceedings were affected by the humanity on these ships. The entire crew on HMS *Comet* and HMS *Lancaster* were exempted from trial and seamen court-martialled from HMS *Inflexible*, *Lion*, *Proserpine*, *Champion*, *Tysiphone*, *Pylades*, *Swan*, *Vestal*, *Isis*, *Agamemnon* and *Ranger* were pardoned by the courts.[4] Unfortunately for William Redfern, Captain Parr on HMS *Standard* showed no such leniency to the 28 men accused of mutiny on his ship – quite the reverse, in fact.

On 22 June 1797, a court martial held on HMS *Neptune* decided the fate of Richard Parker, the President of Delegates on HMS *Sandwich*. It was a foregone conclusion that he would be harshly punished. The case aroused enormous public interest with several newspapers printing the court martial proceedings in their entirety. The trial concluded on 26 June with Parker being found guilty of treason. He was hanged from the yardarm on HMS *Sandwich* four days later in front of the entire crew.[5] On the day of his execution *The Morning Post* wrote:

> There is much public regret for his fate. We can say nothing on the subject; but we earnestly hope that the conduct of Government may restore content and discipline in the Navy.[6]

Another 25 seamen from HMS *Sandwich* were court-martialled, with 15 sentenced to death and six eventually hanged. The court martial of mutineers from other ships followed. William Redfern was among the 28 accused men from HMS *Standard* imprisoned for a month in a London gaol before appearing before a court martial on 17 August 1797. They were charged with:

> … making and endeavouring to make a Mutinous Assembly and Assemblies on board our said Ship *Standard* and on board divers other Ships and Vessels …. on 26th Day of May last and for several days afterwards and for concealing traitorous and mutinous words spoken to the prejudice of His Majesty's Government and for being present at a Mutiny without their using their utmost Endeavours to suppress the same and for behaving themselves with Contempt to their Superior Officers in the Execution of their Duty and for disobeying the lawful Commands of their Superior Officers and for any of the said offences committed on or after the 26th Day of May last.[7]

On the court martial bench was Admiral Sir Thomas Pasley as President, Commodore Erasmus Gower, Captains John Markham, Edward Riou, Francis Laforey and Richard King. Acting in the role of prosecutor was Captain Thomas Parr of HMS *Standard*. In the first hearing, charges against seamen William Holdsworth, Henry Freeman, John Davis, Bartholomew Connery, William Jones, Samson Harris and Thomas Sael were heard. Six men were found guilty and sentenced to death; Harris was deemed only partly involved and sentenced to 200 lashes.[8]

On 22 August 1797 the court martial heard the charges against a second group of men from HMS *Standard*: John Burrows, Joseph Hudson, William Redfern, Thomas Linniss, Bryan Finn and Joseph Gloves. The trial of surgeon's mate William Redfern, the highest-ranking seaman to be court martialed for mutiny and one of the few men to have legal counsel, caused considerable public interest. Redfern was accused of being a member of the ship's delegate committee, carrying a suspicious document and circulating seditious material. When Redfern was arrested, a pair of pistols was found in a carrying bag that was allegedly his. The circumstantial evidence for William Redfern being culpable of mutinous behaviour appeared compelling.

With six men from HMS *Standard* already sentenced to death, Redfern knew that he faced an unsympathetic court and a hostile prosecutor. The court decided to hear the charges against these men separately. Assisted by a counsel, Redfern prepared a defence to refute any likely evidence of the prosecution witnesses – his life literally depended on him proving that he did not willingly support the mutiny.

At the hearing opening, prosecutor Captain Parr presented a letter to the court claiming, without revealing its contents, that it was in Redfern's handwriting and showed his involvement in the mutiny. The letter was unsigned, so Parr needed to prove that Redfern had written it and, in doing so, had colluded with the mutineers. Midshipman Hamilton Fitzgerald was called as the first prosecution witness. When asked by Parr if he had communicated with Redfern during the mutiny, he replied that while at the Nore Redfern asked him if he could get him a brace of pistols, and he had advised him against it. Redfern was then permitted to question the witness. He asked Fitzgerald if he had ever seen him using any weapons and the witness replied 'no'. Parr then asked Fitzgerald if Redfern's request for the pistols was linked to his support for the protest. He replied that when the mutiny was discussed, it 'was always generally condemned by Mr Redfern and every other officer'. Fitzgerald assured the court that Redfern's opposition to the mutiny remained unchanged even after the officers were disarmed and removed from command.[9]

Several additional witnesses were questioned by the prosecutor and cross-examined by Redfern. Parr asked Lieutenant Delafons if he had ever seen Redfern's writing, and, if so, could he tell if he wrote the letter shown in court. Delafons said he recognised Redfern's handwriting but was uncertain about the letter. The court briefly adjourned, and on resuming, the witness was advised that he did not have to 'swear on oath' that it was the prisoner's handwriting. Parr reframed the question as to whether Fitzgerald had sufficient knowledge of Redfern's handwriting to say that he 'believed the paper produced to be his writing'. He answered 'yes'. Redfern then cross-examined Delafons, asking how he knew his handwriting and whether he had knowledge of the letter before it was presented in court. Delafons first denied knowledge of the letter, but later in the trial admitted he had seen the letter before but had not read it.[10]

The next day, 23 August 1797, the seaman Arthur McLoghlan was called as a defence witness to explain how Redfern's actions on the ship may have been misconstrued as direct involvement in the mutiny:

> All hands were turned up upon the forecastle one morning. William Morris and William Holdsworth were standing abaft of the foremast and said to the people that they heard there was a grumbling against Mr Kirkwood acting as Surgeon the people all sung out with one voice turn him ashore and then Bill Holdsworth asked if they had any objection against Mr Redfern doing the duty as Surgeon they all said no that he had behaved very well to the sick since he had been on board the ship then Bill Holdsworth said he did not know whether Mr Redfern would do the duty as Surgeon but he said he Holdsworth would let us know in the evening then the people said that if he would not do it they would make him do it.[11]

McLoghlan added that it took another day before Redfern agreed to assume the duties of ship's surgeon. When he did, a letter, apparently written by Redfern, was read to seamen stating he 'would do as much as in his power to serve the sick'.[12]

Robert Kirkwood, the ship's surgeon on HMS *Standard*, was called as the next prosecution witness. He informed the court that during the mutiny he acted as surgeon only part of the time after being 'told by Mr William Redfern Surgeons Mate that the Ships Company had ordered him to do the duty of Surgeon'. From then on, he remained on board, though there was little to do as most sick were sent ashore. Captain Parr asked if Kirkwood had seen Redfern's handwriting. He replied that he had no recollection of seeing his writing but was acquainted with his style. Redfern then cross-examined the witness as follows:

Redfern	What do you mean by my acting as Surgeon?
Kirkwood	That the Prisoner did the whole duty of Surgeon.
Redfern	Do you think I did that to displease you?
Kirkwood	I don't know what was intended by it.
Redfern	Did you believe what I said respecting having received orders from the Ships company?
Kirkwood	I had no reason then to disbelieve it.
Redfern	Did you from your belief of it cease to act as Surgeon?
Kirkwood	Yes certainly.
Redfern	As you say there were some sick on board. Was it not necessary that some person should attend them?
Kirkwood	It certainly was.
Redfern	Did I ever send for you to attend the sick after you had ceased to act as Surgeon?
Kirkwood	To the best of my recollections the Prisoner did.
Redfern	Did you come in consequence of my application?
Kirkwood	I do not remember whether I did or not I was always in the habit of going up and down.
Redfern	Did I receive any orders from you after that time?
Kirkwood	Yes.
Redfern	What were those orders?
Kirkwood	One day when we supposed the Ships company would go away from the Nore I ordered him to get everything ready in case of accidents.
Redfern	Do you recollect giving any orders with respect to the sick?
Kirkwood	Not particularly.[13]

At this point prosecutor Parr interrupted the cross examination asking Kirkwood whether Redfern had shown any reluctance to displace him from his medical duties. To this Kirkwood replied that Redfern had twice told him that:

> the Ships company had ordered him to do the duty of Surgeon. I took no notice of it then, the next morning he repeated the same words to me and told me that the Ships company would speak to me but they never did. ... He said he was sorry they had done so it was not his wish that he did not want to be Surgeon of the Ship.[14]

In fact, Kirkwood's evidence was more favourable to Redfern

than he had expected. Both men had acted in a way that was more likely to calm than upset the mutineers. Redfern then called seaman Lancelot Nicholson as a defence witness. Nicholson stated that he was being examined by Redfern 'in the presence of a great number of sick' when Kirkwood came into the dispensary:

> While the ship was at the Nore one evening in the cock pit Mr Kirkwood came down said he had got orders to do no more duty as Surgeon. Mr Redfern told him not to think that he was making any interest to get preferment in it for he did not want to have any hand in it and he told him that he was obliged to do it by the consent of the Ships company.[15]

Nicholson said that Redfern had told Kirkwood in his presence that he had 'written for his discharge twice and offered a sum of money to get clear of being Surgeons Mate'.[16]

The prosecution then called Archibald Ingram, second master of HMS *Standard* as a witness. Parr asked him about the pistols found when prisoners disembarked at Gravesend. Ingram said that the loblolly boy had found two ship's pistols and pistol cartridges in a bag that had come from the dispensary where Redfern used to keep his medicine and other items. Parr asked the witness why this bag was searched? Ingram replied that the 'man was searching for some boots and shoes I believe for Mr Redfern which he had sent for' after being removed from the ship. William Redfern now cross-examined the witness, asking him if he had seen the bag being taken out of the dispensary? Ingram replied that he had not. 'Do you know how the arms came to be in the bag?' Redfern asked. 'Was there any lock on the bag' and was the dispensary 'generally kept locked or open?' The witness did not know.

There followed a lengthy questioning of witnesses by the court on whether the dispensary was usually locked or not, what happened there, who owned the bag and what else was in the bag. The court asked Ingram if he knew whether the bag belonged to Redfern. He did not. The witness said the loblolly boy had been sent to get Redfern's boots and shoes and after searching for them had 'brought that bag out' but did not say it was Redfern's. 'What did the Loblolly boy say on taking out the pistols?' the court asked Ingram. 'He asked if they were to go in the bag, I said no, by no means. I took one and the Master Mate took the other they were not loaded at the time'.[17]

Next, seaman Thomas Cheeseman was questioned as a witness

for the prosecution. He was asked if he had ever seen Redfern with the delegate committee of HMS *Standard*? He replied that he had seen him there after they had sailed to the Nore. Redfern parried with the questions, 'Do you know who were reckoned Committee men?' 'Yes, I do', Cheeseman replied. 'Was I ever known to be a member of the Committee?' 'Not that I ever heard of', was Cheeseman's response, adding, 'I never saw him but two times' there. When queried by the court on the reasons why Redfern was present in the committee, Cheeseman replied that it was because of the crew's objections to Surgeon Kirkwood. 'They said he did not properly attend the sick and they would sooner have Mr Redfern for Surgeon'. The attention of the court now focused on the letter allegedly written by Redfern and read to the entire crew of HMS *Standard*. 'What was the subject of the letter?' the court asked. That Redfern 'was agreeable to aid and assist during the time of the mutiny in serving the sick, I think', said Cheeseman. He was then asked whether he had seen, or knew, if the Committee had received any letter from Redfern. The witness responded that he did not know.[18]

This concluded the case of the prosecution, in which not one of their witnesses testified that Redfern had urged or incited mutiny. Much later in Australia Commissioner Bigge and others would claim the court martial trial proved that William Redfern incited mutineers to be 'more united amongst themselves'.[19] That was clearly not the case.

During these lengthy court hearings all prisoners were held on board HMS *Neptune*. In preparing to refute the charges, Redfern and his counsel had spent the whole night preparing a 30-page defence document. The next morning, 24 August 1797, when the martial court resumed, 'Prisoner Redfern delivered in a written Defence which was read by his Counsel'. In the opening paragraph Redfern submitted to the integrity of the 'Military Profession' for an 'impartial ... indulgent hearing'. Stating that, if he was 'found capable of Deliberately exiting Mutiny and Disaffection of inculcating Disorder and circulating Sedition of poisoning the minds and misapplying the strength of brave and honest Seamen', he freely consented to die.[20] He said he was confident that the court would 'Discriminate Infirmity from bad intention'. Redfern declared that the mutiny had commenced without his knowledge and had been carried out to an enormous height without his concurrence 'as appears from the evidence of the Witnesses adduced against me'. After the mutineers took command, he had worked with other officers 'to soothe and palliate' mutineers, prevent 'excess of violence' and to save their own lives.[21] Redfern then pleaded:

> That I alone of all the Gentlemen on board should have any connection with the Mutineers may at first excite some prejudice against me but the nature of my profession when considered will suggest a general and the prejudices for whatever cause entertained against Mr Kirkwood will assign a Particular reason whereby this circumstance may be advantageously explained. Being less known I was consequently less odious to those who imagined they had been healed with neglect and hardship.[22]

He asked the court why:

> I stand charged with making and encouraging Mutiny but what kind of a Mutiny can a man make by carrying a piece of paper concealed about his Clothes let whatever you please be contained in it or written upon it that is indeed a formidable Mutiny which is made in a man's pocket and which he can easily suppress with his Tobacco Box or smother with his Handkerchief?[23]

Redfern then compared his situation to that of the martyr Algernon Sidney, a Whig politician falsely accused and executed for plotting to overthrow the government of King Charles II.[24]

> Algernon Sidney was condemned by Jefferies upon writings found upon him without any proof of their emission and this sentence has since been condemned by Moral and informed Men of all parties.[25]

Redfern opened his defence of the accusations against him with the statement, 'I bear no ill will to any one but am warranted in using every likely mean to save my own life whatever may be the consequence to other persons'.[26] He stated that Midshipman Fitzgerald's evidence had shown that, as a trained surgeon, it had been necessary for him to provide service of 'a professional nature more connected with the Mutineers than any other officer because necessary to attend the sick'. Considering that the mutineers were in power, he reminded the court that the sick 'could not with any Humanity' be neglected. Redfern pointed out that during the mutiny, he had felt very unsafe and wished that the officers on the ship would 'oppose the Mutineers if necessary and to guard me in any attempt to escape on Shore which I have ever since the Mutiny began wished for with the greatest impatience'. Fitzgerald had confirmed that he had 'always condemned the Mutiny in all conversations as much as any other officer in the Ship'.[27]

A lengthy defence statement refuting the prosecution evidence of Lieutenant Delafons followed. Redfern said Delafons had little knowledge of his handwriting, and the letter in question was written in Latin, a language foreign to him. Redfern remonstrated that 'Captain Parr [seems] strangely eager to convict me' and had encouraged Delafons to say the letter was his when he had previously not been willing to swear this under oath. He added

> Captain Parr insists that he has a right to put his inquiries in all possible shapes till he can get out something to the purpose. When I by the advice of my Counsel make an objection which is instantly repelled and the Court is ordered to be cleared. ... this Interval is most unfortunate for me. It seems to have operated like a charm upon the Intellect of the witness.[28]

Redfern then challenged the value of Ingram's evidence. He claimed it proved only that a brace of unloaded ship's pistols with ammunition had been found in a bag, but it was not proven to be his. Additionally, the prosecution had made no attempt to uncover when and how these items had come into the bag, or whether he had used any arms at any time during the mutiny.[29] Redfern moved on to examine the evidence of Cheeseman and said:

> There is no satisfactory evidence that the letter read at the forecastle was very different from the contents of the paper produced in Court – nothing about being a Brother in the cause or in the least Degree of an inflammatory nature or tendency but a simple assurance that I would comply with their order and attend the sick as they desired till matters became composed and restored to their former course.[30]

Redfern concluded his defence thanking the court for 'this Indulgence and commits my life into their hands', pleading that the court be 'preserved from error' and he from an 'undeserved Death'.[31]

The next day, 25 August 1797, the court reconvened to read the verdict of the Judge Advocate for the six prisoners. It read:

Charges fully proved against John Burrows, Joseph Hudson, William Redfern and Thomas Linniss but recommended Joseph Hudson to his Majesty's clemency on account of his having received a wound in his Majesty's service at St Lucia which deprived him of his senses after having drank strong liquor and William Redfern on account of his professional situation leading him more among the Mutineers than the other officers were obliged to be. The Court finding the charges in part proved against Bryan Finn and Joseph Gloves sentenced the former to receive 300 lashes and the latter 250.[32]

It was the verdict Redfern had feared most. His only hope now was that his life would be spared by a King's pardon.

The extensive court martial records of this trial reveal no evidence that Redfern was sympathetic to the mutiny. Of course, it is entirely possible that the whole story of his involvement in the mutiny was never exposed in the court martial for political reasons – the government was sensitive to his Irish connections and to his professional standing. They certainly did not want to make William Redfern a martyr for the Republican cause. This might also explain the odd wording in the verdict, that 'his professional situation leading him more among the Mutineers than the other officers were obliged to be'. Surely that 'obligation' was not in itself reason enough to find him guilty and impose the death sentence. None of the evidence presented appears to show he advised the mutineers, and, throughout his life, Redfern maintained he never had. When 20 years later Commissioner Bigge wrote that William Redfern had been the 'Secretary to the Mutineers', he furiously rejected it declaring, 'I never wrote a line for any Mutineer nor for any person connected with the Mutiny; nor did I ever see Parker'.[33]

What is apparent from the court proceedings is that the Captain of HMS *Standard*, Thomas Parr, was determined to prove Redfern was part of the uprising. Parr's stance was in stark contrast to the humanity displayed by many other ship captains in the fleet, who gave wholesale pardons to crews participating in the protests. This suggests that William Redfern either played a part in the trouble aboard HMS *Standard* or that he had greatly offended the captain in some other way, and Parr was going to make him pay for it. Even at the age of 22, William was not known for his reticence or tact, and his court defence clearly displays a certain intellectual superiority and arrogance. Exhibiting such attributes as a junior rank in the Royal Navy would not have endeared him to those in command, and if Redfern had criticised poor health and victualling standards on HMS *Standard*, it certainly would have raised the ire of Parr, even if he was right. Warships were rigid workplaces where being correct was far less important than respect for senior officers and the navy tradition. The fact that Redfern twice applied to quit the Navy after a month's service suggests that he may have had personal conflicts with the captain or the ship's surgeon, and he realised that remaining on board during the protests would be dangerous on several fronts.

We may never know the true motivation of Captain Parr or, for that matter, of the court martial in convicting William Redfern. On the other hand, Parr showed little mercy to any of his men, when he had 28 of HMS *Standard's* crew prosecuted. Of the 26 warships involved in the mutiny, only six ships had some of their men sentenced to death. Of the 59 men given the death sentence for the Nore mutiny, 10 were from Parr's crew.[34]

In his 1953 talk on *The Life and Work of William Redfern*, Sir Edward Ford, Professor of Preventive Medicine, said:

> But the fact that he [Redfern] was selected for trial from the thousands of seamen in the great fleet … indicates that he played no minor part. … William Redfern, from the evidence of the Nore, stands out as a brave man who was impatient of injustice and ready to support his convictions with his life. He was an adviser of his fellows and was moved by their sufferings. These were characters on which were based his subsequent greatness as a pioneer in New South Wales.[35]

Ford's narrative suggests that Redfern had far more sympathy for the mutiny than the court proceedings, or Redfern himself, revealed. Nevertheless, it was a belief widely held in many Irish Republican circles during the 18th century.

On 4 Sep 1797, ten days after being sentenced, William Redfern was granted a pardon from hanging, as follows:

> John Hudson, William Redfern and Thomas Linniss … to grant them our Pardon for the said Crimes on the following Conditions. That the said William Redfern be kept in Solitary Confinement for one Year, and after the expiration of that Term he be Transported to the Eastern Coast of New South Wales or some one or other Islands adjacent for and during the Term of his natural Life.[36]

Shipmates Joseph Hudson and Thomas Linniss were kept for six months in solitary confinement, followed by four and a half years of hard labour on a hulk. John Burrows received no pardon and was hanged on HMS *Standard*. Unquestionably, Redfern was greatly relieved at his pardon but incensed at being transported to the other side of the world *for life*. Of the 28 mutineers from HMS *Standard* who stood trial in August 1797, ten were sentenced to death but only three were hanged. Six did hard labour on prison hulks – only Redfern's sentence was commuted to transportation for life. The other eighteen seamen received lesser sentences; three were flogged, seven imprisoned and eight were released.[37]

A total of 412 men were court-martialled for the Nore mutiny. Of the 59 sentenced to death, 29 were hanged aboard their ships before a full complement of crew. Nine seamen were given up to 380 lashes, and 29 were imprisoned. The rest were released and promptly sent back to their ships.[38] Many of the punished seamen were unable to cope with the floggings or the mental stress of the imprisonment. The Fleet physician Thomas Trotter noted 'an unusual despondency and dejection of spirits among the patients in the different sick berths. The outrageous fury of late proceedings had subsided; and the horror induced by some awful examples of punishment was now operating'.[39] Some seamen were so ill with frequent fits of hysteria, convulsions and violent outbreaks of weeping characteristic of shock, that they had to be transferred to the hospital ship.

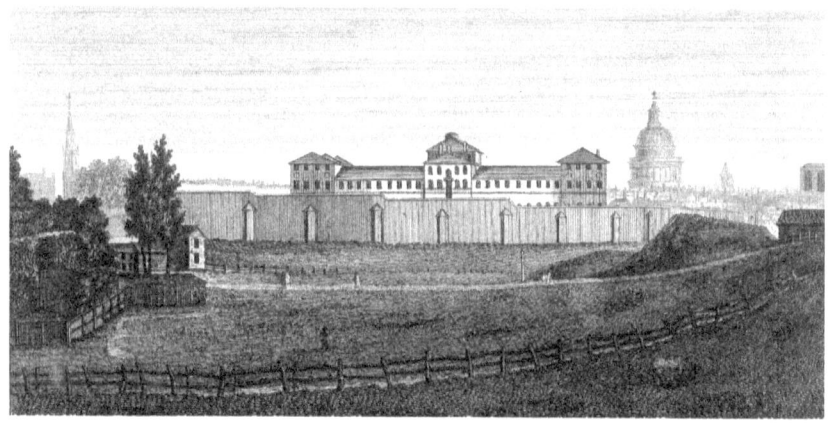

1798 etching of Coldbath Fields Prison located in Clerkenwell London with St Paul's Cathedral viewed in the distance.

On 23 September 1797 William Redfern and other men guilty of mutiny were moved to Coldbath Fields prison in Clerkenwell London.[40] The gaol, run by the local magistrates, opened in 1794 and had 232 small cells for prisoners and debtors. Most of the adults and juveniles held in the prison served only short sentences. By the time Redfern and the seamen were incarcerated, the severity of its solitary confinement cells gave it the reputation of being a 'prison in hell'. The cells were bare stone, without fire or furniture, and only a little straw for bedding. There was no protection from the weather except for a small iron grate, a 'damp cell, not seven feet square, without either fire or candle, chair, table, knife, fork, no glazed window'.[41]

Though there is no direct evidence of it, one can assume that brother Thomas visited William in prison. From such a visit, or perhaps from another prisoner, Redfern acquired the 26 September 1797 issue of *The Whitehall Evening Post*. This is evidenced by entries in his trusty notebook. The *Post* articles were windows to the outside world for the 23-year-old in solitary confinement. An early entry in the notebook was how to make butter, followed by a recipe 'To make Black Gall' a water-based black ink. A medical entry was a 'Recipe for the Gravel and Stone' that used blackberry jelly to breakdown kidney stones. All recipes came from his treasured issue of *The Whitehall Evening Post*.[42] Redfern used his notebook sparingly over the next two months and added only two more recipes extracted from newspapers.[43] During the winter of 1797-8 he stopped adding to the notebook because he was so cold it was 'scarcely possible to exist'.[44]

Redfern's first notebook entries in 1798 were twelve French fables, indicating a change of interest and perhaps another distraction from the horrors of solitary confinement. Each fable is about a page long, written in perfect French. Later entries returned to his previous interest in recipes; in these instances, for destroying bugs, making various gunpowder and how to write with gold or silver. William must have acquired, perhaps from another prisoner or visitor, a book on fishing because there are several pages in the notebook listing fish baits, details of fish, and where and how they might be caught.[45] It would seem that his notebook had become a stalwart for positive thoughts and some planning for the future.

In September 1798 Redfern's year of solitary confinement ended and he was moved to a larger cell where men, women and children were herded together. Throughout his imprisonment he suffered from severe cold and malnutrition. The only thing that kept him sane was the belief that one day he would be transported out of this madness – any place had to be better than this prison.

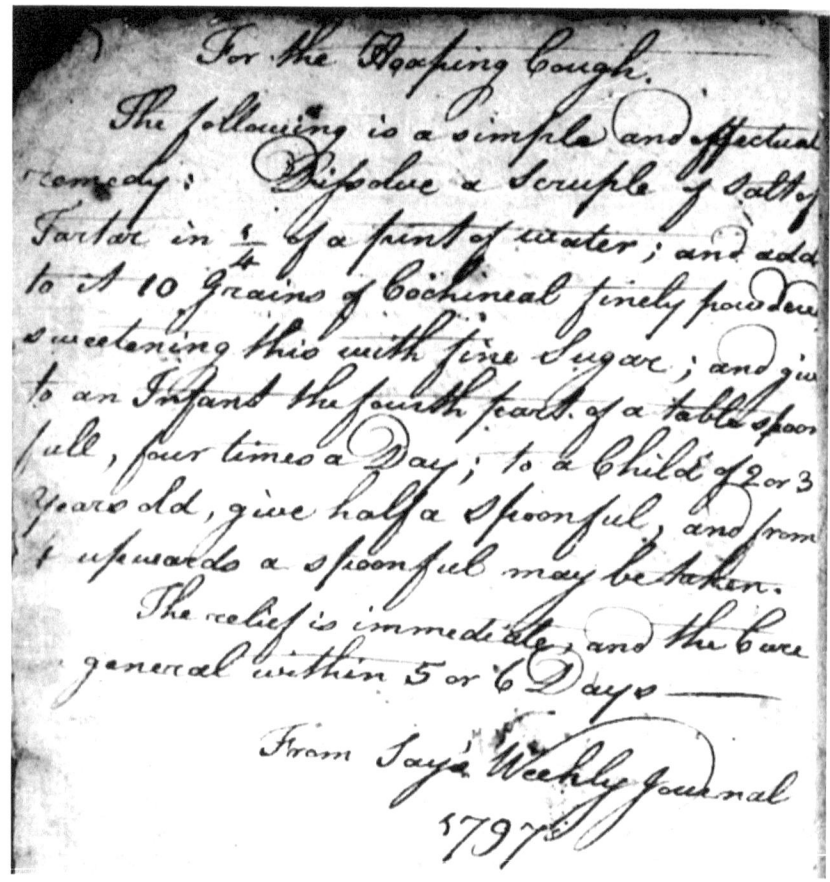

A page from William Redfern's notebook written in 1797 while he was in solitary confinement in Coldbath Fields Prison.

In 1798, a year after the Nore mutiny, there was a major uprising against British rule in Ireland led by the United Irishmen who were encouraged by the American and French revolutions. Only a year earlier William's brother Robert had been charged with treason for belonging to this organisation. The Irish Rebellion was put down viciously by the British military between May and October 1798. During this period, Colonel Edward Despard, an Irish officer in the service of the British Crown, was arrested with 30 other men for joining the London Corresponding Society and the United Irishmen in June 1798. These men were committed to the Coldbath Fields prison on charges of treason without trial.

In December 1798 the deplorable state of the prison was exposed publicly when Despard's wife Catherine, complained about the inhuman conditions her husband was being held in. She lobbied the radical young Member of Parliament Sir Francis Burdett, who, with the support from John Courtenay MP, tabled a paper on the prison conditions in Parliament.[46] Burdett would become a fierce opponent of Prime Minister William Pitt the Younger and an advocate for human rights. It is interesting to note that Edward and Catherine Despard appear as characters in the 2015 popular British television drama, *Poldark*.

The uproar about prison conditions forced William Pitt to visit the Coldbath Fields prison and he found it disgusting. Pitt told the House of Commons on 22 December 1798 that the wardens had 'kindly subjected these prisoners to so much pain in this world, that the less punishment might be inflicted on them in the next'.[47] By then, Edward Despard, who had frostbitten feet, had been moved from solitary confinement to a larger cell with a fire. Four days later, John Courtenay MP told the House of Commons that he had seen solitary cells without fire or candles and prisoners denied of 'every kind of society'. On 5 January 1799, Sir Francis Burdett MP visited the Coldbath Fields prison to see 'first the mutineers, and afterwards the persons committed under suspicion of treasonable practises'. Burdett was taken to the cells 'where nine of the said Mutineers were confined' and found very ill men who had not received any medical treatment. He declared the prison a 'very improper place for a sick person'. Some of the mutineers had told him in detail how cruelly the gaol keeper was treating them. Burdett then met with Edward Despard and his visiting wife Catherine. When departing the prison, Burdett gave the chief gaoler three guineas for the comforts of the prisoners and 'two half crowns to buy tobacco for the mutineers'. Burdett was the first person outside family members to ever leave money for any prisoner.[48]

However, Burdett's visits to the Coldbath Fields prison and his interviews with prisoners were condemned by Parliament, and, for a while, he was barred from visiting any prison in the country. This ban outraged the editor of *The Courier* who reported:

Clamour against Ministers. ... Who will now dare speak or write contrary to the wishes of Ministers? ... Oh! The happy effect of the Cold-Bath-Fields Prison and Colonel Despard's statement![49]

In March 1799 the government appointed a Select Committee to enquire into the conditions at the Coldbath Fields prison.[50] Another year passed without government action and on 11 July 1800 Sir Francis Burdett tabled a report in the House of Commons on *The Inhuman Cruelties discovered in the Coldbath-Fields Prison*. The report, which largely overlooked the putrid conditions and mismanagement in the prison, was written following the visit of a Grand Jury of 18 Gentlemen two months earlier; Burdett was not included. Although their inspection started in the part of the gaol where the mutineers were held, prisoners initially refused to be interviewed in case the gaol keeper got to know of a complaint. After assurances of confidentiality, prisoners revealed that rations were 'not sufficient to support human nature' and they suffered in winter from the cold with 'scarcely a bit of shoe to their feet'. The bedding was on planks topped with a layer of straw and a thin small blanket. The men also reported that friends and family had left money for them at the prison gate, but it had never been passed on.[51]

Many men complained of illness and appeared to be 'worn out by wretchedness and disease'. The necessaries of life were so sparingly given to these men 'as if it was calculated to lengthen out a miserable existence for the purpose of punishment'. One very ill mutineer, James Johnston, could hardly stand up and had to be supported by two men when he wanted to talk to the Grand Jury. He told them that the prison doctor had disregarded his illness and said he was faking it. Johnston said he no longer had the strength to face the cruelty. Burdett noted that the men attributed their many illnesses to bad treatment and want of food. The medicine given was always the same and they believed it was nothing more than vinegar and water – it was later proved to be vitriol (sulphuric acid) and water. These particular observations were clearly made by a prisoner who knew about medicine but was unable to treat fellow inmates.[52] William Redfern is not named in the report, but he was most likely one of the men who spoke to the Grand Jury.

The Parliamentary Grand Jury next inspected the prison sick ward. They found it very clean but with only one patient. The Jury observed that many of the prisoners they had seen in their cells were far sicker than the patient in the sick ward. It was clear that the magistrates in charge of the prison were hiding the poor prison conditions by only allowing visitors to see cleaned up areas. At the close of his speech to Parliament, Francis Burdett concluded that 'The prisoners have a right to complain'.[53]

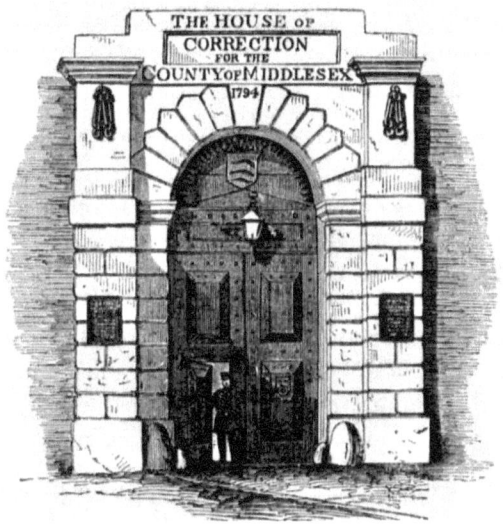

Etching of main gate to the Coldbath Fields Prison.

After this report appeared in the newspapers, prisoners across Britain were encouraged to demand better food and conditions. A month later, on 14 August 1800, a riot broke out in the Coldbath Fields prison. When the keeper proceeded to lock up prisoners for the night, they began to hiss, groan and shout. The noise was so loud that it was heard beyond the prison walls and a large mob assembled at the gate. Emboldened by the shouts coming from outside, inmates overpowered some keepers and threatened the Prison Governor, James Aris. A newspaper reported that the prisoners shouted 'Murder! murder! murder!'. They were starved; 'A fever raged within!' and it was now feared that the riot would spill onto the streets. The military was sent for, but the mob made no attempt to destroy the prison, and the rioters soon released the keepers. By midnight all had returned to their cells.[54]

The Inspector-General of Health, Sir Jeremiah Fitzpatrick, a physician and campaigner for prison reform, inspected the prison shortly after the riot. His visit to the Coldbath Fields prison appears to have profoundly altered William Redfern's prospects of release. Fitzpatrick was also responsible for the sanitary regulations applied to warships and convict transports, and he classified convicts on their suitability for transportation. During his inspection visit, Redfern revealed he was a ship surgeon and spoke with authority about the prison conditions. Redfern may have also told him about the atrocities he had personally suffered at the hands of the prison Governor, James Aris. The following article later appeared in *The Star* newspaper.

> Among those abuses he stated the case of Redfern, which was so atrocious that Aris at first denied it, but when pressed under the testimony of the Surgeon, who had humanity, he was compelled to admit it. This unfortunate man (Redfern) had a piece of cow's udder administered to him as food, which was so bad that the milk was found in it, and proved to be in a state of putrefaction; and this statement was corroborated by the Surgeon. But what was the consequence of such complaint and remonstrance? Redfern was taken, and, without any one charge against him, was threatened to be transported, and was sent aboard the hulks.[55]

The journalist may have exaggerated this report, but it probably reflects the true conditions in the prison. It is unlikely that Redfern resisted being transported. He realised this was his best chance of escaping the Coldbath Fields prison and it was his 'own particular request to Sir Jeremiah Fitzpatrick' that he be transported and work on the ship as a surgeon.[56] On 14 November 1800, the name 'William Redfern' appeared on a list of men who would be transported to New South Wales:

> William Redfern at the Court Martial held on board the Neptune the 22 Aug 1797 for making a Mutinous Assembly on board the Standard and for concealing traitorous and Mutinous Words and for behaving with Contempt to his superior officers in the Execution of their Duty and disobeying their lawful Commands… With his Majesty's intention of Mercy on Condition of their being severally Transported beyond the Seas for the Terms … William Redfern, for the term of his Natural Life[57]

On 25 Nov 1800, the keeper of the Coldbath Fields prison received a letter from the Duke of Portland, the Home Office Secretary, requesting that inmate William Redfern be transferred to a naval hulk moored off Portsmouth to await transportation.[58]

Not unexpectedly, within weeks of Sir Jeremiah Fitzpatrick's inspection of Coldbath Fields prison, conditions there improved markedly, and better food was served; family and friends were allowed to bring food to be delivered to a prisoner.[59]

During the three years and three months Redfern spent in the Coldbath Fields prison, his family remained in contact both with him and his brother Robert, who was gaoled in Dublin. After the British Parliament passed the September 1798 amnesty bill, Robert was pardoned on the condition he lived in another country that was not at war with Britain.[60] He requested to be transported with his wife and three children to America but, at the close of 1800, he was still in prison awaiting permission to board a ship. It was not until April 1801 that he and his family were able to sail to America.

The anxiety of having two sons in prison weighed heavily on Robert Redfern senior who, following the bloodbath of the Irish Rebellion in 1798, feared greatly for the safety of his family. Thomas was securely working in Trowbridge as a surgeon and a farmer, but he worried about 15-year-old Joseph getting into trouble for 'his political opinions'. Ireland was no longer a safe place. As soon as his sons Robert and William were transported out of Britain, Robert senior and the rest of the family took refuge in Porto in Portugal, where they remained until 1808 when the Peninsular War broke out with France.[61]

Chapter 4

BANISHED TO NSW

> *Mr. Redfern, in consequence of the Mutiny at the Nore in 1797 was, at his own particular request to Sir Jeremiah Fitzpatrick, then Inspector of the Transport Service, sent to this Colony in 1801. During the passage, he assisted the Surgeon, and kept the Journal of the treatment of the sick.*
> Macquarie to Viscount Sidmouth, 1821[1]

On a bitterly cold and wet winter day in January 1801, William Redfern was taken from the Coldbath Fields prison with an iron collar on his neck and chained to an open wagon for the two-day 80-mile journey to the Portsmouth docks. On arrival he was rowed out to the prison hulk *Captivity* where his collar was removed. A letter listing his court martial sentence and behaviour at Coldbath Fields was handed to the hulk warden, and he was consequently labelled in the prisoner log as a 'Character Bad Convicted before'.[2] Clearly, the Coldbath Fields wardens were glad to get rid of him – he was far too vocal a prisoner for them to tolerate!

Life for convicts aboard prison hulks was as strictly regulated as the navy and most prisoners were required to do hard labour. The conditions on the *Captivity* were, however, superior to land prisons and this newly refitted hulk was clean, well-ventilated and served decent food. Healthy convicts laboured ashore in the dockyards, while those ailing or convalescent worked on the hulk. In such improved conditions Redfern relished being back on a ship, albeit one that was not sailing anywhere.

In March 1801 Redfern was told he would soon be transported to New South Wales on the convict ship *Canada* and that, prior to embarkation, he would be sent to serve as surgeon on the *La Fortunée* hulk moored in Langstone Harbour Portsmouth.[3] It was a retrograde assignment; the *La Fortunée* hulk had a large hospital ward in a state of decay. The ship's timbers were rotting, and water seeped through the decks into the hospital. The *La Fortunée* was poorly maintained and the 500 convicts on board had insufficient food rations. Straw in the beds was filthy and only changed three times a year. Most portholes could not be opened for ventilation and many convicts were ill and unable to work. The lack of hygiene meant that diseases such as typhus spread quickly and one in four prisoners on this hulk died in 1801.[4] While still recovering from his harsh confinement in Coldbath Fields prison, Redfern was ordered to attend the sick on board. The prospect of soon departing on the *Canada* would have kept his spirits up and he did his best in the decrepit hulk. Redfern expected the conditions aboard the *Canada* to be much better and through an agreement with Jeremiah Fitzpatrick he would be permitted to take some medicine, medical instruments and books with him.

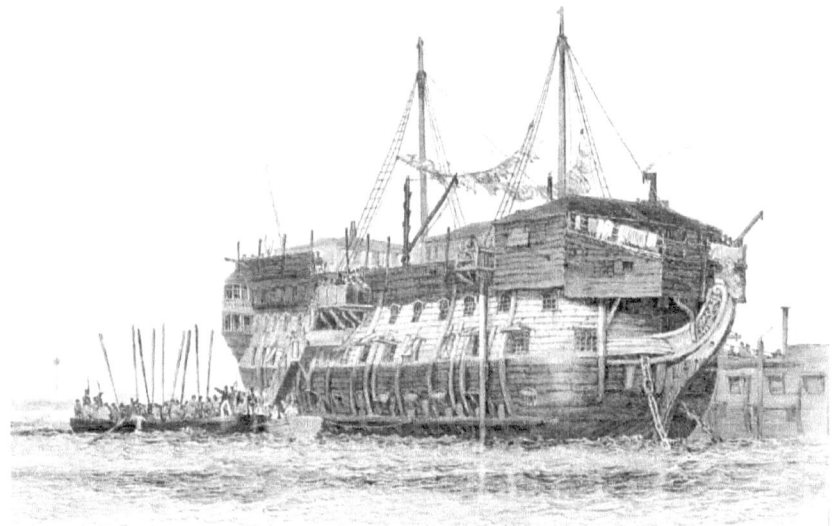

Prison hulk docked in Portsmouth harbour. In 1801 William Redfern was imprisoned on the hulk *Captivity* and served on the hospital hulk *La Fortunée*.

He duly informed his family of his imminent departure for New South Wales, and they were allowed to come and say farewell to him. Since his sentence was transportation *for life*, Redfern assumed he would never set foot in Britain again and believed that this would be the last opportunity to see his beloved family.

In April 1801 the Admiralty chartered three merchant ships, the *Canada*, 393 tons, the *Minorca*, 407 tons, and the *Nile*, 322 tons; each with ten guns, to transport the latest cohort of convicts to the colony. The *Canada* and *Minorca* would carry male convicts and the smaller *Nile* would be for female convicts.[5] The ships were refitted at the Deptford docks to house prisoners and once complete, they would load provisions for the long voyage, as well as items needed by the New South Wales colony.

Government officials declared that every effort was being made to reduce the high convict mortality of past voyages to New South Wales, and the Inspector-General of Health, Jeremiah Fitzpatrick, warned captains that their ships would be thoroughly inspected. Updated regulations stipulating the cleanliness and hygiene on vessels were issued to ship's masters and surgeons, with an order that all convicts must be examined on embarkation and anyone unfit for the long voyage removed. Because ship's masters on previous transportation voyages had been paid for the number of convicts *departing* Britain rather than *arriving* at the colony, health matters were often ignored, and disease among embarking convicts disregarded. Moreover, masters routinely cheated convicts of their rations and sold the surplus food at the stopover ports or when they reached New South Wales.

Just as it had in the slave trade, the profit motives of ship's masters regularly caused high morbidity and mortality on convict transporters. The *Hillsborough* was one such 'death ship' to depart for Sydney in December 1798. When Inspector-General Jeremiah Fitzpatrick inspected the *Hillsborough* at the Thames docks, he ordered some of the sick on board to be transferred to a hospital hulk and prevented the transfer of convicts from the Langstone Harbour hulks where typhus was raging at the time. But the *Hillsborough* captain and surgeon ignored his instructions and 95 of the 300 convicts died on the voyage.[6] William Redfern's future wife Sarah Wills, along with her mother Sarah and convict father Edward were on that ship and they would tell him in later years of their dreadful experiences.

Because of the *Hillsborough* tragedy, Fitzpatrick and his officials required future convict transport ships to strictly adhere to health regulations. In May 1801, he personally inspected the newly refitted *Canada*, *Minorca* and *Nile* docked in the Thames and listed deficiencies needing rectification before departure. These included more water kegs and antiscorbutic remedies such as lemon juice, additional hospital utensils, clothing, barrels of tar, vinegar and brimstone, and various medical ingredients.[7] The day after Fitzpatrick's inspection, female convicts boarded the *Nile* and male prisoners from the hulks at Woolwich embarked on the *Minorca*. Soldiers of the newly formed New South Wales Corps and free emigrants with their families boarded all three ships. The passengers included several husbands, wives and children of convicts, as well as 21 settlers and their children sailing to a new farming life in the colony.

On 18 May 1801 the three ships sailed from the Thames docks to Spithead, an anchorage outside of Portsmouth harbour. On arrival four days later, the ships took on further provisions, water and cargo, including goods ordered by Governor King in New South Wales.[8] On 6 June 1801, 75 male prisoners from the *La Fortunée* hulk, among them William Redfern, were chained together and rowed to the *Canada*. The next day, 29 convicts from other prison hulks were transferred to the ship.[9] Convict James Lowe, alias James Vaux, described his embarkation on the *Minorca*:

> Having entered the ship, we were all indiscriminately stripped (according to indispensable custom) and were saluted with several buckets of salt-water, thrown over our heads by a boatswain's-mate. After undergoing this watery ordeal, we were compelled to put on a suit of slop-clothing. Our own apparel, though good in kind, being thrown overboard. We were then double-ironed, and put between-decks, where we selected such births, for sleeping, etc. as each thought most eligible.[10]

The Transport Office instructed the surgeons on the three ships to keep diaries during the voyage listing 'not only relative to the Sick and Medicines, but also to the Daily number of Convicts admitted upon Deck', when the decks were scraped, the beds washed and aired, the ships fumigated and any other circumstances affecting the health of those on board. The masters were informed that on arrival in Sydney, Governor King would examine the surgeon's diaries and that only after he had certified that the surgeon had done his duty would he be paid for his 'Assiduity and Humanity'. Any neglect in duty would have consequences.[11] Such conditions were in stark contrast to those William Redfern had just experienced on the *La Fortunée* hulk.

Three days after Redfern boarded the *Canada*, Jeremiah Fitzpatrick arrived at Spithead and inspected all three ships.[12] On board the *Canada* he spoke to convict Redfern and Ship Surgeon John Kelly. He instructed Redfern that during the passage, 'he assisted the surgeon and kept the journal of the treatment of the sick'.[13] To the masters and surgeons of the ships, Fitzpatrick reiterated the importance of maintaining the good health of the convicts.[14] This included the need for each person to use soap, combs and razors; the means of fumigation, ventilation, scrubbing and cleansing, and the purification of drinking water. Fitzpatrick stressed that surgeons were obliged to record all medical events in their diary, and reminded them that:

> You are to see that the between-decks, as well in the sleeping apartments as hospital, are kept in a perfect state of cleanliness, by sweeping and scraping them every day, and once a week at least by moistening the planks (if necessary) with wet swabs, so as to render it more easy to disengage in the scraping any matter which may foul them; but it is by no means intended to wash those decks or bed spaces in the usual manner, except where the air may have free access to carry off or remove the moisture, that being one of the agents of putrefaction. However, in such parts of the passenger's births where the air may have access they may be washed, but the bottom boards of all the births, as well those of the passengers, guards, as of the convicts, and also those in the hospital, shall twice a week be brought on deck, washed with salt-water, and dried before the laying of them again; and, without any excuse or apology whatever, the bedding of every of the aforesaid persons shall every day, or at such time of the day as is fair, be brought upon deck, there to be opened out and properly aired.[15]

These new regulations were also promulgated in *The Caledonian Mercury* and the newspaper editor wrote that the ships had 'been regularly supplied with every necessary [*sic*], on a plan superior to any other since the colony of New South Wales was first established, under the immediate direction of Sir Jerome Fitzpatrick'.[16] After inspecting the ships, Fitzpatrick removed one male convict from the *Minorca* and four from the *Canada*.[17]

The duties of the ship's surgeons were various and included the trimming of windsails placed over open hatches. These small canvas sheets served to channel air below to displace the foul bilge air that accumulated below deck when windows and gun ports were closed. The deck hatches had to be closed during storms and this left those below in dark putrid conditions. The ship's sickbay had its own passage to the upper deck, but surgeons needed permission to release convicts from irons for treatment. Recovered patients could not return to their bunks until their clothing had been fumigated with 'the vapour of burning brimstone and the oxygenec [*sic*] gas'. Surgeons were also required to ensure each convict be admitted to the upper deck at least twice in every 24 hours. Without exception, nobody was allowed to wash or dry clothing below deck and fumigation was preferred to scrubbing floors with vinegar. Rations for the convicts were fixed but 'lemon-juice, sugar, sago, rice, oatmeal, peas, and bread, with a certain proportion of wine and tea' may be given to anyone showing signs of scurvy, fever or ulcers.[18]

Aboard the *Canada*, Redfern's strength gradually returned and with the resumption of medical duties his appalling memories of Coldbath Fields prison began to fade. Although the 26-year-old remained a prisoner on the ship subject to the same regulations as other convicts on board, he no longer wore irons. Also, his berth was close to the sickbay away from other convict cells, giving him a level of privacy he had not experienced in years. Important to his recuperation was that he was kept busy and within days of boarding five men were confined to the sickbay. Unfortunately, the surgeons' diary on the *Canada*, of which two copies were kept, has not survived, though Captain Wilkinson's logbook does record some details on how the health regulations were adhered to and how the convicts exercised.[19]

The imminent departure of the three ships for their remote destination generated both exhilaration and remorse among convicts on board. Altogether, 541 people were about to sail; 299 convicts, 88 crew, 32 NSW Corps soldiers and 122 passengers (23 men, 37 women and 62 children).[20] Most of the convicts on board were being transported for committing theft or burglary. Many petty crimes had been reclassified as capital offences and could be punished by hanging. These offences now included burglary, highway robbery, housebreaking and picking pockets above one shilling, shoplifting above five shillings and stealing items valued at over 40 shillings. For these offences transportation was often the only escape from the noose.

Inspector Fitzpatrick, who had been administering convict ship departures for six years, wrote that the ships *Canada*, *Minorca* and *Nile* were the first to fully meet the governmental health standards and was satisfied he was 'sending Useful & Healthful Members to colonize New South Wales'. In his departure report, he listed the ages of convicts, and the trades of the male convicts. Half the females were under the age of 25, and half the men had a trade as bricklayers, tile makers, stone masons, carpenters, smiths, sawyers, painters, cabinet makers, shoemakers, weavers, bakers, butchers, fishermen, saddlers, sailors, wig makers – and one surgeon. The last, William Redfern, was the most educated of the convicts.[21]

This blend of convict tradesmen and labourers was exactly what the colonial governors in Sydney had been requesting for years, and Fitzpatrick's efforts for them to arrive healthy was even more important. Previous transports had come to New South Wales with so many sick and disabled convicts that the colony's hospital and medical supplies were overwhelmed, and the men were unable to contribute to the colony's desperate need to grow more food. Farmers in the colony preferred new arrivals to be fit young men with rural experience, but such skills had become rare since petty felons increasingly came from urban areas. On the other hand, if 'urban convicts' had a trade, they contributed to the workforce of the construction industry and other businesses of the colony. Interestingly, 14 convicts on the *Canada* and *Minorca* had been transported for mutiny but only two, William Redfern and Thomas McCann, had been sentenced for the Nore mutiny. They were the only men from this mutiny to ever land in Australia.[22]

On 21 June 1801 the *Canada*, *Minorca* and *Nile* departed Portsmouth bearing southwest in the English Channel towards the Atlantic Ocean. The only port of call on the voyage to New South Wales would be Rio de Janeiro Brazil, some 6500 nautical miles (12,000 km) away. The small flotilla sailed south on a well-known route towards the Island of Madeira, taking full advantage of the trade winds and elemental Atlantic currents. Occasional heavy seas and strong winds were encountered, and many convicts and passengers at sea for the first time were sick. But eventually all adapted to the daily routine of shipboard life dictated by the ship's bells. Redfern kept the *Canada*'s medical diary up to date and performed the tasks Surgeon Kelly assigned to him. Apart from seasickness, there were few illnesses on board. Weather permitting, groups of 30 or so convicts exercised on deck, their bunks were aired, and their cells were cleaned and fumigated. On 29 June, the seven men being treated in the sickbay recovered within a week.

When the *Canada* sailed past the Island of Madeira on 11 July

1801, Captain Wilkinson signalled the *Minorca* and the *Nile* that a strange sail had been sighted on the horizon. Since Britain was still at war with France, there was a flurry of activity on the ships to prepare for a possible attack – the cannons were primed, and the passengers and convicts confined below decks. Fortunately, the distant ship turned out to be British, as were all other sightings on the voyage. This was a nervous time because of the many enemy and pirate ships in the Atlantic, which captured vessels and crews for ransom. Shipboard illnesses were inevitable and despite the efforts of Surgeon Kelly and assistant Redfern a male convict on the *Canada* died of fever on 1 August.[23] Another convict also died on the *Minorca*.

As the flotilla neared the equator, heavy seas battered the ships, and, with huge waves breaking over the gunwales, hatches were quickly battened down to limit flooding below decks. The tropical storms were so fierce that sails and riggings were damaged on all ships, and Captain Leith on the *Minorca* reported losing a topsail.[24] For most convicts, soldiers and passengers on board the heat, humidity and rain was distressingly oppressive. Between storms those below were released from their dark noxious quarters and the hatches were opened so that fresh air could be forced below with a windsail installed by surgeons Kelly and Redfern.

However, the tropical heat and humidity frayed many tempers and the combination of confined quarters and regular rum rations fuelled friction among the soldiers. The lack of privacy, even for married couples, meant every verbal conflict was shared. Sheets were hung between bunks, but these were of little help. On 11 August, Sergeant Brumlow and Captain Earley reported to the ship's master Wilkinson that Sarah McHenry was often abusing her soldier husband, James McHenry, and this made it difficult for others living close by. They requested the couple be separated.

The reason for Sarah McHenry's behaviour is unknown but, since she would later become William Redfern's companion, this episode is pertinent to the story. It is also possible that Redfern intervened in the quarrel and discussed this with Surgeon Kelly because, later in the day Kelly argued with Sergeant Brumlow who had been drinking and pushed him off the quarterdeck. Captain Wilkinson then ordered the enraged Brumlow and Kelly to their quarters. After further confrontations, Sarah and James McHenry, as well as Captain Earley, were transferred to the *Minorca*.[25]

On 28 August 1801, the three convict ships entered the Rio de Janeiro harbour, the *Canada* firing an 11-gun salute that was returned by the harbour fortress. On anchoring, longboats were immediately sent ashore to purchase fresh food and water, and carpenters, caulkers and riggers set about repairing masts and sails, and sealing leaks in the hulls. All on board received a large ration of fresh beef and vegetables and this quickly restored everyone's spirits. Even so, escape was never far from the minds of convicts. When several were caught trying to cut off their irons, the ships' watch was doubled while in harbour.[26]

Captain Wilkinson's wife Elizabeth had accompanied him on the voyage. She was pregnant and a week after arriving in Rio gave birth to a healthy boy. Surgeon Kelly and assistant Redfern most likely delivered the baby.[27] On the day of the birth, a second convict died of alcohol poisoning. Although convicts were not entitled to alcohol, some were assigned to serve the rum ration to the free passengers as part of their duties on board. These men had been taking their share. Wilkinson ordered that the rum supply be diluted so convicts were less tempted to steal it.[28]

After four weeks in Rio de Janeiro, the flotilla was ready to sail for New South Wales. The long stopover had replenished the ships' supplies and given crews ample time to make crucial repairs. Just prior to departing, Captain Wilkinson heard from Portuguese ships moored in the harbour that several French privateer vessels were close by and had already captured a Portuguese vessel. He decided that the *Canada*, *Minorca* and *Nile* should accompany a departing Portuguese convoy.[29] On reaching the open seas, the Portuguese sailed south, and the convict ships bore east on their 10,300 nautical-mile (19,000 km) journey over the Atlantic, Indian and Southern Oceans to New South Wales.

Initially sailing conditions suited the ships' eastern bearing but within days the weather changed dramatically. For the next week they were buffeted by violent storms, heavy squalls, thunder and lightning. Rough and powerful seas broke over the gunwales and, even with hatches battened down, flooding occurred below decks. All but the sailors on duty were confined below in the frigid darkness and the putrid bilge air. It got icier the further south they sailed; ice crystals hung from the riggings and the convicts' thin clothing and blankets gave little protection against the bitter cold. On 4 October 1801, convicts on the *Canada* appealed to Captain

Wilkinson for better clothing – their well-composed letter was most likely written by Redfern.

> We in general take the Liberty of Addressing you on the Subject of our present uncomfortable Situation for wants of Cloaths for what was served out to us in England are entirely worn out and coming from a warm Climate Occasions us to feel the Cold to a great degree. We therefore humbly hope kind Sir that in consideration of our present distress you will supply our wants which probably will enable us to live the remainder of the fatiguing voyage.[30]

After Fitzpatrick's admonitions Wilkinson realised this was a health issue that he may be held accountable for and within two days convicts received new warm clothing. On the occasional calm days, convicts were allowed on deck to wash and the cells below deck were thoroughly fumigated. In November Redfern was urgently transferred, mid-ocean, to the *Minorca* to help Surgeon George Longstaff treat a very sick female passenger and a young seaman. Both died and Redfern remained on the *Minorca*.

The consistent pelting rain, hail and heavy gales now gave the ships their first taste of the fabled Roaring Forties. Driven by fierce winds, the ships were tossed about by mountainous waves. The conditions were so fierce that veteran seamen were fearful – for everyone else it was the most frightening experience in their lives. Seasickness was rife, and in the drenching icy storms, sailors were wet most of the time. When possible, they stayed in their bunks, but this gave little respite from the bitter cold.

On 30 November 1801 the green-grey silhouette of the southwest coast of Van Diemen's Land appeared on the horizon. With considerable difficulty the three ships had managed to stay together and now bore east around the southern tip of the island and headed north up the east coast of Australia to the entrance of Port Jackson. Few on board had any idea what to expect in this strange new land, but when they sailed into Port Jackson they were astounded, both by the beauty of the deep-water harbour bordered by woodlands and the prosperous settlement of Sydney. On 15 December 1801, after a voyage of six months, the ships dropped anchor in Sydney Cove.[31] The passengers and soldiers almost immediately disembarked, but it was two days before government officials boarded the ships to examine the convicts.

During the voyage only two male convicts died on the *Canada*, and one male convict, one female passenger and a crewman died on the *Minorca*. There were no deaths among the female convicts on the *Nile*. Over the next three days, 296 convicts were escorted ashore: 101 men from the *Canada*, 99 men from the *Minorca* and 96 females from the *Nile*. Among them was William Redfern, who disembarked from the *Minorca*.[32]

Governor Philip Gidley King received the muster record of the incoming convicts, along with the captains' logbooks and the surgeons' diaries. He examined all documents, and later reported to the British Colonial Office Under Secretary John King that 'The passengers were all in good health, and the convicts the healthiest and best conditioned that ever arrived here, being all fit for immediate labour'.[33] He also complimented 'the great attention shown by the Masters of those Ships, to those under their Care, who were all landed in high health'.[34] The captains and surgeons had easily passed the new stringent salary requirements and were promptly renumerated. William Redfern was not paid but he had come to the favourable notice of the governor, and this would benefit him in the future.

Within days of disembarking, the majority of convicts were transferred to Parramatta. However, the surgeon's assistant, William Redfern, was about to be sent to a remote settlement on Norfolk Island, a small landmass in the Pacific Ocean 900 nautical miles east of Sydney. It was one of the most isolated places in the British Empire.

Chapter 5

NORFOLK ISLAND

> *The excellence of Redfern's work in the convict hospital at Norfolk Island – his kindly sympathy with his fellow unfortunates there incarcerated under appalling conditions, his extraordinary capacity for hard work, his exemplary conduct, his technical and practical skill, his loyalty to the Governor and the Administration, so won the admiration of Lieutenant-Colonel Foveaux that he recommended Absolute Pardon for Redfern.*
> John Antill et al., *The Emancipist*, 1936[1]

On 30 December 1801 eighteen of the recently disembarked convicts from the *Canada* and *Minorca* were escorted on board the small two-masted *Harrington* about to sail for Norfolk Island. The men included seven mutineers, one of whom was William Redfern. The settlement at Norfolk Island was one of Britain's remotest outposts and the *Harrington* arrived there on 8 January 1802. The island had no harbour or dock, so offloading people and supplies involved the hazardous use of longboats over the rocky reefs and through surf. William Redfern brought with him a single chest containing clothing, medicine, instruments and books.[2] Another passenger on the *Harrington* was Sarah McHenry, the lady who had argued violently with her soldier husband James McHenry on the *Canada*. Possibly the McHenrys had now separated, as James remained in Sydney for another ten months before being transferred to the island.[3]

Norfolk Island is a small rocky landmass 5 miles (8 km) long and 3 miles (5 km) wide, bounded by steep cliffs. It would be Redfern's home for the next six years. The main town on the island was Sydney (today known as Kingston) located at Slaughter Bay on the south coast. The settlement had no natural harbour and the large waves coming off the vast expanse of the Pacific Ocean often prevented ships from offloading cargo across the limestone reef at Slaughter Bay. Even in calm weather, ships needed to anchor well off the coast and bring goods and people ashore on longboats. Cascade Bay, another landing place northeast of the island, was just as hazardous in windy conditions.

The British had occupied Norfolk Island in March 1788 shortly after the First Fleet had arrived in New South Wales. They had taken possession of the island primarily to discourage the French who were busy at that time establishing colonies in the South Pacific. Lieutenant Philip Gidley King RN was sent to Norfolk Island aboard HMS *Supply* with 23 people, including nine male and six female convicts who were to grow cereal crops and raise pigs to feed the colony. They also planned to grow flax for making sails and to use the large straight native conifer (*Araucaria heterophylla*) for ship spars, but that was never successful. In the first two years, the sole purpose of the island was to supply grain and pork to the struggling settlement on the mainland.

When famine threatened the mainland colony, Governor Arthur Phillip sent more men to grow crops on the island. In March 1790 HMS *Sirius* and HMS *Supply* arrived at Norfolk Island with 280 people on board, including Corps Major Robert Ross who was to replace Lieutenant King as commandant of the settlement. A major storm raged when the two warships arrived at Slaughter Bay making the unloading of people and cargo nigh on impossible. During an attempt to do this, *HMS Sirius* struck a reef and was smashed beyond repair. No lives were lost but attempts to salvage cargo proved futile and Captain John Hunter and his crew were stranded on Norfolk Island for almost a year. Lieutenant King managed to return to Sydney on HMS *Supply* and was promptly ordered to take dispatches detailing the colony's food crisis to the Home Office in England. King reboarded HMS *Supply*, which was being sent to China to purchase food for the colony. King disembarked *en route* in Batavia (now Jakarta) and boarded another British ship to England. On arrival in London, he quickly completed his courier duties and immediately sailed back to Sydney, arriving in September 1791, to resume his duties as Lieutenant Governor of Norfolk Island.

In December 1792 Arthur Phillip resigned as Governor of New South Wales to seek medical treatment in England, probably for kidney stones. Major Francis Grose of the NSW Corps, and later Captain William Paterson from the same regiment became interim governors of the colony and they immediately instituted major administrative changes on the mainland and Norfolk Island. Grose transferred legal authority of civil courts to Corps officers, permitted convicts to buy alcohol and allowed rum to be used as payment for convict labour. These changes allowed Corps officers to quickly take control of the burgeoning rum trade. Grose also curtailed direct government participation in cereal production, instead granting farmland to Corps officers, officials and free settlers. Profits from the rum trade, generous land grants and free access to convict servants were a bonanza for the military but left many others struggling and short of food. The main benefactor of Grose's preferential governance was John Macarthur who became a rich and powerful landowner and, for many years, would prove to be the nemesis of later governors.

In the meantime, Norfolk Island flourished under Lieutenant Governor King's leadership, and its farm surpluses were offered for sale to the mainland. But Grose refused them because they would reduce food prices in Sydney and lower Corps officers' profits. In later years Norfolk Island would become a prison for reoffending convicts, but until 1814 the island's primary purpose was to grow food for the mainland. When King needed to return to England in October 1796 for medical treatment, the island had about 1000 inhabitants, many of whom were ex-convicts and ex-marines who had decided to remain there as settlers and farmers.

In 1792 Captain John Hunter sailed back to England with his crew from the shipwrecked HMS *Sirius*, and in 1795 he returned to Sydney as the second Governor of New South Wales. By then Grose's misadministration had facilitated the Corps' domination of many businesses in the colony and they fiercely opposed any curtailment of the rum trade. Without military backing, reform attempts by Hunter were unenforceable and his restrictions on the rum trade were ignored. Corps officers not only obstructed Hunter's administration, but they complained constantly to the Home Office that the governor was stifling business. This eventually led to Hunter's early replacement, but he only learnt of his dismissal in April 1800 when Philip Gidley King returned to Port Jackson as the third Governor of New South Wales.

King was, of course, already familiar with problems in the colony and itched to institute much-needed reforms. But Hunter was not in a hurry to hand over leadership, and it was not until September 1800 that he sailed for England. King's first actions targeted the two greatest problems in the colony, alcohol trading and the high cost of imported goods. He knew that Corps officers would oppose any changes that challenged their monopoly, and that their spokesperson, Lieutenant John Macarthur, was 'the master worker of the puppets he has set in motion'.[4] His proposed reforms were also resisted by a group of businessmen heavily involved in the importation of spirits and other goods.

This influential cartel included the principal surgeon of the colony, William Balmain. In fact, most surgeons in the colony were involved in retail trading, and they strongly opposed the reforms. Disagreements with the government became so bitter that Macarthur insisted that all Corps officers refuse social interactions with Governor King. This edict angered the Corps Commandant Lieutenant Colonel Paterson, and he fought a duel with Macarthur in which he was seriously wounded. Lieutenant Macarthur was subsequently imprisoned until Paterson had partially recovered. In November 1801 King banished Macarthur to England to face a court martial for the duel.[5]

As Governor of New South Wales, King maintained a special interest in Norfolk Island affairs. Since his departure from the island in 1796, three Corps officers had been appointed Lieutenant Governors of Norfolk. The last appointee, Captain Thomas Rowley, strictly opposed the trade in spirits and tried to stamp out drunkenness. He was a good administrator, but his seizure of illicit stills caused outrage on the island, and in May 1800 he was accused of unlawful confiscation of property. Rowley had King's support but resigned his post claiming ill health.[6] King realised that the next Norfolk appointment needed to be more resilient and in June 1800 offered the post of Lieutenant Governor to 33-year-old NSW Corps Major Joseph Foveaux.[7]

Foveaux had arrived in the colony in 1792 on the *Pitt* as part of the NSW Corps regiment commanded by Major Francis Grose. William and Ann Sherwin arrived on the same ship and, after the death of their son a year later Ann left her husband and became Foveaux's partner.[8] When Foveaux took up his post on Norfolk Island accompanied by Ann Sherwin, he found it dilapidated and short of commodities. Alcoholism among residents was rife. King ordered Foveaux to restrict alcohol imports and to open a government store that would undercut the inflated prices of goods sold by private traders. He also gave Foveaux permission to grant land to encourage farming but not to allow the construction of boats that might be used for convict escapes.[9]

In 1800 the first ships transporting convicts who had participated in the Irish Rebellion reached New South Wales. Some were senior United Irishmen charged with treason prior to the rebellion.[10] The majority of Irish convicts considered themselves political prisoners and deeply resented having to work as labourers or servants. On the mainland many tried to escape and were subsequently sent to Norfolk Island. Foveaux believed that the isolation of the island, and lenient treatment, would rehabilitate these convicts, many of whom were well educated. It was wishful thinking. In December 1800 a group of Irish planned a mass breakout. The escape never eventuated because one of the convicts considered the plan to kill soldiers, and if necessary their families, as unacceptable and he informed Foveaux. Furious that his efforts at rehabilitation had been abused, Foveaux promptly hanged the two leaders in front of everyone on the island. Four Corps soldiers who had been bribed to assist the plot received 500 lashes and were expelled from the regiment. Other instigators were flogged and committed to hard labour in chains. The informer was pardoned and returned to the mainland. Despite the undue swiftness of the punitive hangings, Governor King sanctioned Foveaux actions and the Colonial Office praised him for preventing another Irish revolt.[11]

Joseph Foveaux's instant justice for the plotters has earned him an ugly reputation in Irish historical annals. Claims of his excessive brutality appear in Robert Jones' *Recollections* and Joseph Holt's *Memoirs*, both accounts published after their deaths. In Foveaux's defence Reg Wright wrote in 1998 that both these published critiques had factual errors, and do not convey the true character of the man.[12] Even more emphatic support comes from Anne-Maree Whitaker, who writes in her biography *Joseph Foveaux*:

> Contrary to the depiction in works such as Manning Clark's *A History of Australia* and Robert Hughes's *The Fatal Shore*, Foveaux's period on Norfolk Island was not marked by him slavering over the flogging of naked women, nor subjecting convict men to concentration-camp-style forced labour.[13]

The extensive records describing Foveaux's time on Norfolk Island suggest he was an approachable, intelligent and ambitious soldier who adhered strictly to the military norms of the period. In fact, Foveaux's behaviour compares more than favourably with that of most military officers at that time, and he was well liked and respected. It is also relevant to note that, unlike most Corps officers who refused contact with emancipists and convicts, he was accessible to all island residents, free or otherwise. Nonetheless Foveaux was first and foremost a soldier not averse to using his authority to personal advantage. He quickly recognised merit in others and befriended anyone, independent of rank or status, who might help advance his own career and wealth. This will become more apparent later in the story when he grants convict surgeon William Redfern a full pardon and takes on the role of leading the colony for a time following the Rum Rebellion.

Major Joseph Foveaux was in command of Norfolk Island when convict William Redfern arrived on the *Harrington* on 8 January 1802 with his few possessions. Redfern's first impressions on landing may have been tinged with disappointment; the rugged wind-swept coastline and sparse landscape dotted with a few pine trees would not have been as inviting as the lush vegetation along the shores of Port Jackson. With so few residents, there was an eerie loneliness about the place. He marched with other convicts to an assembly point in the settlement and lined up for muster. Here, officials ascertained the skills and training of each convict and decided where they would fit into the island's workforce. Educated convicts were assigned to government duties, others to settlers wanting farm labourers and the remaining prisoners were sent to work on building projects.

As a trained naval surgeon, William Redfern was promptly assigned to James Mileham, the assistant surgeon in charge of the hospital. Mileham arrived in New South Wales in 1797 as a colonial assistant surgeon and since October 1799 had been doing rotational duty on the island. Surgeon Thomas Roberts, who was stationed on Norfolk with the NSW Corps guards, would soon replace Mileham.[14]

The governor's house was at the centre of the settlement overlooking Slaughter Bay. Small granaries, storehouses, barracks, a prison and a row of convict huts along the shoreline surrounded it. Close by was the island's hospital comprised of two buildings and the surgeon's house. William Redfern joined a hospital staff composed of surgeons Mileham and Roberts, several female nurses and the physician Bryan O'Connor. The latter had been transported for life for taking part in the Irish Rebellion, and after a year on the island was pardoned by King to practise medicine.[15] Learning of O'Connor's quick release would have given Redfern cause for optimism. In any case, his hospital duties were a giant leap forward from solitary confinement in Coldbath Fields prison. He was now free to roam the little island without irons, practice medicine, sleep in a warm bed and receive a weekly ration of 8 lb flour and 7 lb of fresh pork. With this glorious rise in status, he resolved to "play by the rules" and avoid at all costs the miserable existence he had endured over the past five years.

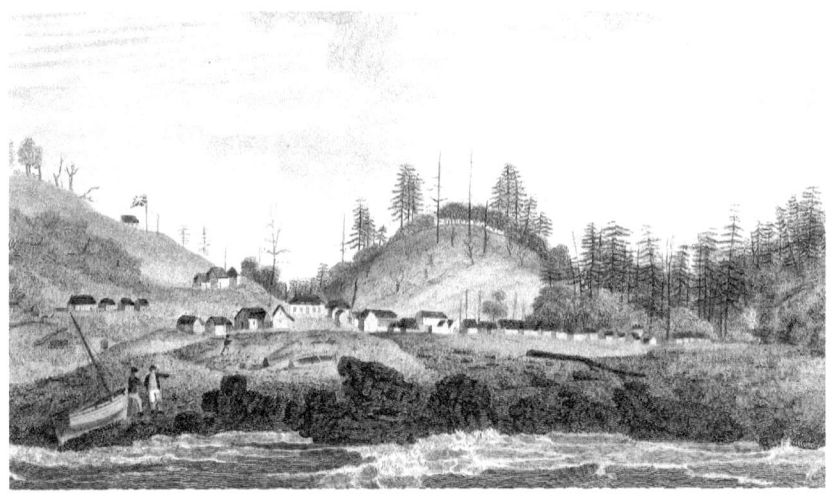

1798 view of Sydney settlement on Norfolk Island. The Government House is surrounded by storehouses, administration and accommodation buildings. The row of convict huts along the shoreline lead to the hospital on the right.

When the hospital surgeon James Mileham returned to Sydney on 12 March 1802, Thomas Roberts replaced him, and Redfern was to become his unofficial assistant. But a tragedy was about to favour Redfern. In June 1802, when disembarking personnel from HMS *Porpoise* at Slaughter Bay, a longboat smashed onto the reef and surgeon Thomas Roberts, returning from professional duties on the warship, drowned.[16]

Roberts' sudden death left the Norfolk hospital without an assistant surgeon, and Lieutenant Governor Foveaux appointed convict surgeon Redfern as his temporary replacement. This was unexpected – it was unusual to fill a skilled post with a convict even when no qualified free person was available. But Foveaux had monitored Redfern's work at the hospital and knew he had the necessary medical skills. He informed King that Redfern 'conducted himself in such a manner as to merit my perfect approbation'.[17] Despite the shortage of surgeons in the colony, no convict or ex-convict had previously been offered such a medical post, or had administered a hospital before, even temporarily.[18]

Earliest record of William Redfern as the 'Officiating Surgeon' at the Norfolk Island hospital, listing the sick, death and birth between May and Aug 1802.

The search for a permanent assistant surgeon for Norfolk was promptly initiated in Sydney. Redfern would have been fully aware that he needed to take advantage of his temporary role and tackled his hospital duties with the energy and dedication he later became well known for. He was determined to use this opportunity to demonstrate his capabilities, and to impress Foveaux.

Redfern occupied one of the small houses close to the hospital and was assisted in his duties by Bryan O'Connor, as the 'Assistant at Dispensary', and by the seven female nurses.[19] Although still officially a convict, William Redfern was now renumerated as an 'Officiating Surgeon' at the rate of 4s 4½d per day (£68 annually for a 6-day week), with full rations, free firewood and a convict servant.[20] His new position meant he was now rated as an 'Overseer' and received an additional 10 lb of maize on top of his weekly food ration of 4 lb of flour and 7 lb of fresh pork.[21]

His clothing allowance was also higher. Redfern's shoes were so worn out when he landed on the island that surgeon Mileham had arranged for two new pairs of shoes to be made by the island boot maker and charged to the government. In late April 1802 the 36 overseers on Norfolk Island, including surgeon Redfern, received a set of new clothing from the stores: '2 White Shirts, 1 Duck Frock

[coat], 1 Pair Material for Shoes, 1 Hat'. This followed with the notice of the clothing allowance for December, when Redfern received: '2 White Shirts, 1 Blue Jacket, 1 Pair Trousers, 1 Hat'.[22]

This must have seemed like a cornucopia to the 27-year-old, who only a year ago was locked in a decrepit prison. He may still be a convict, but he was a well-dressed and well-fed one – small rewards perhaps for a man with his education and skills, but a bonanza compared to the torments of the past few years.

Most arable land on Norfolk Island was used for farming, and the majority of residents were involved in food production. Fresh or salted pork was the main produce, and this was either consumed on the island or sold to the mainland. Many of the farmers were retired soldiers and ex-convicts who had decided to remain on the island. Occasionally, their number included surgeons. By 1802, 700 acres of maize and the same of wheat were cultivated on the island. There were 4000 pigs, 360 goats, 850 sheep, 24 cattle, 6 horses and 11 donkeys.[23] All cattle and three of the horses belonged to the government. With few animals suitable for ploughing, convict servants did most tilling by hoe or spade.

William Redfern was to remain the assistant surgeon in charge of the hospital until a free surgeon could be found to replace him. Because this might happen quickly, and unexpectedly, Redfern appears to have questioned if medicine was really the most secure career for a 'convict lifer'. However, what were the alternatives? Although becoming a farmer may not have appealed to him, Redfern began inspecting farmland on the island that he thought might be suitable as a future home and occupation. During his medical visits to farmers on the island, he listened to their experiences and considered buying some land with a house. If a permanent surgeon post was out of reach, being a part-time farmer with a private medical practise seemed like an attractive alternative.

Civil laws in the colony were similar to England. One major difference was that convicts could own property and Redfern took full advantage of this. On 9 July 1802 he bought 48 acres of land and based on its later sale price, his purchase price was probably over £140.[24] The land was 1.2 miles from the main settlement on the road to the village of Queenborough. D'Arcy Wentworth had previously owned the land when he served as a surgeon at the hospital from 1790 to 1796. Even with his good salary this was an expensive purchase for Redfern. It is unlikely he had saved enough to pay for the farm and there is no record of him arriving in the colony with any funds. Redfern wrote, sometime later, of making great exertions 'to better My condition' with the 'assistance & remittance in goods I at various times had received from my relatives in Europe'.[25] Even with family help and savings, he almost certainly would have needed to borrow money for the land purchase. Although no banks existed in the colony, there were always men willing to lend money at exorbitant rates.

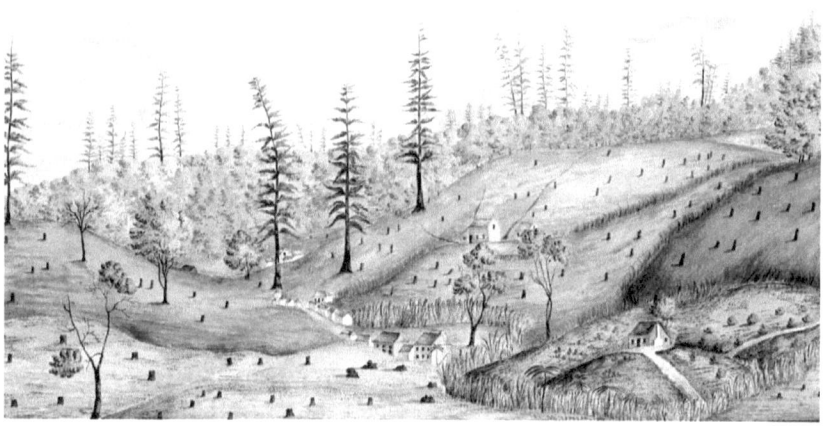

1804 painting of the Queenborough village on Norfolk Island.

William Redfern's life on the island had altered in other ways – Sarah McHenry appears now to have become his companion. She arrived on Norfolk on the same ship as Redfern, but no official records connect them until she departs the island accompanying Redfern as his 'wife'.[26] There seems little doubt that Sarah had become William's common-law wife, and that they had first met on the *Canada* and *Minorca* travelling from England. It is likely that she was at the hospital before becoming Redfern's housekeeper and partner.

Few personal details are known of Sarah McHenry and the only records of her on Norfolk Island are from the victualling lists. We know from a letter Redfern wrote to D'Arcy Wentworth in 1807 that he had a partner he referred to as 'My Lady'.[27] Somewhat ironically, if Sarah had come to the colony as a convict rather than a soldier's wife, more records of her would have existed. Typically, colonial documents and newspapers provide little information about free females, even for fashionable ladies married to prominent men.

Many unmarried couples lived together on Norfolk Island – it was common practice across the colony. *De facto* relationships existed for a variety of reasons, but mainly because prior marriages in England could not be annulled. Even when a spouse lived in the colony, as Sarah's husband James did, getting a divorce was almost impossible – most could only remarry when their spouse died. Common-law unions had become the norm both for convicts and military officers. Lieutenant Governor Johnston had a large family with his companion ex-convict Esther Abraham. When Philip Gidley King was Lieutenant Governor on Norfolk, he cohabited and had two children with his convict housekeeper Ann Inett. Lieutenant Governor Joseph Foveaux maintained a *de facto* relationship with Ann Sherwin, a Corps soldier's former wife.

Back on the mainland, finding a permanent assistant surgeon for Norfolk Island was proving difficult. The principal surgeon in the colony, William Balmain, was on leave in England and, in his absence, James Thomson was acting as his deputy. This changed on 28 June 1802 when Thomas Jamison returned from England and became the new acting principal surgeon. Thomson was then instructed to take the Norfolk Island post, but he instead sought leave to go to England.[28] Until he returned, Surgeon Charles Throsby was designated as his replacement.

When, on 4 July 1802, Surgeon D'Arcy Wentworth learnt that he had been overlooked for the well-paid Norfolk post, he sought the appointment based on his seniority. Governor King was delighted at the interest because the post would give Wentworth an opportunity to use his proven talents, and he offered him the appointment if taken up within three weeks.[29] King was also trying to eliminate the lucrative alcohol trade in the colony and knew that Wentworth had recently bought 3000 gallons of spirit. New regulations had fixed the prices on retail items and sales now required King's approval. Consequently, surgeons Wentworth and Balmain had problems selling their alcohol and faced heavy losses.[30] Wentworth sought permission to take his unsold merchandise to Norfolk Island and sell it there, but it was refused.

Wentworth then requested that his goods be sold in Sydney during his absence. Again, King said 'no'. Faced with financial ruin, Wentworth favoured his purse over his surgical aspirations and on 9 August informed King he would not be going to Norfolk.[31]

While the search for a replacement surgeon continued, William Redfern remained in charge of the Norfolk hospital and treated most sickness on the island. In August 1802 Lieutenant Governor Foveaux conducted a census that revealed the demographics on the island. There were 1007 inhabitants: 556 men, 172 women and 279 children, with three adult males to every female. Free inhabitants outnumbered convicts four to one. There were 201 convicts (196 male) on the island, guarded by 107 soldiers. The medical report of the 'Officiating Surgeon' is the first official record written by William Redfern in the colony. It showed that dysentery had been the most common illness in the last four months, with an average of 13 adults and 3 children being sick, half were male convicts. Two free men and one male convict had died, and there were eleven births.[32]

On 10 September 1802, Charles Throsby was selected to be the assistant surgeon on Norfolk Island. However, he never took the post because a month later he was appointed as the medical officer and magistrate at the newly established government prison farm at Castle Hill in the Hawkesbury farming district.[33] Since the colony was short of qualified medical practitioners, King had to place them where they were most needed. Redfern would remain in charge of the Norfolk Island hospital and Throsby was sent to Castle Hill where the 350 convicts doing hard labour needed frequent medical attention.

William Redfern's medical competency may well have exceeded most other surgeons in the colony, but his convict status precluded him from permanency. His posting as an Officiating Surgeon had already angered Corps officers opposed to rehabilitating convicts. Governor King, who regularly excluded the Corp officers from his administration and cultivated collaboration between emancipists and free settlers, ignored such views. But King fully understood that a military presence was essential for a penal colony, and he carefully exercised his civil authority while maintaining a working relationship with Corps officers. He was particularly pleased with the performance of Lieutenant Governor Foveaux on Norfolk

Island, reporting that 'it appears that officer is doing his utmost to reduce the expenses of that island, and to draw it from the neglected state it has been in'.[34]

Unobtrusively, King reinforced his own personal support base in the colony by pardoning large numbers of educated and well-behaved convicts and, in doing so, created an influential block of emancipist men and women who were loyal to the government. Among this group were two Irish emancipists on Norfolk Island: Redfern's assistant Bryan O'Connor and Chaplain Henry Fulton, a protestant clergyman transported for life. Both were implicated in the Irish Rebellion and had been granted conditional pardons by King. William Redfern would soon find himself in the same circle of men advising the Governor.

Governor King trusted Joseph Foveaux to such an extent that he had sent him four signed *blank* pardons, in which only the name of the person had to be filled in. Foveaux used one of them on 21 November 1802 when he granted Redfern a *conditional* pardon.[35] With the stroke of a pen, 27-year-old William Redfern became a free man with all legal rights except permission to leave the colony. He had been emancipated after serving only five years of his life sentence and less than a year on the island. Redfern was indebted to Foveaux for his release and for other kindnesses – they would remain friends for the rest of their lives.

When informed by Foveaux of the pardon, King replied on 25 December 1802 that he supported William Redfern's appointment as assistant surgeon and was glad 'he has merited your approbation'. He noted, however, that 'the Establishment will not allow of his continuing in that situation' and a new assistant surgeon would be needed.[36] This would have disappointed Redfern, but he understood the protocols of government appointments; an emancipist was an ex-criminal, and the social norms of the time limited their acceptance in certain circles.

Redfern's medical duties on Norfolk Island had established his reputation as a skilled surgeon, physician and a valued member of the community. In December 1802 he reported to Foveaux on the hospital staff and patients.[37] His assistant at the dispensary remained Bryan O'Connor and there were five female nurses and four men fetching wood and guarding the buildings. In the last two months the hospital staff had cared for 18 patients who suffered mainly from dysentery. All had recovered. During the same period two children were born. There were 25 births on the island in the last year, all assisted by his nurses and midwives. Redfern practiced medicine using the latest remedies and techniques from England but most of his treatments would be considered primitive by today's standards. Indeed, the common practice of bloodletting offered no benefit at all, and, apart from laudanum and alcohol, no anaesthetics were administered to patients needing major surgery or limb amputation.

On Norfolk Island convicts and farmers routinely cleared large pine trees, dug out stumps and tilled rocky soil with spades and hoes. It was physically demanding work that resulted in broken bones, wounds, burns and infections. The food rations issued to convicts, soldiers and officials contained few vegetables or fruit, and the constant diet of salted meat often led to chronic sickness. Dysentery due to malnutrition and poor hygiene was a common illness. It is unknown how Redfern treated this but the typical remedy at that time was an enema of ipecacuanha (dried root of a Brazilian plant) and water. William Balmain, the assistant surgeon on Norfolk Island in 1796, used the bark of local trees instead. When D'Arcy Wentworth was surgeon, he first bled his patients with leeches or an incision in the arm, and then dilated the bowels with castor oil followed with large doses of opium and calomel (mercurous chloride).[38]

Other diseases treated in hospital were fevers, colds, ulcers, inflammations, bruises and skin rashes. Often Redfern would crisscross the island visiting the sick who could not get to the hospital, and he regularly did this on foot – the island was only five miles long and three miles across. He also performed post-mortems on deaths outside of the hospital or if they were considered suspicious. In addition to his daily hospital rounds, Redfern routinely checked the health of 200 convicts, who were only exempted from work if he certified that they were sick. He also attended floggings and could halt a punishment to avoid undue pain. Similarly he could order the removal of leg-irons if a convict was suffering or developed sores. Across the island Doc Redfern was 'well liked for his many kindnesses and liberal ways'. He had a reputation for being 'blunt and outspoken', but he always listened carefully to anyone who required his medical attention.[39]

Desperate to find a permanent surgeon for Norfolk Island, King asked D'Arcy Wentworth on 8 February 1803 to take up the post.[40] Again Wentworth refused. In the same month, Lieutenant Governor Foveaux, having served in the colony for twelve years, applied for leave to visit England. King granted him leave and put Lieutenant John Bowen in command of Norfolk Island during his absence. At the same time Jacob Mountgarrett, the ships surgeon on HMS *Glatton*, volunteered to act as surgeon on the island. But the incessant juggling of this post continued, and a week later these assignments changed again. Bowen and Mountgarrett were instructed to sail to Van Diemen's Land and serve in Hobart Town, a settlement on the Derwent River.[41] Bowen's new assignment made the granting of leave to Foveaux impossible, and with no replacement surgeon for Norfolk Island, King advised him on 18 April 1803 that he would grant William Redfern an *absolute* pardon if he continued to 'behave well'.[42] On 7 June 1803 a further letter to Foveaux advised that, if Mr Redfern was 'so Useful in doing the Duty of Surgeon', he had no objection to him using one of the blank pardon forms. Foveaux did as advised and completely absolved William Redfern of his life sentence. This was published in *The Sydney Gazette* on 19 June 1803.[43] Redfern was now a free man who could do as he pleased, and even return to England if he wanted. Such freedoms were implicit to most skilled people gaining an absolute pardon, but the reality for a medical practitioner in the colony was very different.

On Norfolk Island William Redfern had joined the many farmers on the island producing fresh and salted pork for the mainland colony. His hospital duties prevented him from putting much time into farming, but he had an assigned convict servant managing the pigsties. His farm was productive, and records show that on 3 September 1803 Redfern sold 1450 lb of 'Swine Flesh' to the government store. Across the island farmers delivered 47,000 lb of fresh pork and 55,000 lb of salted pork to the store between July and September, receiving vouchers as payment. Although these vouchers entitled holders to prompt reimbursement from the British Treasury, the payments were notoriously slow.[44]

With no decision on a permanent surgeon replacement, Redfern's responsibilities remained unchanged. There were 1109 people on the island and dysentery was still the most common illness in the hospital. Between May and June 1803, 27 men, women and children were hospitalised. Two of the nine sick convicts died, as well as one soldier and one child.[45] Redfern also had a more prominent patient. Lieutenant Governor Foveaux had suffered from asthma all his life, and it flared up to such an extent in early September that he was confined to bed. Redfern attended him daily and was on call around the clock. On 21 September 1803 the brig *Dart* anchored off Norfolk Island and was due to return to Sydney with farm produce within two days. Desperate to relieve his persistent asthma, Foveaux asked Redfern if he should get a second medical opinion in Sydney. The next day Redfern wrote an assessment report of Foveaux's health.

> Being called upon by Colonel Foveaux, Lieutenant Governor, to give my advice and opinion concerning the state of his Health, and the probable relief which could be offered him by Medical aid and having very maturely considered the nature of his disease, (a complicated asthmatic complaint) the violence of its attack, the rapid progress it has made, together with other alarming symptoms, which have several times manifested themselves, I am of opinion that all medical aid on this Island is rendered ineffectual, and that a removal to Port Jackson is a measure indispensably necessary for the preservation of his Life; not only from the more possibility of his obtaining further advice, but also from the favourable effects to be expected from a sea voyage and change of Climate.[46]

Foveaux had initially intended using this report to request leave for the recommended sea voyage.[47] But the asthma worsened suddenly and, since he had received prior permission to leave the island, Foveaux decided on 23 September to immediately leave for Sydney on the returning *Dart*. With his partner Ann Sherwin, their two-year-old daughter Ann, their servants and families, and, most importantly, with his now personal physician, William Redfern, they boarded the *Dart* and set sail.[48] Foveaux left NSW Corps Captain Ralph Wilson in charge of the island and physician Bryan O'Connor to run the hospital.

Foveaux and his entourage arrived in Sydney a week later, much to the surprise of Governor King who became greatly concerned about Foveaux's health. The sights and sounds of the busy Sydney settlement would have been a revelation for Redfern. Two years earlier he had seen it only briefly when disembarking as a convict from the *Minorca*, but now as a free man he could go wherever he wanted in this bustling town. No records have survived of Redfern's duties or movements during his four months in Sydney. He would have resided close to Foveaux's accommodation ready for an emergency call, and he most likely visited the hospital. As a free man, Redfern could now meet other surgeons, professionally and socially. However, the British class system thrived in Sydney, especially among the military, business and professional ranks. In rural districts, class and rank had little relevance, especially among small settlers where men of all backgrounds supported each other. This was also true on Norfolk Island where Redfern attended officers' houses as their doctor and would occasionally be invited to dinner. But in Sydney the social status of emancipists could not be taken for granted and class distinctions were still observed.

In October 1803 Governor King received a letter from Captain David Collins RN who was sent out from England to establish a settlement at Port Phillip (Melbourne). This site was unsuitable and with King's approval, Collins sailed to Van Diemen's Land to establish a settlement in the south of the island on the Derwent River.[49] It was at the time the British government baulked at the high cost of maintaining the Norfolk Island settlement, especially when valuable ships and men were lost offloading there. King had long been aware of this concern and, two months earlier, had advised that 'a principal part of the people and Establishment' at Norfolk Island be moved to Van Diemen's Land. Nevertheless, he reminded the Home Office that the island had been a valuable source of food at times of need and had 'been of the greatest assistance to this Colony in providing entirely for its numbers since 1794'.[50] King discussed this with Joseph Foveaux during his stay in Sydney, seeking his opinion on the possibility and feasibility of the island's exodus.

On 3 January 1804 just before the Foveaux party returned to Norfolk Island, King once again appointed D'Arcy Wentworth as surgeon at the hospital – this time it was an official command that he could not disobey.[51] The medical advice Joseph Foveaux received for his asthma in Sydney had not noticeably improved his health and, on 19 January 1804, he and Redfern departed for Norfolk Island on the *Union*.[52] They arrived on 9 February to find the island administration in chaos. Captain Wilson, who Foveaux had left in charge, had not followed his detailed orders. Items taken from stores had not been recorded and the construction of Government House had stopped with labourers and materials diverted for use on Wilson's private property. Wilson was arrested and charged with maladministration.[53]

In Foveaux's absence, the convict John Morris had injured two people during a robbery in January and when arrested he was severely beaten by Captain Wilson. Redfern examined Morris and found that he had been beaten with a stick, flogged and had salt water thrown on his back. As 'additional torture', leg irons had been attached with hot rivets that burnt his legs. Foveaux deemed this punishment excessive and in March 1804 when a court sentenced Morris to death, Foveaux recommended to the Colonial Office that he be shown mercy.[54] He was never hanged, and one suspects Redfern's humane advice had been given and followed.

A severe outbreak of dysentery had also occurred on the island in Redfern's absence and was still rampant when he returned. The convicts were most affected but through the efforts of Redfern and the hospital staff the outbreak was curtailed. In the next six months, 6 men and 4 children died, and 14 children were born.[55]

While Redfern was in Sydney, Sarah McHenry had been left in charge of his farm, and it had flourished. The March 1804 records of the Norfolk Island 'Return of Number of Acres of Land' show that Redfern owned 48 acres and had six goats and 130 hogs – the most pigs owned by any military and civil official on the island. They were, however, only a small fraction of the 6237 pigs on the island.[56] Redfern now had a new salt house on his property, and from April to June 1804, he delivered to the government store 1862 lb of fresh pork and 1068 lb of salted pork.[57] The doctor had not only retained his cherished surgeon position at the hospital but had, with Sarah's help, become a successful pig farmer.

In these more secure times Redfern renewed his habit of recording information that intrigued him in his notebook. His entries show diverse practical interests that focus on "how to make things", especially medical remedies. They describe how 'To clean the Tops of Boots', a 'Recipe for getting the stain of Wine out of White or Yellow Leather Breeches' and how to use 'Marseilles Vinegar' as an antidote to putrid fever. Other notes explain how to make cement for mending broken glass, china and earthenware; a recipe for 'Vitriolic Acid from Sulphur', followed by one to use diluted Cognac-brandy to rinse 'Weak Eyes'; a 'Process of Making Port Wine'; how to waterproof leather; how to make a cork waistcoat for swimming; and how to accelerate the separation of churning butter. More technical entries record how to make 'Silver Looking-glasses' and give instructions for making 'an alarm by sand in place of clock-work', and an 'Aeolus Harp' (small harp played by the wind).

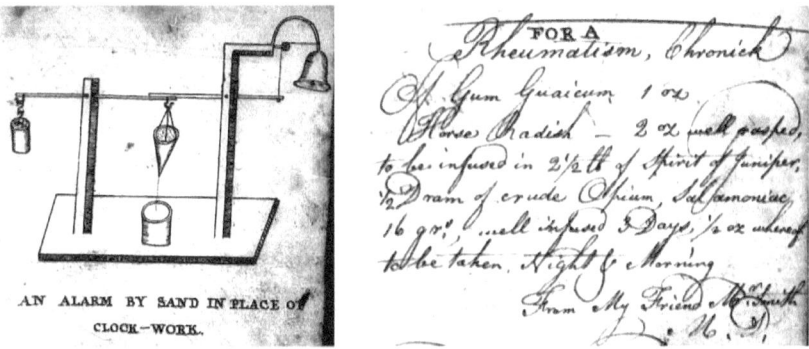

Two excerpts from Redfern's notebook showing a "sand clock alarm" and a remedy for chronic rheumatism.

Redfern's notebook is a fascinating memento of how an inquisitive individual kept information at his fingertips 200 years before the advent of Internet search engines.[58]

Chapter 6

NORFOLK FARMER & TRADER

I do hereby Certify that Mr. William Redfern, having been landed on Norfolk Island some time in January, 1802, performed the duty of Assistant to the Surgeon until the 19th June following, when he was appointed to the charge of the Hospital, and acted as Surgeon to the Settlement until the 12th May, 1804; in the duties of which office, he conducted himself with such diligence and attention as to merit my perfect approbation. Foveaux, 1804[1]

On 12 May 1804, D'Arcy Wentworth arrived on Norfolk Island to become the assistant surgeon in charge of the hospital, a post William Redfern had held temporarily for over two years.[2] The two men had met and become acquainted during Redfern's recent visit to Sydney, and though they differed widely in character, their Irish upbringing and medical interests led to a close life-long friendship. Both men had also experienced the sharp end of British justice and shared the distaste of social exclusion.

William Redfern had been raised in a close stable family that nurtured honesty and service in the children. He had grown up to be a serious young man who spoke his mind, and his repudiation of injustices probably upset authorities. Redfern also abhorred unearned privilege and this, with his blunt matter-of-fact manner, conveyed an openness that appealed to patients wanting an honest diagnosis but not to those seeking a friendly bedside manner.

Born in 1762 in Belfast, D'Arcy Wentworth arrived in Sydney as a free man but only sailed to New South Wales as a surgeon to avoid being convicted of highway robbery in the Old Bailey. Although D'Arcy's father was an innkeeper, the Wentworth family was influential politically and they included the Marquess of Rockingham, a past British Prime Minister. When the Marquess died in 1782 his vast estate passed to his nephew Lord William Wentworth Fitzwilliam. In 1778 D'Arcy became apprenticed to Surgeon Alexander Patton in Tandragee, Northern Ireland. After completing his medical training in 1785, he moved to England under the patronage of Lord Fitzwilliam. In December that year

Wentworth qualified before the Court of Examiners for the Company of Surgeons in London, with an intention to work for the East India Company. In the meantime, he led a frenetic social life in London that exceeded his modest income and earned him a reputation for extravagance and gambling in doubtful company.

Lord Fitzwilliam attempted to have the young rake serve as a surgeon on the First Fleet flotilla sailing for New South Wales. To do this Wentworth needed naval qualifications and in July 1787 he passed exams to be a third-rate naval surgeon, but by then the First Fleet had sailed. D'Arcy subsequently resumed a dissolute life and six months later faced three charges of highway robbery in the Old Bailey. He was found not guilty on two charges and acquitted on the third because of insufficient evidence. In a concurrent trial, his mistress Mary Wilkinson was charged with receiving stolen goods but was also acquitted.[3]

Convinced that Wentworth would soon be jailed, or worse, his family tried unsuccessfully to find him a position on the continent. In desperation, John Villiers, the 2nd son of the Earl of Clarendon, wrote to the Colonial Office in October 1789 advising them that D'Arcy was 'extremely desirous of going to Botany Bay' and that his training as a surgeon might prove useful to the colony. Villiers revealed that 'if he continues in this country, it is scarcely possible for him to return to any honest course of life'. The Colonial Office declined the offer – they already had many such men in Botany Bay.[4] Two months later Wentworth was again arrested for robbery. At a hearing on 9 December 1789, he pleaded for leniency of the court so he could depart for Botany Bay to work as a surgeon. After a controversial trial involving accusations of bribery and perjury, the jury acquitted him. However, the Judge questioned the verdict and advised D'Arcy to promptly pursue his profession overseas. He was released a free man with a tarnished reputation.[5]

Wentworth repaid his debts to Mary Wilkinson and in late December 1789 boarded the transport *Neptune* about to sail for New South Wales.[6] On seeing his quarters Wentworth would have undoubtedly been shocked at the cramped putrid conditions he would have to endure for the next six months. In addition to the 502 male and female convicts on board, there was a battalion of NSW Corps soldiers destined to replace the Royal Marines in the colony. Prior to departure, one of the Corps officers, Lieutenant John Macarthur, insulted the ship's captain, John Gilbert, and this led to a duel. No one was injured but Gilbert was replaced by Donald Trail, a change that would cost many convicts' lives.

On 19 January 1790 the Second Fleet, comprising the *Surprise*, *Neptune* and *Scarborough*, sailed for New South Wales with 1095 convicts on board. Unlike the First Fleet, the ships were privately contracted to owners who were paid according to the number of convicts embarked, not the number delivered. Consequently, the ships were crammed to the gunnels with chained convicts who were rarely allowed to exercise on deck. Scurvy was rife and in late April an epidemic of typhoid devastated the convicts in their filthy, lice-infected and vermin-ridden cells. Despite his training, Wentworth was not allowed to interfere with the medical practices on the *Neptune*. By the time the Second Fleet reached Port Jackson in June 1790, 270 convicts were dead, 486 required hospitalisation and 124 died later. The mortality of convicts on the Second Fleet was the worst in the history of transportation to Australia.

Despite the trauma of the *Neptune* passage, Wentworth had managed to befriend the 17-year-old convict Catherine Crowley, who was being transported for stealing clothes. It would prove to be an enduring relationship. Six months after landing, D'Arcy Wentworth was sent to Norfolk Island to assist the hospital surgeon Thomas Jamison and was accompanied by Catherine and their newborn son William. The couple would eventually have three sons, William, D'Arcy and John. In 1796 Wentworth and his family returned to Sydney where, in 1800, Catherine died during childbirth. Subsequently D'Arcy Wentworth formed a relationship with the convict Maria Ainslie, who raised his sons. In 1802 the two older boys, William and D'Arcy, were sent to England to further their education.

In May 1804 the 42-year-old D'Arcy Wentworth returned for a second time as surgeon at the Norfolk Island hospital while Maria and 9-year-old John remained in Sydney. A week prior to Wentworth arriving on Norfolk Island the Secretary of the Colonial Office, Lord Hobart, instructed Lieutenant Governor Joseph Foveaux to move some of the island's residents to Port Dalrymple (Launceston) in Van Diemen's Land. The relocated settlers were to be compensated for every acre of land they owned on the island with four acres in the new settlement and to be fully victualled for one year.[7] Foveaux informed island inhabitants of

Hobart's order and asked who was prepared to make the move in September. According to his first report to Governor King, the settler's initial response was positive. However, this changed when they heard of the conditions at Port Dalrymple, which most residents considered worse than those on Norfolk. Many of the ex-convicts and soldiers who had created farms on the island saw no benefit in moving and told Foveaux they had been young men when they first settled on Norfolk but were now too old to start again, or to chance the uncertainties of the new settlement.[8]

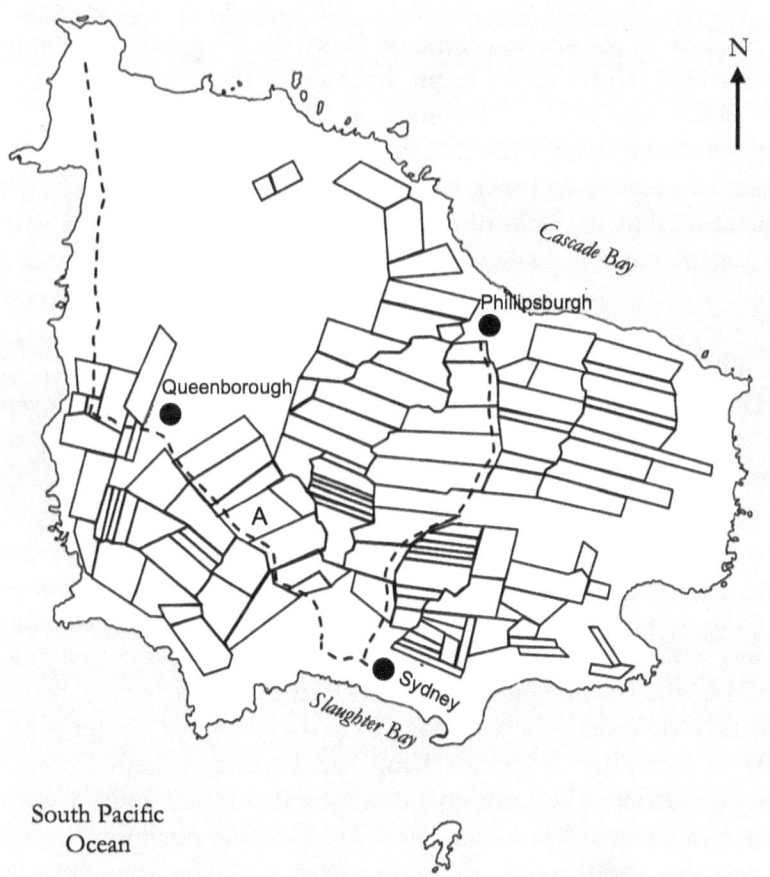

View of Norfolk Island showing the main settlement areas and the freehold farm divisions. In 1802 William Redfern bought farmland (A) on the road to Queenborough.

On hearing the islander's objections, King initially considered vetoing Lord Hobart's order. However, since Lieutenant Colonel Paterson had already been sent to command Port Dalrymple, the relocation order would be hard to reverse.[9] He pressured Foveaux to convince settlers of the benefits, and on 19 July 1804 he was informed that 41 of the 135 settlers on Norfolk had agreed to relocate.[10] King instructed Foveaux that once the evacuation of the island had begun, the role of the hospital surgeon would 'be performed by a junior assistant, and the eldest assistant now acting as surgeon at Norfolk Island would need to be removed to Port Dalrymple'.[11] If acted upon, this meant William Redfern would stay put on the island and D'Arcy Wentworth should be relocated.

Because of his previous time on Norfolk, King fully understood the settlers' reluctance to leave. In August 1804 he told Foveaux that older residents could remain, as younger people were better suited to start new lives. However, King warned Foveaux that those who agreed to move would need to be assessed so 'idle and worthless' settlers could not claim the liberal compensation. King envisaged that farmers remaining on Norfolk would continue to supply meat and grain to the colony and assist visiting whalers. In addition, convicts staying on Norfolk had to be trustworthy so that the military presence could be reduced, and a Corps officer could replace the Lieutenant Governor. Pending on the return of Joseph Foveaux to England, Governor King appointed Corps Captain John Piper to be in charge of Norfolk Island.[12]

The evacuation of residents to Port Dalrymple now preoccupied many on Norfolk Island. However, for those who remained, the hospital was about to provide a welcome service – vaccination against smallpox (*variola virus*). This virulent disease was much feared in the colony, but so far there had been only one outbreak. The first vaccine, lymph of cowpox, arrived in Sydney on 8 May 1804, a year after Governor King had requested them from the Colonial Office. The London Cow-Pock Institution and the Royal Jennerian Society led a campaign to eradicate smallpox through vaccination and had provided the vaccines. The following day Surgeon John Savage performed the first smallpox vaccination in Sydney. Savage, a member of the Royal Jennerian Society, had experimented with cowpox since coming to the colony in 1803. It turned out that the only effective lymph of cowpox was the one sent from his Society. Over the next few weeks Savage, along with Principal Surgeon Thomas Jamison and Corps Surgeon John Harris, successfully inoculated close to 400 children. After their success, vaccines for 320 children were sent to Norfolk Island.[13]

Foveaux reported on 10 August 1803 that surgeons Wentworth and Redfern had used these vaccines to inoculate the island's children, but it had been unsuccessful because the lymph was no longer active.[14] It would be another year before Lieutenant Thomas Davis arrived in early 1805 with his recently inoculated children from Sydney. In this way Davis' children brought 'live' cowpox to the island, and Redfern and Wentworth used *variolation*, taking the lymph from the skin blisters of Davis' children, to successfully immunise the islands' children.[15]

In August 1804 Foveaux's asthma flared up again and, because of his 'very ill state of heath', surgeons Redfern and Wentworth advised him to go to England for further treatment.[16] Foveaux agreed but before departing, he wrote a 'Testimonial in favour of Assistant-Surgeon Redfern' who had 'conducted himself with such diligence and attention as to merit my perfect approbation'.[17]

One of Foveaux's last official duties on the island was to conduct a general muster of settlers, listing their land, animals, family relationships and houses owned. This shows William Redfern with a 'Wife' (no name), no children, one servant, 25 acres under cultivation, 23 acres fallow, 3 sheep, 6 goats and 66 pigs. The housing of settler families varied greatly, 44 lived in huts of 'no value' and 88 had houses valued from £4 to £110. D'Arcy Wentworth's house, the fourth most expensive on the island, was valued at £36. William Redfern's house was worth only £4.[18] Redfern's home was a 24 x 12 ft (7.3 x 3.7 m) lath and plaster house with a shingled roof, a cellar, a staircase to the attic and an adjacent 30 x 10 ft barn.[19] His 'Wife' could only have been Sarah McHenry; her former husband was now stationed in Parramatta.

On 7 Sep 1804 Joseph Foveaux, Ann Sherwin, their 3-year-old daughter Ann and servants sailed for England on the whaler *Albion*.[20] Redfern would miss the professional support of Foveaux. Moreover, contrary to the social norms of the time, he had also become a friend. Foveaux greatly valued Redfern's medical skills and, in 1806 when suffering gout in England, he lamented not having his trusted surgeon at his side. He wrote to John Piper that

'I shall be very glad to find that Mr. Redfern is still with you' when I return to the colony.[21]

On 8 September 1804, a day after Foveaux's departure, Redfern sold his farm for £160 to emancipist William Thompson, a settler who had been living on Norfolk since its first settlement in 1788.[22] Thompson was one of the older residents not prepared to relocate to Port Dalrymple. And nor was William Redfern; his aim was to eventually return to either Sydney or England, but he knew the latter destination would be difficult while surgeon appointments remained the pawns of the Governor. In any case, his plans were about to be thrown awry by Captain John Piper, the new island Commandant. Whereas Joseph Foveaux had been a good administrator who was well liked by residents, Piper soon showed his utter disregard for regulations and ex-convicts. Within weeks of arriving he permitted the import of spirits and allowed residents to leave the island without Governor King's approval.

On 6 January 1805 King reprimanded Piper and ordered that he obey orders. In the same communication, Piper was told that the ships *Investigator* and *Harrington* would soon arrive to take inhabitants to Port Dalrymple. In late February these ships relocated 45 convicts, 49 soldiers with families, and 4 settlers with families.[23] Thereafter few settlers agreed to relocate, and in August there were still 770 people living on the island.[24]

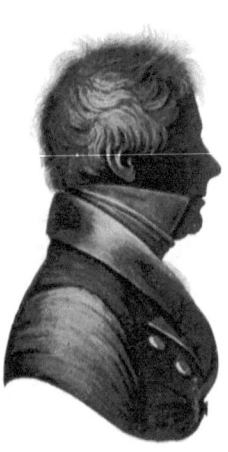
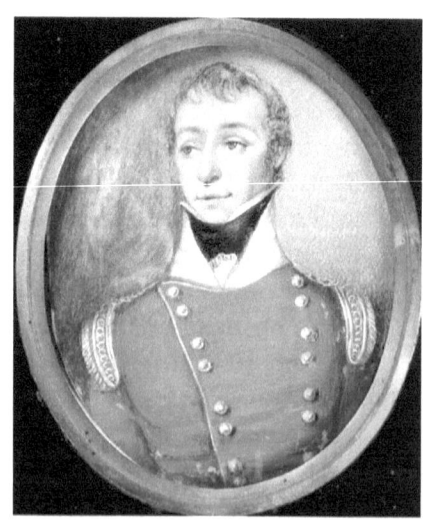

1815 silhouette portrait of Principal Surgeon D'Arcy Wentworth.

1815 portrait of John Piper, Norfolk Island Commandant (1804-1810).

As an assistant to D'Arcy Wentworth, Redfern's hospital salary was small, and he was not paid for treating military patients. Without any farm income William sought D'Arcy's advice on how to improve his financial situation within the trading constraints of the island, which were both complex and cumbersome. No bank or regulated monetary institution existed in the colony because the Colonial Office had deemed it unnecessary for a penal settlement. Cash payments were made either in pounds Sterling or Spanish dollars, but such transactions were difficult since visiting traders removed coinage from the colony. The lack of hard currency meant that local payments relied heavily on government bills, store receipts, promissory notes and barter. Barter, or payment in grain, goods or services was the most common way to settle debts. Promissory notes aided a cash-strapped system, but these risked forgery and non-payment.[25]

The salaries of military and civil officers stationed in the colony were usually paid in England and cashed in Sydney by drawing bills on private agents in London. D'Arcy Wentworth's London agent, Charles Cookney, settled his bills, collected his pay, bought him goods and supervised his sons' education. Many in the colony depended on this tedious and expensive process. Traders refused to accept private salary bills as payment for goods, unless endorsed by a prominent colonist. Local agents or merchants commonly paid military officers and later cashed their salary bills with the officers' agents in London.[26] Wentworth acted as a local agent, a practice he had continued on Norfolk Island with merchant Simeon Lord as his partner in Sydney.

In July 1805, on Wentworth's advice, Redfern began trading in local farm produce. He acted as an intermediary for other small farmers, reimbursing them with either promissory notes, goods bought from trading ships, or medical services. A hired butcher prepared 798 lb of fresh pork that Redfern sold to the government store. Two months later he sent 625 bushels of maize and 10,468 lb of fresh pork valued at £311 to the store.[27] His 'Store Receipt' for these goods was accepted as currency in the colony, passing from person to person with each transaction. Most receipts ended up with Corps officers, merchants and shipmasters or with 'Dr Redfern', who would have arranged with D'Arcy Wentworth to have them converted to cash in London.

In November 1805 pork production on Norfolk Island faced a

major crisis when the salted pork in the island's store was declared unfit for human consumption. The meat was rancid and pork feet and heads were found in storage casks. It is likely that Surgeon Redfern issued an alert following a case of food poisoning. He had had previous experience with rancid food in the Royal Navy and at the Coldbath Fields prison where he had been fed a cow udder still filled with curdled milk. The presence of rotten meat endangered the island's food exports and Piper promptly ordered examination of all products in the government store. It found leaking casks of 1118 lb of pork 'rotten, stinking and unfit for men to eat'.[28] By then, it was too late to for the 30 casks of 16,090 lb of salted pork already sent to Van Diemen's Land. An inspection in Hobart showed the entire shipment of Norfolk pork was inedible. In May 1806 Governor King required Piper to inspect all salted pork before shipment and stipulated that pigs' feet or heads must not be included.[29] After this incident, Redfern and Wentworth temporarily stopped selling pork to the store.

In February 1806 D'Arcy Wentworth was informed that Surgeon John Connellan would replace him at the hospital, and that he should return to Sydney on the next ship. Wentworth tolerated Piper's lax standards much better than Redfern and did not relish returning to the mainland where governance was much stricter. He had already applied to his patron Lord Fitzwilliam for leave to visit his sons in England but had not received a reply.[30] On 30 March 1806 D'Arcy Wentworth and Maria Ainslie sailed for Sydney.

With his colleague's departure, Redfern took over Wentworth's business dealings and occupied his substantial house and property. The house was 33 x 12 ft with a shingled roof, plastered lath walls and a cellar. There was also a 20 x 14 ft salting house, a small shed and a privy.[31] Redfern continued trading in the salary bills of local officials, forwarding them to Wentworth in Sydney for remittance by his agent in London.[32] He also sent casks of salted pork to D'Arcy in Port Jackson.

Redfern was not the only senior official on the island trading in produce. The new surgeon John Connellan also formed a business arrangement with Simeon Lord and D'Arcy Wentworth in Sydney, and with the Norfolk settler James Mitchell. Another local trader was emancipist Michael Hayes, who was an agent for Principal Surgeon Thomas Jamison exporting wheat and pork. Commissary

William Broughton and the collector of duties, Aaron Davis, were other Norfolk officials trading in island produce.

There is no indication that William Redfern was unhappy with his current duties at the Norfolk hospital, but there is little doubt he hoped to be eventually transferred to Sydney. The change in leadership on the island had made his life difficult. The hospital received less support from John Piper and the relationship between the two men was fragile at best – it had suffered in the absence of Wentworth's diplomacy. Whereas Foveaux praised Redfern's abilities and treated him civilly, the Commandant did neither. Captain John Piper had arrived in New South Wales on the same ship as Major Grose who, as temporary Governor of the colony, had reinstated all the trappings of the British class system. Piper was also a friend of John Macarthur; both men maintained that ex-convicts should have no place in respectable society.

The comfortable serenity of social life on the island disappeared with Piper's arrival. Alcohol consumption was excessive and single females were seriously disrespected. Piper hosted fellow officers to nights of bawdy entertainment with young girls at the military barracks. Redfern was not invited to these affairs, but Wentworth sometimes participated.[33] After copious rum had been served at these parties, numbers were painted to the girls' bare backs before they performed 'the dances of the mermaids' to excite the men.[34] Piper fathered at least four children as a consequence of these nights. In April 1806 Redfern delivered a son, John, to 14-year-old Margaret Eddington, and in August 1806 another John to 16-year-old Mary Ann Sheers. In November 1806 a girl, Mary Ann, was born to Sarah Hughes and in 1807, a daughter Rebecca to Mary Power. Piper had already fathered a child in Sydney with a teenage girl and would father at least 19 children with five different females while in the colony. In 1816 he married Mary Ann Sheers who bore him 13 children.[35]

According to the British Articles of War, government surgeons did not attend childbirths; this was the responsibility of midwives. Normally government surgeons would only treat someone 'not victualled by the Crown' if they paid a fee. Nevertheless, it had become an accepted practice since Governor Phillip's time that surgeons assist everyone, independent of their status. The issue of medical responsibility was tested in May 1805 when Principal Surgeon Jamison prosecuted surgeons James Mileham and John

Savage for not attending the birth of a child. A settler's wife had died after Savage refused to visit their house. The civil court found the men guilty of negligence.[36] Mileham received a reprimand and Savage was sent to England where the charge was dropped because midwifery was not required within the Articles of War.[37] This case challenged the legal obligations of government surgeons to treat residents who were no longer the Crown's responsibility. An increasing number of free emigrants and emancipists required medical care and there was an urgent need for doctors who could act in a private capacity.

John Macarthur returned to Sydney in June 1805. His court martial in London had been quashed because documentary evidence of his behaviour submitted by Governor King had been stolen *en route* to England. Quite unfairly, the Colonial Office rebuked King for wasting the court's time. Macarthur had promptly resigned his NSW Corps commission and been privately told by an informant in the Colonial Office that King would soon be recalled.

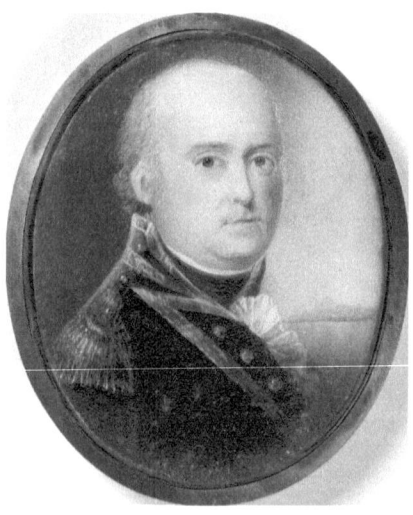
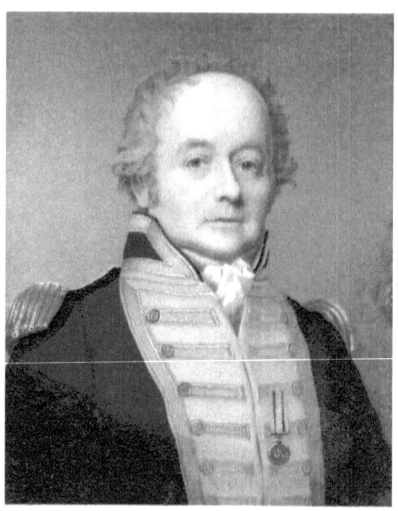

Portrait of Philip Gidley King, third Governor of NSW (1800-1806).

Portrait of William Bligh, fourth Governor of NSW (1806-1808).

Governor King was mortified when he heard that Macarthur and others had convinced the Colonial Office he was incompetent and had disrupted Corps duties. Records show that King was a hardworking diligent administrator who tried to eradicate rampant profiteering in the colony. Despite the injustice of his imminent recall, King continued to encourage better food production and to assist settlers who struggled after major flood losses. In March 1806 he informed the Colonial Office that 25 soldiers would stay on Norfolk Island to guard the few remaining convicts. No one else wanted to leave the island 'where they had been so long and so comfortably settled'.[38] Knowing the importance of these settlers to food self-sufficiency, King requested there be no further relocations to Van Diemen's Land.

Unfortunately, the Colonial Office had received contradictory advice from Joseph Foveaux in London who recommended Norfolk Island be completely evacuated. He claimed that, although removal costs were high, they would be less than maintaining the island.[39] This issue remained unresolved when Captain William Bligh was appointed the next Governor of New South Wales. In fact, Bligh sailed with orders to follow Lord Hobart's plan to partially evacuate Norfolk Island, only to be instructed on arrival in Sydney that the British now wanted to relocate *all* island residents, as per Foveaux's proposal.[40]

Captain William Bligh and his daughter Mary arrived on the ship *Sinclair* on 6 August 1806. Mary's husband, Lieutenant John Putland, commanded the escort ship HMS *Porpoise*. Bligh was a veteran mariner who was famous for several reasons: he sailed a longboat from Tahiti to Batavia following the HMS *Bounty* mutiny; Nelson praised him for bravery in the Battle of Copenhagen and he advised the Admiralty during the Nore Mutiny. Bligh had a reputation for strict discipline, intolerance of disobedience and use of strong naval invective. Sir Joseph Banks saw Bligh's qualities as necessary to meet the challenges in the colony and had endorsed his nomination as Governor. Bligh was well briefed on the NSW Corps' intransigence with past Governors but was supremely confident he could instil discipline into this military rabble.

In February 1807 Philip Gidley King and his family boarded HMS *Buffalo* to return to England. Most residents were sorry to see him go; he had been a popular man who had strived to make the colony self-sufficient. As a humane governor he fostered convict rehabilitation and encouraged emancipists to participate in private enterprise. King had rewarded Redfern's service to medicine with an absolute pardon and a promotion. Unquestionably Redfern's rise in professional status owed much to both Foveaux and King's belief in equality and meritocracy.

William Bligh's installation as the third Governor of New South Wales took place on 14 August 1806 after recent major floods in the Hawkesbury district. He continued government assistance to devastated farmers and, in doing so, gained enormous personal support in the district. Bligh reinforced this by promising to protect farmers from the unfair trading practices of NSW Corps officers and their cronies. He infuriated the Corps by appointing civilians as new officials rather than military officers. Undeterred by protests, Bligh pressed ahead with reforms benefiting ordinary residents, especially the smaller settlers.[41] Unsurprisingly, Bligh's reforms galvanised opposition among the business elite who had previously suppressed similar reforms by previous governors. They now supported John Macarthur and Corps officers who opposed any changes that eroded their profits. Surgeon D'Arcy Wentworth and businessman Simeon Lord were among those who strongly resisted Governor Bligh's new regulations.

For years the excessive fees charged to transport Norfolk Island products to and from Sydney had been a serious impost on trade. Prior to 1797, local boat building was disallowed in the colony to prevent convicts from escaping. However, in 1798 Governor Hunter permitted the first ship to be constructed in Sydney and in 1802 Governor King endorsed boat building for the Hawkesbury River trade. In 1806 Norfolk traders convinced Commandant Piper that a locally constructed boat was needed, and a consortium was formed to build a 50-ton schooner.[42] It included William Redfern as the chief financier and planner, the beachmaster John Drummond, boatbuilder Thomas Ransome and convict superintendent Robert Jones. On 9 September 1806 Piper informed King that he had granted permission to build the boat.[43] By the time this letter reached the mainland, Bligh was governor and had just issued port regulations controlling incoming ships, cargoes, crews and passengers. Heavier fines were to be imposed if convicts escaped on ships, and vessels could only be built with the Governor's approval. Piper was told that the ship should not have been constructed without his or Governor King's permission and if already built, it must immediately sail to Port Jackson to be registered before being allowed to trade.[44]

On 15 April 1807, Surgeon D'Arcy Wentworth was put in charge of the Parramatta hospital. Within months of his appointment, Captain Abbott, commanding Corps officer at Parramatta, arrested Wentworth for using convalescent convict patients to work on his farm. The Parramatta Chief Constable Francis Oakes was sent to investigate and found 'invalid' convicts labouring on Wentworth's property. They were returned to the government camp and three days later Abbott directed a constable to take two of the ill men back to the hospital for re-admission. When Wentworth refused to accept them, he was charged with insubordination.[45]

On 18 July Wentworth's case was scheduled for a hearing. This did not concern him unduly because he knew the officers on the court bench and considered the Judge Advocate, Richard Atkins, weak. He was right; the court found Wentworth guilty, but Atkins only sentenced him to a reprimand. Bligh was furious and suspended Wentworth from duties pending advice from the Colonial Office. Wentworth applied to take leave in England but was refused. The sacking of such a prominent medical official unsettled many in the colony, but Bligh wanted to send a clear message that no one was above the law. The misuse of assigned convict labour had become a major rort in the colony and this was a wakeup call for the military, business and medical fraternity.[46]

Farming on Norfolk Island was difficult in the summer of 1806-7. There had been a drought for five months and by March 1807 the island's wheat and maize fields were parched. The lack of feed for pigs brought pork production to a standstill, and the island's few supplies were sold at inflated prices. The situation was so dire that Governor Bligh sent the *Lady Nelson* with provisions to relieve the settlement.[47] With little opportunity to trade, Redfern sold his pork meat to the local government store and received bills of £175 to be converted into treasury bills.[48] The inflated prices on the island encouraged D'Arcy Wentworth and Simeon Lord to ship William a cask of sugar and a box of tea for sale. They also informed Piper that Redfern would offer him up to 200 lb of the sugar and some tea for a bargain price.[49] One is left to ponder on how the usually fastidious Redfern justified this sweetener! Or had the ingratiation of authorities now become accepted practice in the colony?

In June 1807 HMS *Porpoise* captained by John Putland docked off Norfolk Island to offload supplies.[50] Putland suffered from

Phthisis pulmonalis (tuberculosis) and sought medical advice at the island hospital. Putland remained on the island for a month and surgeons Connellan and Redfern tried to help him. Although no cure existed then, there were a few standard palliatives – cod liver oil, vinegar massages and the inhalation of hemlock or turpentine. Connellan, who had only recently finished his medical studies, was the senior doctor, but Redfern was more experienced in common diseases and probably took charge.

In September 1807 Redfern received a letter from Wentworth describing his dismissal by Bligh and claiming to be an innocent victim of his autocratic rule. Redfern replied he 'felt much shocked at the unworthy treatment' and rather foolishly condemned Bligh for punishing his friend's illegal behaviour, writing:

> ... as lamented a species of depravity as can possibly be attendant on the most degenerate state of Human nature, is strongly marked in the present instance: namely, that the Man who has been most ungenerously and iniquitously offended and injured is the last Person that can be (if I maybe allowed the expression) forgiven by the Parties so offending.[51]

Redfern should have known of William Bligh's admirable treatment of the crew following the Nore mutiny. However, one also suspects that as a longstanding resident of Norfolk Island, he did not understand the extent of business malpractices in Sydney. It is unlikely that Wentworth told Redfern that Bligh was trying to impose fairer trading regulations in the colony or that he was assisting the less privileged settlers. Fortunately, Redfern resisted further treasonous chatter and wrote that 'your Brother Officers have perfectly concurred in the proprietary of your conduct' and that on proper application to His Majesty's Ministers would obtain 'ample redress for the indignity' he had suffered. His letter then focused on financial matters. He concluded the letter with a matter of personal concern – he sought Wentworth's advice on how he might best return to Sydney.

> Let me entreat you to favour me with all the Information you have been able to obtain relative to the coming out or detention of Colonel Foveaux: His arrival here is expected with the utmost impatience, being destined, in the public opinion to bring the ultimate Fiat of Government respecting the fate of this Island. Do you think the Evacuation will be total or partial? I should be glad

to know your opinion of my success, if as soon as I can settle my affairs, I will return to Port Jackson – and what pursuits would be the most eligible. I hope you will answer this letter as pointedly as you possibly can.[52]

The letter finishes with greetings from Sarah, 'My Lady desires her Best Respect to you and Maria and wishes me to inform Maria that she has sent two small cases of Bananas marked D. W'.

The Colonial Office's order to evacuate Norfolk Island arrived in early September 1807. Bligh informed Piper that HMS *Porpoise*, HMS *Lady Nelson* and the *Estramina* would be sent to take residents to Port Dalrymple or to the Derwent River (Hobart Town). Evacuees could choose their preferred destination.[53] The order shocked everyone on the island, and especially traders with large investments in property and stock. Some inhabitants were heavily indebted to James Mitchell, William Redfern, William Broughton, Aaron Davis and Michael Hayes to a total of £15,000. Redfern alone was owed £4200. With little hard cash accessible, payments had to be made either as promissory notes, bills or farm produce.[54] Settlers needed to suddenly sell their devalued farm produce and animals to settle debts. Considerable stock ended up with Redfern as debt repayments, and he delivered 2913 lb of pork to the store over the next five months.[55]

In late October 1807, HMS *Lady Nelson* arrived to begin the exodus but only 34 residents embarked. A month later HMS *Porpoise* docked, departing the island on 26 December 1807 for the Derwent settlement with 182 people on board.[56] It was the last time Redfern saw Lieutenant Putland; he died on 4 January 1808.

In Sydney there was much dissatisfaction with the government. Bligh's insistence that his reforms be complied with "to the letter" had caused opposition beyond the business and military circles. Paradoxically most of Bligh's new reforms were at Whitehall's insistence. John Macarthur was again the most recalcitrant and vocal critic, and, in November 1807, Bligh saw an opportunity to get rid of him. A convict had escaped to Tahiti on the schooner *Parramatta* owned by Macarthur and Garnham Blaxcell. When the ship returned to Sydney it was impounded and Macarthur was required to pay a bond. He refused and abandoned the crew of the confiscated vessel. John Macarthur was jailed, given bail and committed for trial on 25 January 1808.

The year 1808 opened with the colony in high dudgeon. Although most small settlers revered Bligh, there was seething discontent in the larger settlements. Merchants in Sydney and Parramatta claimed the Governor was ignoring their businesses and helping only the farmers. They asserted Bligh's blunt demeanour and crude manners better suited illiterate settlers than the educated people of Sydney. On 1 January 1808 Bligh was presented with a Loyalty Address with 833 signatories of free and emancipist settlers in the Hawkesbury district. The address thanked Bligh for improving their lives and pledged their loyalty at the risk of their lives and lands to support a 'Wise and Patriotic Government'.[57]

Those against the governor denigrated the signatories of the Address as ignorant farmers who knew no better. In any case John Macarthur had more immediate issues to deal with. On 25 January 1808 he appeared before a court on the convict escape charge with Judge Advocate Atkins adjudicating and six Corps officers on the bench. At the opening of the hearing Macarthur demanded Atkins be disbarred from presiding because he was suing him for an unpaid debt. Atkins immediately withdrew from the bench and, in his hurried exit, left his court papers behind. The Corps officers on the bench then, quite illegally, released Macarthur on bail.

The next day Governor Bligh ordered that John Macarthur be re-arrested and summoned the court officers to Government House to return Atkins' court papers. Macarthur claimed this latter order was an attempt to arrest the six Corps officers for treason. On this pretext he prepared a petition calling on Commandant Major George Johnston to arrest William Bligh and take charge of the government. Macarthur's improvised arrest petition was initially only signed by six other men. The final version was circulated after Bligh's arrest and 151 signatures were collected, some at gunpoint. The signatories included the Corps Surgeon John Harris, Principal Surgeon Thomas Jamison and the Assistant Surgeons D'Arcy Wentworth and James Mileham.[58]

In the early evening of 26 January 1808, a troop of 300 Corps soldiers marched to Government House accompanied by the civilians John Macarthur, Simeon Lord, D'Arcy Wentworth and Henry Kable.[59] At Government House William Bligh presided over a dinner celebrating the 20th anniversary of the colony. The soldiers detained the dinner guests and Bligh was placed under house arrest. Major Johnston then took command of the colony as the self-appointed Lieutenant Governor. To avoid a countercoup, Corp soldiers scoured the rural districts confiscating firearms. A multitude of reprisals followed. Bligh civil appointees were dismissed from office, and many were placed in prison. John Macarthur was appointed Colonial Secretary, a post that enabled him to oversee most business matters in the colony and restart the trade in alcohol to pre-Bligh levels.

Macarthur wasted no time in rescheduling a trial to clear his name of the convict escape charge, and a court session with the bench full of friends was quickly convened to find him not guilty. Encouraged by the rebel's new judicial flexibility, D'Arcy Wentworth requested another court martial to clear his name. On 17 February 1808 he was found not guilty and reinstated as assistant surgeon.[60] Corps officers resumed their control over imported retail goods that, ironically, severely disadvantaged private Sydney merchants and supporters, such as Simeon Lord. With Macarthur as Colonial Secretary, rebels now had easy access to government stores and animal herds from which quantities of food, material and cattle were stolen for their personal use.

Initially, Bligh's overthrow and the rebel administration had little impact on Norfolk Island and the relocation to Van Diemen's Land proceeded as planned. In any case, when Piper eventually heard of the rebellion, he would have known that Macarthur and the rebels would support him. HMS *Lady Nelson* docked at Norfolk in late January 1808 and departed for Hobart Town on 14 February with another 50 people on board.[61]

By now William Redfern and John Piper were at loggerheads. Redfern had never approved of Piper's shambolic lifestyle but in April 1808 any semblance of civility vanished for quite bizarre reasons. A Tahitian missionary, James Elder, had come to Norfolk looking for a respectable young woman to marry and the 13-year-old Mary Edge from the orphan school had been strongly recommended by Captain Piper. On enquiring further, Elder heard discouraging remarks about the girl's character and, knowing of Piper's antics in Sydney where he had 'tried to seduce every woman that came in his way', Elder suspected that Piper had had an affair with the girl. The missionary sought an independent opinion from the hospital surgeon. Redfern sympathised with this decent man seeking a lifetime partner and told the missionary that his suspicions were justified. He also told him that Mary Edge had been acquainted with Thomas Gorman who had been flogged 'on account of criminal connections with her'. At the time it was rumoured that the sentence given by Piper was more out of jealousy than as a punishment. The next day Elder told Piper that he had heard of Miss Edge's dubious past and was no longer interested in her.[62]

Piper was furious and under pressure Elder eventually disclosed his sources. The missionary said that a girl named Mary Power, who had had a child with Piper, claimed that he was in the habit of meeting Mary Edge every morning. For saying this, Piper had Mary Power's head shaven, and an iron collar placed on her neck.

Elder also revealed that he had sought the advice of the hospital surgeon. Summoned before Piper, Redfern admitted having spoken to Elder but denied telling him about Piper's relationship with Mary Edge. In a rage, Piper instantly dismissed Redfern as hospital surgeon, cancelled his daily rations and ordered him to leave on the first ship sailing to the Derwent. Piper also insisted Redfern relinquish his share in the schooner *Endeavour* that was close to completion. If he did not sell his share, Piper threatened to stop the launch of the ship.[63]

Few other details of this episode exist but one can be certain that Redfern did not take Piper's threats without a fight. He was a free man, and he could do what he wanted within the law. In late April 1808 the whaler *Sarah* anchored off the island and Redfern requested a passage to Sydney, to which Captain Bristow readily agreed. Since all residents needed a permit to leave the island, Redfern informed Piper that he was about to sail for Sydney. Piper refused him a permit to sail on the *Sarah* and ordered him to leave on the *Estramina* sailing to the Derwent. Redfern immediately wrote to Wentworth and Captain Bristow secretly agreed to deliver the letter when he reached Sydney. The letter explained what had happened and asked his friend to get permission from the rebels for him to leave the Derwent and sail to Port Jackson. Redfern had no idea if this would be achievable.

Before the *Estramina* weighed anchor, Piper compiled an embarkation list of the settlers eligible for compensation in Van Diemen's Land and listed their land, livestock, grain and dwellings owned on Norfolk Island. William Redfern, his wife (Sarah

McHenry) and servant were listed with no land, two buildings, 62 pigs and 4730 lb of corn of a total worth £88. Piper remarked on Redfern's claims for compensation: '£50 is the value of this man's claims. He is a dangerous Character to Society'.[64]

The *Estramina* departed Norfolk Island on the 19 May 1808 with 62 people, their animals and baggage on board, docking in Hobart Town on 7 June 1808.[65] What transpired on arrival in Hobart is unclear, but there is no record of the Redfern family disembarking. It is unlikely that Lieutenant Governor David Collins would have taken Piper's warning that Redfern was 'a dangerous Character to Society' seriously and not let him come ashore. It is more probable that Redfern, a free man not appointed to a government post, was allowed to remain on the *Estramina* until it sailed for Sydney.

In any case, on 21 June 1808 the *Estramina* docked in Port Jackson with William Redfern, Sarah McHenry and their servant on board.

Chapter 7

MEDICAL QUALIFICATIONS

We have examined Mr. William Redfern touching his Skill in Medicine and Surgery, and the other necessary collateral Branches of Medical Literature, and that We find him qualified to exercise the Profession of a Surgeon. And consequently to fill the Situation of an Assistant Surgeon in any Department of His Majesty's Service. Thomas Jamison *et al.*, 1 Sep 1808[1]

William Redfern's decision to defy Piper's orders and sail to Sydney before hearing from Wentworth was bold and headstrong – although a free man, disobeying a direct military order carried serious consequences. Redfern must have been very confident that Wentworth could gain rebel support in Sydney and that Joseph Foveaux would remove any other legal obstacles when he returned from England. The gamble paid off. Two weeks earlier Captain Bristow had delivered Redfern's letter to D'Arcy Wentworth as soon as the *Sarah* docked in Sydney. When Redfern disembarked from the *Estramina*, a messenger was waiting for him with the necessary entry papers signed by Wentworth's rebel associates.

Much had changed politically since Redfern last visited Sydney in 1803. The rebel government was increasingly chaotic and there was growing uncertainty across the community about the legality of Bligh's arrest. The pros and cons of his overthrow were split roughly along urban-rural lines. Redfern listened carefully to the views of D'Arcy Wentworth, Simeon Lord and their friends. Men who had supported the rebellion five months earlier, and even marched with the soldiers to arrest Bligh, now doubted the competency of the rebels and the legitimacy of the insurrection. This may have included D'Arcy, even though the rebels had restored him as assistant surgeon at the Parramatta hospital.

Unsurprisingly, enthusiasts among the business elite who had encouraged the overthrow of Bligh were starting to appreciate the full legal consequences of a 'mutiny' – it was a treasonable act punishable by hanging. And when the rebel administration, composed mostly of military officers, failed to improve their lives and businesses, a general sense of distrust pervaded the colony. Rivalry also surfaced among rebel leaders who realised that only a few would benefit materially from the overthrow. Without the prospect of personal gain, support faded. Even within military ranks, dissatisfaction with John Macarthur as Colonial Secretary grew by the day and the rebel cause was rapidly losing its base.

As early as April 1808 settlers complained to Major Johnston that Macarthur was the cause of constant quarrelling in the colony and that he had 'violated the Law, violated public faith, and trampled on the most Sacred and Constitutional Rights of the British Subjects'. They demanded his dismissal. But Johnston's future was bound to Macarthur, and he was never going to dismiss him. He told disgruntled rebels to put up or shove off, telling the most troublesome men to leave the colony.[2]

Confined to Government House, Bligh refused rebel demands to return to England. He was secretly kept well informed of the squabbling among rebels and of the rumour that William Paterson would soon come from Port Dalrymple to reinstate him as the lawful Governor.[3] In fact, this was most unlikely since the ship sent to collect Paterson from Van Diemen's Land had returned on 26 May 1808 without him. It was rumoured he was reluctant to commit to the rebellion because Bligh was still resident in the colony. Almost certainly Paterson would have also realised that it was far too dangerous to try and reinstate Bligh as Governor without the Corps' backing.[4] As far as he was concerned, this was a political mess of John Macarthur's making and, since he loathed the man that he had duelled with in 1801, Paterson wanted nothing to do with the whole affair. He had heard that Joseph Foveaux was soon due back in Sydney – let him sort it out.

During his first weeks in Sydney, Redfern cautiously canvassed people's views on Bligh's arrest. Many had quite different opinions about the rebel administration to Wentworth and Lord. He quickly realised it was risky to discuss these matters in public; the rebels were nervous, and they were sending dissenters to the Coal River prison settlement in chains. For this reason alone, most men kept their loyalty to Bligh a secret. One such man was the Reverend Henry Fulton whom Redfern had known when he was chaplain on Norfolk Island from 1801 to 1805. Fulton had previously lauded Bligh for helping Hawkesbury flood victims and was present at

Government House when Bligh was arrested. He was interrogated by the rebels and subsequently removed as chaplain.

Another loyalist, Andrew Thompson, a wealthy Hawkesbury farmer and ship owner, was a close friend of Simeon Lord. Thompson had been Chief Constable and spokesperson in Green Hills, Bligh's farm bailiff and a government official. The rebels interrogated him for evidence of corruption at Bligh's farm, and then dismissed him from all official positions. Thompson and Fulton were among the men picked by Bligh to go to England for the tribunal about his dismissal. John Macarthur was particularly hostile to loyalist settlers and launched a litany of accusations that led to trials and bizarre acts of retribution.[5] Redfern observed the turmoil and, for once, kept his head down and mouth shut.

On 28 July 1808 Lieutenant Colonel Joseph Foveaux returned to Sydney aboard the *Sinclair*. He expected to resume command of Norfolk Island and oversee the resettlement of inhabitants to Van Diemen's Land. His return fuelled hope among some loyalists that he would reinstate Bligh, and a delegation of Commissary Palmer, Secretary Griffin and Reverend Fulton planned to board the *Sinclair* and invite Foveaux to meet with Bligh. But as soon as the ship docked, Macarthur and Johnston barred them from boarding and spent the day explaining to Foveaux why they had deposed Bligh. They managed to convince him that Bligh had a 'plan to destroy and ruin the better Class of Inhabitants'. Foveaux met with Bligh the next day at Government House, but the meeting was fruitless, and he refused to reinstate him.[6]

During the next week Foveaux had Wentworth and Redfern update him on Norfolk Island affairs and discuss Redfern's future prospects as a colonial surgeon. Wentworth had received news that surgeon James Thomson had died while on leave in England. This provided an opening at the Sydney hospital for Redfern and a possible senior assistant surgeon appointment for Wentworth. Supported by Wentworth, Foveaux was prepared to recommend Redfern's appointment to the permanent government medical staff pending proof of his qualifications. As a free man Redfern was already eligible to establish his own private practise in the colony but he was attracted to a hospital post where the most challenging medical cases occurred. Since Redfern had no documentary evidence of his 1797 medical qualifications, he requested another examination before a medical board.[7]

Because of William Paterson's reluctance to leave Port Dalrymple and take command of the rebel administration, Joseph Foveaux, as the senior Corps officer on the mainland, was pressed to take charge of the entire colony. On 31 July 1808 Foveaux agreed to be Lieutenant Governor of New South Wales 'until His Majesty's pleasure shall be known'. Bligh's arrest had been reported to the British government and Foveaux wisely declined to judge the legitimacy of the rebel takeover – only His Majesty's ministers could rule on this. Even so, he dismissed John Macarthur as Colonial Secretary and appointed his adjutant, Lieutenant James Finucane, in his place.[8]

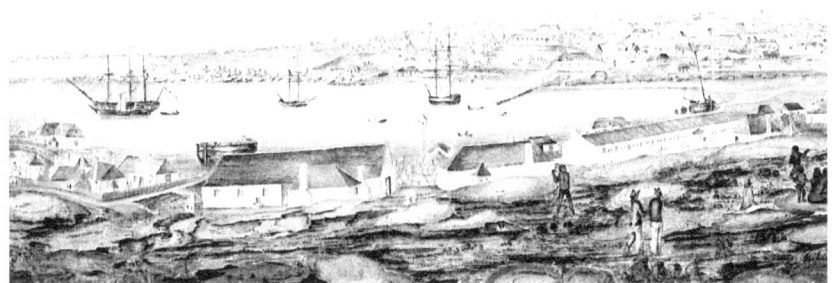

1803 view of Sydney looking east across the Cove with hospital buildings in the foreground. The building on the right is the 1790 prefabricated hospital.

On 1 August 1808 Lieutenant Governor Foveaux made William Redfern the assistant surgeon in charge of the general hospital in Sydney.[9] This was a major decision for Redfern and an important precedent for the colony. Emancipists struggled to gain official and social recognition, and Foveaux appointing an ex-convict to this prestigious medical position would have raised eyebrows in Sydney and led to grumbling among the elite. Rather oddly, while promoting the emancipist Redfern to be a surgeon in the main hospital, Foveaux criticised Bligh for having the emancipist Reverend Fulton as an adviser. He wrote to the Colonial Office:

The astonishment I felt at the report of the Governor's Arrest was increased on observing that, in naming the persons he had deputed to wait upon me, he had spoken of a Mr. Fulton (a man whom I had known in Norfolk Island in the condition of an emancipated convict) as his friend; and this circumstance strongly tended to confirm the information I had at first received – that the Governor had been chiefly guided by persons of that Class, in following whose advice.[10]

Foveaux's views on class equity were, at best, inconsistent. On one hand he supported the creed that a crime, no matter how trivial, excludes anyone from the society of gentlemen and officers. On other occasions his views were unmistakably egalitarian. Possibly listening to Redfern and emancipists Thompson and Lord, made him appreciate that ability was far more important than past vicissitudes or birthright. During his first weeks in Sydney, Foveaux also learnt a great deal about the past activities of Macarthur and Johnston and became convinced that there was scant evidence of Bligh being a 'corrupt tyrant'. He also realised that heading the rebel administration was fraught with personal danger, and he strived to govern in a way that any future judicial assessment of the rebellion would find his leadership fair and equitable. In an attempt to relinquish the rebel "hot seat" as soon as possible, Foveaux sent the *Estramina* to Port Dalrymple on 21 August 1808 to try and coerce William Paterson back to Sydney.[11]

In October 1808, with an examination of his medical knowledge only a month away, William Redfern studied all the medical literature he could lay his hands on. In the navy, as well as in the colony, a government assistant surgeon was required to serve as a surgeon, a physician and an apothecary. Since there were no libraries, universities or medical schools in the colony, most books were borrowed from colleagues. Medical facilities at the Sydney hospital were rudimentary, but superior to what Redfern had experienced in the Royal Navy. Separated from the latest medical advances in Britain and Europe, colonial medicine depended mostly on the skill and innovation of individual surgeons and their access to adequate medical supplies. Professionally, Redfern had gained much experience over the past decade and was confident of receiving a license to practise at the hospital. One also suspects that he probably believed he knew more than his examiners!

MEDICAL QUALIFICATIONS

On 1 September 1808 William Redfern was examined on aspects of medicine and surgery by a board composed of Principal Surgeon Thomas Jamison, the Corps Surgeon John Harris and the NSW Corps Assistant Surgeon William Bohan. Redfern passed and was awarded the first medical diploma issued in Australia.

> We whose Names are hereunto subscribed do hereby certify that We have examined Mr. William Redfern touching his Skill in Medicine and Surgery, and the other necessary collateral Branches of Medical Literature, and that We find him qualified to exercise the Profession of a Surgeon &c. And consequently to fill the Situation of an Assistant Surgeon in any Department of His Majesty's Service.
> Given under Our Hands at Sydney in New South Wales this first day of September, 1808.
> THOS. JAMISON, Principal Surgeon
> J. HARRIS, Surgeon, New South Wales Corps
> WM. BOHAN, Assistant Surgeon New South Wales Corps[12]

This examination of William Redfern initiated a qualification system that remained the standard in Australia for many years. Medical boards were convened as deemed necessary to examine a person wanting to practice in the colony and anyone failing was ordered to desist from practising medicine.[13] Redfern would later become a member of the board.

On 6 September 1808 Foveaux wrote to the Colonial Secretary Lord Castlereagh seeking confirmation for Redfern's appointment:

> The distress'd State of the Colony for medical aid, and the expression of your Lordship's wish to provide such as could be obtain'd in this country, has induced me to appoint Mr. Wm. Redfern to act as Assistant Surgeon. As his skill and ability in his profession are unquestionable, and his conduct has been such as to deserve particular approbation, I beg to solicit for his confirmation.[14]

A week later Foveaux offered appointments to three surgeons: D'Arcy Wentworth as assistant surgeon in Parramatta; James Mileham as assistant surgeon in the Hawkesbury district and 'Mr. W. Redfern is approved to act as Assistant Surgeon in the Colony, and is to do duty at Sydney'.[15]

Redfern's new position entitled him to a salary of 7s 6d daily (£117 yearly for 6 days work a week), a servant, 6s per week for

MEDICAL QUALIFICATIONS

firewood and a rent-free house.[16] He and Sarah McHenry moved into the assistant surgeon's house north of the hospital, adjacent to the house of Thomas Jamison, the colonial principal surgeon. The principal surgeon's role in the hospital was mostly administrative, reporting to the Governor and managing hospital administration. Assistant surgeons treated the patients, helped by a predominately convict staff comprised of nurses, overseers, wardsmen, gardeners, guards, clerks and boatmen. Redfern commenced duties at the general hospital in September 1808 when Sydney's population was about 6000. Although the number of sick admitted to the hospital steadily increased, its facilities had not changed since 1790.

The hospital was located on the west side of George Street in the Rocks district, today bounded by Globe, George, Harrington and Argyle streets.[17] Only metres away, on the east side of George Street near the head of Sydney Cove was the 'Market Place' known today as First Fleet Park. The bustling area close to the hospital wharf was where many merchants, traders and ship owners lived and had their shops, taverns and warehouses. Between the wharf and the Tank Stream bridge was a ship builders' yard, a post office, a prison and the female orphan school. Convict transport ships off-loaded their human cargo at the hospital wharf from where they were marched to the nearby gaol yard for inspection and work allocation. Small local vessels continuously docked to deliver provisions to the town: livestock, fish, grain, fruit and vegetables. The area teemed with pigs, cattle, poultry, men offloading ships, convicts marching single file to and from work, and finely dressed merchants inspecting their ships and cargos.

The Sydney general hospital admitted sick from every walk of life – convicts, settlers, soldiers, sailors and Aboriginal people. The hospital facilities had improved markedly since first settlement in January 1788. Early medical accommodation was an assembly of canvas tents with 80 beds.[18] In June 1790 a prefabricated hospital arrived with the disease ridden Second Fleet. This building was distinctive because of its wooden walls and copper roof. Extra patient rooms were later added and by 1800, the hospital complex comprised three main buildings and several supplementary houses.

In August 1806 Governor Bligh deemed that most buildings in Sydney were 'sinking into decay' and many public offices were unacceptably decrepit. Inspectors decided the prefabricated hospital building was irreparable and that other buildings needed new fittings or a complete renovation. Bligh declared 'the Hospital and Premises in ruinous State'. Over the following years they were renovated, and the wooden building were repaired.[19]

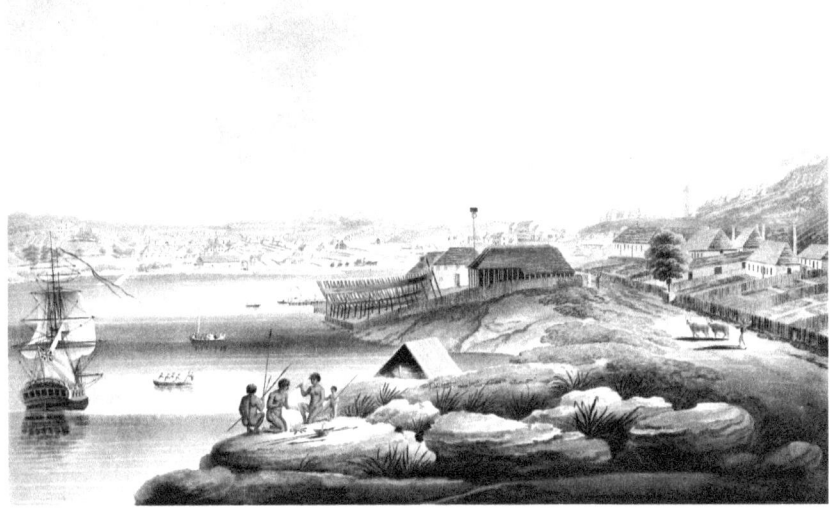

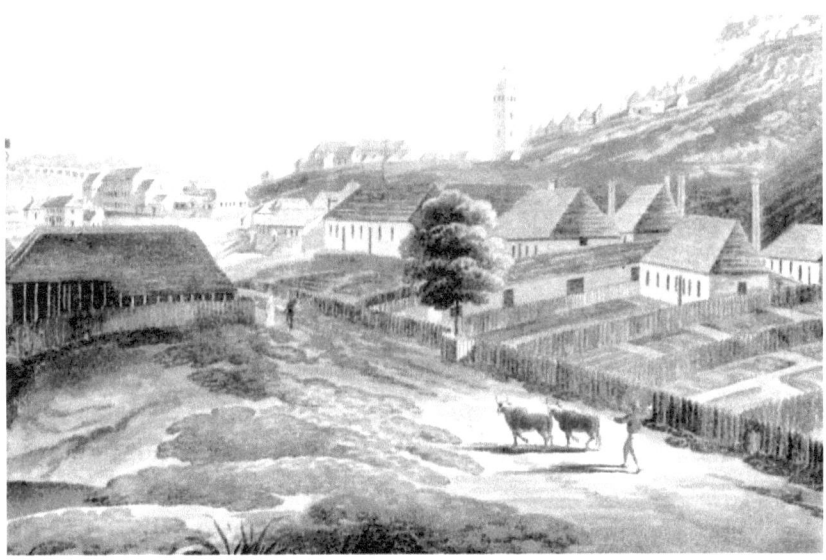

1802 painting of Sydney Cove viewed from Dawes Point, shown in full above and below as an enlargement. The principal surgeon's cottage is to the far right and the assistant surgeon's cottage and the hospital buildings are adjacent. The wharf was used to land hospital goods and convicts. Surgeons boarded convict ships from the small boathouse in the foreground.

MEDICAL QUALIFICATIONS

Inadequate staffing at the hospitals was another major problem. Principal Surgeon Jamison complained of an urgent need for more surgeons, nurses and victualling, as well as additional medications and instruments. Bligh supported Jamison and forwarded his requests onto the Colonial Office. However, facilities and staffing had not improved when Assistant Surgeon Redfern joined the hospital two years later.

By late 1808 Lieutenant Governor Foveaux's attitude to the rebels had clearly hardened and his actions show a heightened awareness of the danger the rebel leadership posed for him personally. He attempted to reduce the colony's financial burden on the British government and to mitigate Macarthur's and the Corps' control over trading in the colony. Despite these welcome changes, Bligh loyalists maintained their opposition to the legitimacy of the rebel administration, and Foveaux routinely met with hostility from those suffering from rebel fines, prison sentences, foreclosures and banishment to the Coal River mines. Many complained of personal abuse from the Corps, of property theft and injustice in the courts.

Encouraged by Foveaux's increasingly disenchantment with the rebels, D'Arcy Wentworth attempted to change camps as well. On 12 September 1808 he wrote to his patron Lord Fitzwilliam:

> ... there is not an officer in the King's Service who could govern this Country in opposition to the Whims, and Caprice of the Officers of the New South Wales Corps and I have no hesitation in assuring Your Lordship that it [is] useless to expect Quietness in this Country so long as that Corps is suffered to remain.[20]

Wentworth's allegiances had clearly shifted since marching with Corps soldiers to arrest Bligh's eight months earlier. His letter also contradicts what he told Fitzwilliam in April about his acquittal in the second mock trial in which he had unashamedly admitted to employing convict patients for personal benefit. He trivialised the charges against him as frivolous, claiming he was simply following accepted codes of conduct. What he did not tell his patron in April was that support for the rebels in the colony was evaporating.[21]

On 12 October 1808 the *Estramina* returned from Port Dalrymple without Paterson. This time he claimed that poor health prevented him from coming to Sydney. Foveaux was furious. He was now convinced that commanding the rebels would lead to a charge of treason and, at short notice, announced his departure for England on the *Albion*. However, the *Albion* master Cuthbert Richardson told Foveaux he could not be quartered on the ship at such short notice. This may have been true, but Richardson was also a Bligh loyalist and would not have wanted to assist him. Nevertheless, this forced Foveaux to rethink his strategy and he now instructed the warship HMS *Porpoise* to sail to Port Dalrymple and convince William Paterson to take charge in Sydney. Foveaux pointed out in an accompanying letter that, as senior Corps officer, Paterson had a duty to take charge of the colony, as he was about to return to England now that only 250 people remained on Norfolk Island and his presence was no longer needed.[22] However, Foveaux's arguments were still not persuasive enough and it would take another two months before Paterson left the safety of Port Dalrymple to assume leadership of the rebels on the mainland.

One of Redfern's medical duties as a government surgeon was to monitor the health of the ex-governor, who was now confined to Government House. Few people were allowed to talk to Bligh and medical visits had to be approved by the rebels. It is also somewhat surprising that Bligh agreed to be treated by someone involved in the 1797 Nore mutiny, the naval episode in which he was ousted as Captain from the mutinous HMS *Director*. Bligh certainly would have known of the surgeon's mate on HMS *Standard* who was sentenced to death and was probably fully aware that William Redfern was one of the two Nore mutineers to have ever been transported to the colony.

On the other hand, William Bligh had shown compassion for the mutineers on his own ship, and he may have extended that to Redfern. In any case, the 'mutineer surgeon' William Redfern was preferable to surgeon D'Arcy Wentworth who had marched to Government House with the Corps to arrest him! Also, Bligh would have heard from his daughter Mary that Redfern had cared for his son-in-law, John Putland, on Norfolk Island. Despite his formidable reputation, the Governor was a strong family man and Mary's wellbeing would have been a serious concern after her husband's death. Lachlan Macquarie later observed that Redfern was 'One of the Most Loyal and Useful subjects to the Government in this Country … Exerted himself in preserving an Existence most dear to him [Bligh], that of His own Daughter, the

Governor's only Companion in that Hour of Horror and Misery'.[23]

On 29 November 1808 the recently built Norfolk schooner *Endeavour* arrived in Sydney with a cargo of salted pork and soap. Redfern had helped finance the construction of the *Endeavour* and would have had mixed feelings when she sailed into Port Jackson. If not for John Piper's vindictiveness, he would still be a part owner of the ship.[24] Some of the *Endeavour's* cargo belonged to Redfern and three days later he sold 11,547 lb of salted pork to the Sydney government stores, for which Foveaux issued bills worth £577 on His Majesty's Treasury as payment.[25]

Since becoming the assistant surgeon in charge of the hospital, William Redfern's social standing in Sydney had improved. Nonetheless, his appointment was considered by some Exclusives as further proof that colonial society was "going to the dogs". The unpredictability of official promotion practices and the increasing influence of emancipists upset those in military and elite business circles – indeed, the appointment of ex-convicts to government posts was eroding decent society. Because the medical fraternity was highly respected in the colony, Redfern's success was seen as a particular affront, and many let Foveaux know that it was unacceptable. In this respect, it is interesting to note that there is no record of Redfern ever having personally dined with Foveaux while serving as his doctor. It is quite likely he did, but Foveaux may have concealed it from public knowledge and treated Redfern more as a valuable servant than a close friend. Nevertheless, behind closed doors, their interactions were most likely familiar.

In general, Redfern appears to have kept private matters quite separate from his medical responsibilities. He is known to have mixed socially with like-minded men such as Andrew Thompson, Simeon Lord and D'Arcy Wentworth. None of these men would have expected to socialise with Exclusives, except perhaps Wentworth who, despite frequent court appearances, had aristocratic connections that surmounted social barriers. On the other hand, commercial interactions in the colony often breached the social divide – the need to make money overrode most prejudices. Such was the hypocrisy of the times.

One suspects that if Joseph Foveaux could have avoided the recriminations of social peers in the colony, he would have greatly relished a raucous dinner with the three thieves and the mutineer.

Chapter 8

SYDNEY HOSPITAL SURGEON

> *Mr. Redfern's singular abilities are well known here, and I believe there are few families who have not availed themselves of his services. His duty in the General Hospital has been laborious, and most certainly fulfilled with a degree of promptitude and attention not to be exceeded. — I have heard many poor persons, dismissed from the Hospital, thank him for their recovery; but have never known a patient complain of his neglect.*
>
> Macquarie to Sidmouth, 1821[1]

On New Year's Day 1809 HMS *Porpoise* docked in Sydney with Colonel William Paterson on board. He had finally agreed to leave Port Dalrymple and take command of the rebel administration. Paterson had never fully recovered from the gunshot wound received in the duel with John Macarthur in 1801 and would have much preferred to convalesce in Van Diemen's Land. But as the senior NSW Corps officer, he was persuaded to do his duty and take command in Sydney. He knew from his brief tenure as Lieutenant Governor of New South Wales before Governor Hunter arrived that the colony was difficult to administer. Additionally, he now had to contend with the political machinations of a rebel administration and the recriminations of loyalists who wanted Bligh reinstated. Paterson expected to find the colony in a mess and, most likely, he already regretted his decision to try and sort it out.

To facilitate a fast transfer of power, Joseph Foveaux promptly resigned as Lieutenant Governor. However, the infirm Paterson soon realised that he was physically incapable of taking on such a turbulent administrative task and asked Foveaux to share the duties with him. After several inconclusive meetings, Foveaux applied for leave on 5 January 1809 to return to England to discuss the Norfolk Island evacuation. Several islanders who had recently been sent to the Derwent had protested over the conditions and demanded a return to Sydney.[2] However, Paterson denied Foveaux leave and suggested that the two men control the colony jointly –

Foveaux should oversee the Sydney settlement and he would shoulder official matters from the Parramatta Government House. This shared arrangement appealed to Foveaux because he retained authority in Sydney while official responsibility, which might later be deemed treasonable, sat squarely on Paterson's shoulders. Foveaux had also recently become more confident of his future in the colony – his equitable treatment of settlers had gained him a following among the Bligh loyalists, who wanted him to remain in the colony. This support had blossomed when he replaced John Macarthur with Lieutenant James Finucane as Colonial Secretary. If for no other reason, the loyalists wanted Foveaux to stay just to keep a lid on Macarthur!

Even more fuel was about to be added to the Macarthur-Foveaux fire. Two weeks after Paterson's arrival Foveaux discovered that £500 could not be accounted for while Macarthur was Colonial Secretary, and he had ordered him to be repay this amount to the treasury. Macarthur took this as a personal insult and challenged Foveaux to a duel. Foveaux ignored the challenge, but Macarthur persisted and publicly slandered him by having his friend George Johnston pay £500 directly to the 'gallant Colonel' rather than the Treasury. Foveaux agreed to the duel and the two men faced off with pistols at Johnston's Annandale property on 19 January 1809.[3] Macarthur won the toss and taking 'deliberate aim' fired first but missed. Foveaux then lowered his pistol without firing, signalling that Macarthur was not worth wasting a bullet on.

Foveaux then told Macarthur and Johnston that he was grossly offended at being 'obliged to account in that manner' for decisions made in his service to the government.[4] Macarthur repaid the £500 and thereafter the two had no further contact, verbally or by letter. Foveaux remained Macarthur's bitter enemy for the rest of his life.

William Bligh had now been imprisoned in Government House for over a year. However, the governor's support in the colony had far from diminished during his confinement; the number of loyalists multiplied as the rebels' incompetence became more obvious. There were rumours that the British would soon intervene militarily and, officially at least, Governor Bligh was still Commander of all Royal Navy ships in the South Pacific. HMS *Porpoise* was anchored in Port Jackson and its captain, Commander John Porteous, could soon be ordered by the British to release

Bligh. Such an action appeared imminent when Porteous ignored an order by Paterson on 26 January 1809 to transport the last Norfolk Island inhabitants to Van Diemen's Land. Paterson asked Bligh to relinquish control of HMS *Porpoise* and return to England or be imprisoned in the military barracks. Bligh refused, and on 30 January he was taken to the barracks, along with Mary, who was placed an adjacent room.[5]

Paterson later threatened Bligh with forcible removal on the convict transport *Admiral Gambier*. This ship was to soon take John Macarthur and George Johnston to England. Again, Bligh refused to budge – he was certainly not going to sail anywhere with those scoundrels! But on 4 February 1809 Bligh finally agreed to depart on HMS *Porpoise* provided certain residents could accompany him, and he and Mary could reside in Government House until departure.[6] A week later Assistant Surgeon Redfern went to check on Bligh's health. As thanks for his services, Redfern was presented with a book entitled *An assay on the scurvy* written by naval Surgeon Frederick Thomson. It contains the inscription: '*From His Excellency Gov. Bligh to Mr Will Redfern, 13 Feby 1809*'. A 'W. Bell' had given the book to Bligh in 1791.[7]

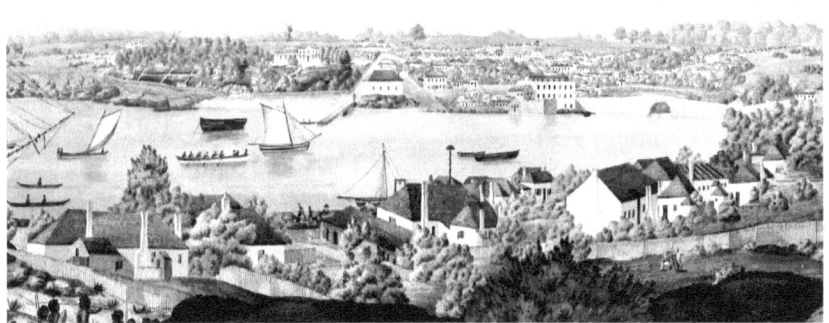

1806 painting of Sydney looking east across the Cove with the George Street hospital buildings in the foreground. Government House is on the distant hill on the east bank of the Cove.

William Bligh boarded HMS *Porpoise* as its commander on 20 February 1809 and the ship was readied for departure. A crucial condition in Bligh agreeing to leave was that he could take selected men to England with him for the dismissal tribunal. However, within a day of boarding HMS *Porpoise*, Paterson, at the request of Johnston, barred John Palmer, one of Bligh's witnesses, from leaving because he refused to alter his account books in favour of rebel transactions.[8] Bligh protested vehemently as Palmer was his leading witness and restricting him violated the departure agreement. The remaining witnesses now wondered if and when they would be asked to board HMS *Porpoise*.

George Johnston and John Macarthur were also assembling witnesses to support their case at the tribunal in England. On 24 February Principal Surgeon Thomas Jamison was ordered to be a witness for Johnston. D'Arcy Wentworth was instructed to replace him in Sydney and Edward Luttrell became the assistant surgeon in Parramatta.[9] William Redfern and Sarah McHenry would have been delighted to hear that D'Arcy Wentworth and Maria Ainslie would soon move back to Sydney.

Reports now circulated that the rebels were about to try and stop HMS *Porpoise* from sailing. Bligh decided his pact with Paterson was now defunct and ordered HMS *Porpoise* to sail to the harbour entrance and drop anchor.[10] Here they could prevent the *Admiral Gambier*, with Johnston, Macarthur and others on board, from departing. These men wanted to reach London first so as to convince British parliamentarians on the legitimacy of Bligh's arrest. Johnston became increasingly concerned about the tribunal and sought to have four of the men Bligh had selected as witnesses to change their allegiance to him. But the men refused, and Paterson declined to intervene.[11]

On 17 March, with HMS *Porpoise* still blocking the harbour, Bligh made it known to his supporters that he would remain in the area until he had orders from the British government. He issued an edict forbidding shipmasters from transporting anyone involved in the rebellion from the colony. The proclamation identified all of the Corps officers along with the names of 15 civilian and public officials, including John Macarthur and the surgeons John Harris, Thomas Jamison, James Mileham and D'Arcy Wentworth.[12] The document sent shock waves through the rebel community and reminded everyone involved in the overthrow that they could soon be charged with treason. Many felt the noose tightening around their neck and even those remotely connected to the rebels started to worry about future implications. Some men quickly shifted their allegiances to the Bligh loyalists.

There was now a heightened belief aboard HMS *Porpoise* that Corps officers would soon try to storm the ship. Reluctantly, Bligh weighed anchor and sailed out through the harbour entrance into the Pacific Ocean and took a southerly bearing. However, days later instead of sailing through the Bass Strait on a westerly route to Cape Town and England, the ship continued onto the Derwent River settlement on Van Diemen's Land. A resolute Captain Bligh was not about to abandon his promise to stay in the region.

On 29 March 1809 the *Admiral Gambier* left Port Jackson to sail for England. On board were George Johnston, John Macarthur, a group of rebel supporters and the surgeons Thomas Jamison and John Harris.[13] On that same day, HMS *Porpoise* anchored in the harbour of Hobart Town where Bligh planned to stay until military support arrived from England. The Lieutenant Governor of Hobart, David Collins, immediately sent a letter to Sydney telling Foveaux of Bligh's unexpected arrival. On receiving the news, Foveaux dispatched a fast ship on 10 April with an order prohibiting all contact with HMS *Porpoise*.[14] Collins tried to comply with the order by cutting off supplies to the ship, but Bligh was not an easy man to deny. Hobart residents who had resettled from Norfolk Island supported Bligh and rowed food out to the ship. When Collins punished several for doing so, Bligh blockaded vessels entering the harbour and requisitioned provisions for his crew.[15] HMS *Porpoise* would continue to control incoming ships until Bligh returned to Sydney in January 1810.

The departure of George Johnston and John Macarthur for England strengthened Joseph Foveaux's hand in Sydney, and to a certain extent aggression against the rebels lessened across the colony. Though Paterson still officially led the colony, his infirmity and excessive drinking meant Foveaux was really in charge and inhabitants looked to him for leadership. Realising that this was only a brief respite before British intervention, Foveaux insisted all subsequent administrative decisions were strictly "by the book". When grain losses due to floods threatened the colony, he gave generous support to cereal farmers and, to the bewilderment of Sydney traders, curtailed spirit trafficking by forbidding the barter of grain for rum. He demanded that magistrates fully enforce the law and issue penalties for any offence.[16]

Foveaux was not alone in foreseeing the changes ahead. There was a growing realisation in the community that the benefits of being a rebel supporter were about to end. D'Arcy Wentworth declared no further interest in politics but nonetheless was granted 1300 acres of grazing land for past services. Some of the civilian and military rebels helped themselves to as much largesse as they could lay their hands on. Following the 1809 Hawkesbury floods, Paterson, at Foveaux's advice, opened up large tracts of land and was swamped with applications. He awarded land grants totalling 67,475 acres. Between 1788 and 1806 only 85,000 acres had been granted by Governors. Lachlan Macquarie would later claim that William Paterson had been 'such an easy good natured thoughtless man that he latterly granted Land to almost every person who asked them, without regard to their Merits or pretensions'.[17]

In January 1809 William Redfern claimed compensation for the buildings and stock he had owned on Norfolk Island. He asked to be compensated in cash, but Paterson offered him cattle from the government herd instead. He received 15 heifers; three for the house and two 'as a reward for his exertion in carrying on the Inoculation of the Cow-Pock'.[18] Redfern had no land to graze cattle and in May 1809 Paterson granted him 500 acres at Cabramatta 20 miles from Sydney as payment for his service to the military on Norfolk Island.[19] Almost certainly, this would have been at Foveaux's recommendation.

For many years Britain had provided few funds for maintaining infrastructure in the colony. Consequently, public buildings were in a poor state of repair unless paid for locally. By 1809 the Sydney cemetery had been damaged by roaming animals and funds were sought to finance a wall and gates for the burial ground. Among the residents who contributed to building the wall was William Redfern, who donated £1 1s on 4 June 1809. The cemetery was important to Sydney residents and many people donated 2s 6d – the amount a labourer earned in two days.[20] Redfern's cemetery donation was relatively modest, but it initiated a lifetime commitment to philanthropy. He supported the underprivileged residents at the Rocks, the rocky district behind the hospital where mostly poor convict and ex-convict families lived. Government support for the aged, poor, orphaned and indigenous residents was almost non-existent, and they depended on charity to fill the gap. William Redfern would become an active member in societies assisting those in need: the Orphan Institute, the New South Wales Philanthropic Society, the Native Institution, the Bible Society and the Benevolent Society. He also donated to the Female School of Industry, various relief programs and contributed to the construction of roads, buildings and monuments.[21]

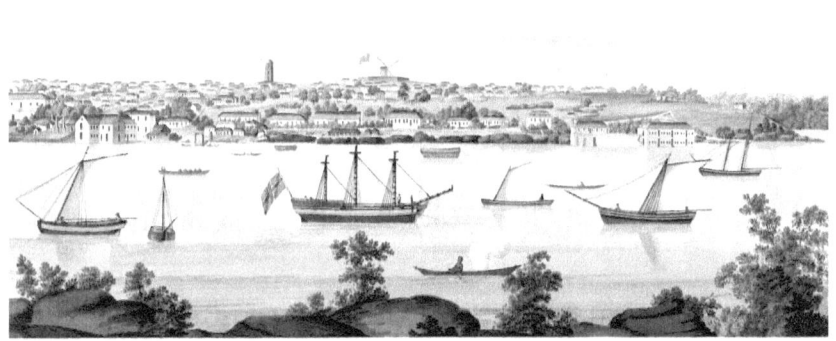

1808 painting of Sydney looking west across the Cove showing the three hospital buildings and the two surgeon houses on the western waterfront.

In September 1809 Lieutenant Governor Paterson secured a new supply of smallpox vaccine. On 16 October 1809 surgeon Redfern reported its successful application to the public.

> It is with extreme pleasure I at length feel myself enabled to state, with a degree of certainty, that my Endeavours to establish the Vaccine Inoculation with the Virus I had the honor of receiving from you, have perfectly succeeded. The re-introduction of so great a blessing to the rising Generation, as an infallible, safe, and mild Preventive of one of the most fatal diseases to which the Human Species is liable, the Small Pox; and which, fortunately for the Inhabitants of this Colony, has not yet made its appearance among them, will, I am confident, afford the most heartfelt satisfaction, and highest gratification to your benevolent and philanthropic mind.[22]

Redfern apologised to Paterson that his report was late because 'it was with the utmost pain and difficulty I was able to carry on my experiments, from a very severe inflammation in my right hand, which commenced the very day after I had received the Virus, and totally incapacitated me from writing'. He had also delayed reporting on the effectiveness of the vaccines until he was certain of their success, which 'I am happy to say, is now the case'. Redfern recommended ways to vaccinate the poor, as 'those in the Superior Ranks of Life' had already received every support. Two hundred years before today's Corona virus pandemic, Redfern issued not unfamiliar advice: 'it becomes highly necessary to impress on the minds of the poorer orders of people, whose ignorance renders them but too susceptible of the grossest and most unfounded prejudices, the usefulness, safety, and superior advantages of this new plan of Inoculation'. He stressed that the potency of vaccines deteriorated with time, saying there was always 'a considerable risque of the Virus becoming effete' before reaching the colony. He suggested that 'inoculating but a few at a time' would assure the supply of vaccine. Paterson was so impressed by the advice he had it published in the 22 October 1809 edition of *The Sydney Gazette*.[23]

A week later *The Sydney Gazette* reported that Mr Redfern had made considerable progress with smallpox inoculations. It praised his success and urged parents to get their children vaccinated, 'No pain attends the operation; no danger, and no possibility of future blemish'. The readers were told that Mr Redfern would provide vaccination to all settlements across the colony. 'His exertions are liberally patronized; and it is sincerely to be hoped will meet with no impediment, as humanity, and more immediately the preservation of our children is its great and only object'.[24]

One of Redfern's private patients was the emancipist farmer and businessman, Andrew Thompson, who was treated for respiratory problems. Thompson, who lived in Green Hills (Windsor), had recently built an imposing house in the centre of Sydney, not far from Government House. The former chief constable suffered from a lung infection he incurred after being drenched for three days while rescuing settlers from the massive Hawkesbury floods in 1809. Redfern treated Thompson's until he died in late 1810.

Many of Redfern's private patients were children from poor families, who after the age of six worked as servants and labourers. Schooling was relatively inaccessible to most of them. This was certainly not the case for John Macarthur's 17-year-old daughter, Elizabeth, who was also a patient of Redfern's. She had been very ill in 1808 when it was feared she would die. On 13 October 1809, while Macarthur was in England, his wife wrote to him that their daughter Elizabeth might never walk again. This was the prognosis before Redfern examined her in Parramatta. It seems likely that he recognised her symptoms as those of a new disease identified by the London surgeon Michael Underwood and published in his book *Treatise on the Diseases of Children* in 1789. This book would have been in Redfern's library and the unnamed disease is known today as the highly infectious virus *poliomyelitis*.[25] Because of her fragile health and slow recovery, Elizabeth and her mother moved to Sydney for several months to be under Redfern's care. In 1810 Elizabeth wrote to Miss Anne Marsden, daughter of Reverend Samuel Marsden, that she was confident that Redfern was the best 'Medical Gentleman' in the colony because the treatment she had received provided 'such extraordinary benefit'.[26] There is no record of his treatment, but it may have involved a metal support frame.

Since arriving in the colony Redfern had written regularly to his brother Thomas in Trowbridge, Wiltshire. After improvements to Elizabeth Macarthur's condition in late 1809, he asked Thomas if he would inform her father, John Macarthur currently residing in Bath ten miles from Trowbridge, of the treatment. Redfern wanted his brother to seek Macarthur's support for his confirmation as a government surgeon. When the letter reached Thomas six months later, he sent his 17-year-old son Thomas junior to see Macarthur in Bath. On 3 May 1810, just one day after John Macarthur had received a letter saying that his daughter may never walk again, Redfern's young nephew Thomas was 'kindly sent by his father with a letter from Mr. Redfern' with news of his daughter's gradual recovery.[27] Macarthur wrote to his wife thanking Redfern and offering to support a hospital appointment for him.

> I think I need not tell you, that if I had as much power as I have inclination, Mr. Redfern's reward for the service he has rendered Elizabeth should be as great as the skill he has manifested in discovering and applying an efficacious remedy to her extraordinary disease. I hope he will have been informed that no pains were spared on my part to ascertain how far it might be practicable to obtain a confirmation of his appointment; and I beg you to assure him that whenever Mr. Bligh's affair is settled,

whatever little interest I may have shall be exerted in his favor.[28]

On 20 Jul 1810 Macarthur wrote again to his wife.

> Inform Mr. Redfern that nothing can be done in his business here, but everything must depend on the report of Colonel Macquarie. Let him know I saw his brother and nephew at Trowbridge, and that I shall feel the greatest pleasure if it should be in my power to aid their exertions to serve him.[29]

Delays in the 19th century postal service meant that Elizabeth Macarthur received this letter well after the next governor had made the new surgeon appointments in the hospital.

Around this time Redfern renewed his interest in recording various useful bits of information in his notebook. His medical remedies are recorded as almost 115 pages of tightly handwritten notes. These illustrate just how simple medicine was at a time when there were few cures for many common illnesses. Doctors mostly used remedies made from the 225 plant, animal and mineral substances listed in the English pharmacopoeia. Over 5000 substances are described in today's edition of the pharmacopoeia.[30]

Modern pharmacological and medical knowledge makes these notes appear oddly whimsical, but one needs to remember that Redfern was considered the leading medical practitioner in the colony. Medicine has made enormous strides in the past two hundred years. Many of Redfern's notes were about common illnesses such as asthma. For a cold it was recommended that one take syrup of garlic, honey and vinegar twice a day with brandy and water. Another remedy for 'Cancer' (presumably skin cancer) uses Turkey figs boiled in hot milk placed onto the affected skin as hot as possible several times a day for three to four months. A cure for 'the Evil' (*scrofula*, or tuberculosis of the neck) involved rubbing the sores with the legs cut from a live toad. Redfern noted that this application would 'cause the parts to swell very much for about 12 hours, and give Violent pain'. Once the swelling decreases, apply an ointment of 'yellow basilicum' daily. He wrote that a person who had this illness for several years was cured after being treated thus for three weeks.[31]

More conventional remedies included instructions for making a tincture of opium and red onion juice to treat baldness; instructions for making eyewash from lead, opium and white vitriol; and the use of peppermint oil for toothache. A remedy for chronic rheumatism, given to him by his friend Mr Smith, recommended taking, twice a day, an infusion of *gum guaicum*, horseradish, opium, *sal ammoniac* (ammonium chloride) and gin. In the latter part of Redfern's notebook, the entries delve into more vicarious matters; alchemy notes on how to make gold. These are written in an unfamiliar hand and were probably recorded by one of his apprentices or clerks.[32]

The news of Governor Bligh's overthrow reached London in September 1808 at a time when the British were busy with the Peninsula War in Spain and the containment of Napoleon's army. A new governor for New South Wales, Lieutenant Colonel Lachlan Macquarie, was appointed in March 1809 and had sailed for Sydney in July. Before departing, the Colonial Office briefed him on the reforms needed to restore confidence, improve morals, encourage marriages, improve education, prohibit the use of alcohol and increase agriculture. Colonial Secretary Castlereagh claimed that past efforts had failed because of the lack 'of Example and Co-operation in the higher Classes of the Settlement'.[33] Similar instructions had been given to William Bligh and other governors but with the decommissioning of the NSW Corps, Macquarie was expected to have a much better chance of achieving reforms.

On 28 December 1809, HMS *Hindostan* and HMS *Dromedary* sailed into Port Jackson. The new Governor, 48-year-old Lachlan Macquarie, and his wife Elizabeth were on board HMS *Dromedary*. When the vessels dropped anchor, Lieutenant Colonel Joseph Foveaux came on board and welcomed Macquarie, and Lieutenant Governor William Paterson travelled from Parramatta to greet the party as they disembarked. Three days later, Sydney residents watched, with a mixture of relief and delight, as the new Governor, his wife and officials, accompanied by the Scottish 73rd Regiment of Foot, proceeded by coach to Government House with a brass band playing 'God Save the King'. Lieutenant Governor Paterson, Lieutenant Colonel Foveaux, 'Gentlemen of the Settlement' saluted the new governor. Among them was Surgeon Redfern.[34]

The Colonial Office had instructed Macquarie to temporarily reinstate William Bligh as Governor before officially assuming office. On hearing that Bligh was still on HMS *Porpoise* moored in Hobart Town, Macquarie decided to take control immediately and he did so on 1 January 1810. While this deprived Bligh of the satisfaction of reinstatement, the rapid resumption of stable governance was considered much more important to the colony.[35] Macquarie had been instructed to arrest Major Johnston and send him back to England for trial. John Macarthur, the leader of the mutiny, was also to be arrested, charged with criminal acts against the government and tried in the colony for his mutinous conduct. The NSW Corps regiment was to be disbanded and sent back to England along with Lieutenant Colonel Foveaux. Colonel Paterson would be allowed, if he wished, to return to Van Diemen's Land.[36]

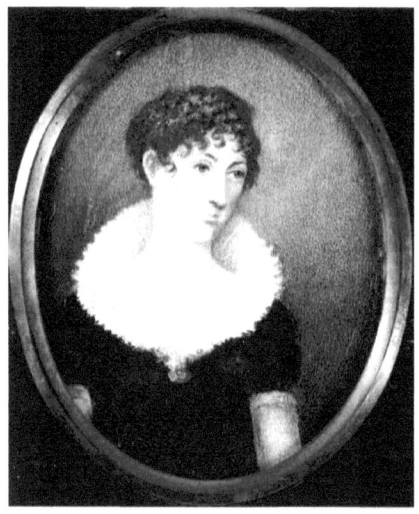
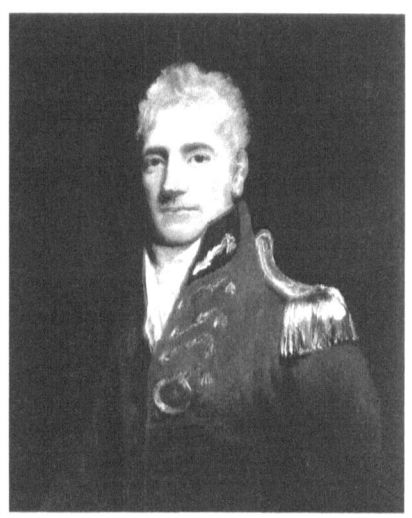

1810 portrait of Elizabeth Macquarie, the wife of Governor Macquarie.

1805 portrait of Lachlan Macquarie, fifth Governor of NSW (1810-21).

In the era of sailing ships, orders given in distant places rarely matched the actions needed at the time of execution. NSW Corps soldiers not wanting to stay in the colony departed on 12 May 1810. Macarthur and Johnston had already left for England of their own accord. Joseph Foveaux would prove himself invaluable to Macquarie and remained in the colony for months before returning to pursue a successful career in the British army.

Under Macquarie's governorship, Redfern's star was to shine even brighter. The new governor, who was a humane egalitarian, surrounded himself with the cleverest men in the colony, independent of class, background or rank. Redfern would join a select band of men on whom the governor relied heavily upon.

Chapter 9

THE RUM HOSPITAL

On my taking the Command of this Colony, General Foveaux personally introduced, and recommended Mr. Redfern to my notice in the strongest terms, as to his conduct, character, and professional abilities, stating, that in order to secure to the Settlement the advantages of his professional skill, he had appointed him Assistant Surgeon in the Colony, and solicited Lord Castlereagh for his confirmation. Governor Macquarie, 1821[1]

On 1 January 1810 Colonel Lachlan Macquarie was officially sworn in as the fifth Governor of New South Wales. In his first official proclamation, Governor Macquarie expressed His Majesty's greatest regret for the mutinous conduct against the former Governor William Bligh. He promised to restore order, law and discipline in the colony, saying that 'the honest, sober, and industrious Inhabitant, whether Free Settler or Convict, will ever find in me a Friend and Protector'.[2] Some in the audience probably thought his speech a bit too ambitious but he would prove to be an energetic pragmatist who meant what he said.

On the same day Lieutenant Colonel Maurice O'Connell was sworn in as Lieutenant Governor and Captain Henry Antill as Macquarie's Aide-de-Camp. The newly arrived lawyer Ellis Bent was made Judge Advocate. Lieutenant Colonel Joseph Foveaux was given command of the military in Sydney and would continue to supervise public works.[3] As the former leader of the rebel administration, Foveaux appreciated his precarious situation, and he wasted no time in making himself indispensable to the new governor. At their first meeting on 28 December 1809 on board HMS *Dromedary*, Foveaux claimed he had led the rebels only because he was duty bound to follow orders from his superior officer Colonel William Paterson.[4]

Foveaux sought to impress Macquarie with his good work over the past 18 months and offered to acquaint the Governor with Sydney and its residents. Macquarie listened cautiously to his views on the 'true interests of the Colony' and which 'principal inhabitants' might best serve him.⁵ It must have intrigued him to hear Foveaux speak so glowingly of the emancipists' contribution to the colony's prosperity. Among the ex-convicts Foveaux praised were Andrew Thompson, Simeon Lord and William Redfern. In fact, shortly after Macquarie's arrival Foveaux 'personally introduced and recommended' William Redfern in the strongest possible terms for 'his conduct, character, and professional abilities'.⁶ Undoubtedly, Macquarie would have been wary of accepting the counsel of a Corps officer who had led the rebels, but he urgently needed local advice before initiating his reforms.

The re-establishment of proper governance in the colony demanded Macquarie's immediate attention, and he acted quickly by declaring that all court trials and investigations initiated after the rebellion were null and void. All convictions were to be quashed and any recent convict pardons revoked. Land grants and leases issued by the rebel administration were cancelled and landholders had to surrender their title deeds, with the Governor reserving the right to ratify any considered worthy.⁷ Public officers appointed by the rebels were dismissed, except for the assistant surgeons Wentworth, Redfern, Mileham and Luttrell, as there was no one with medical experience to replace them. They were returned on 3 January 1810 to the government employee list with William Redfern receiving an annual salary of £136 17s 6d.⁸

On 12 January Macquarie announced that Andrew Thompson would be the next magistrate of the Hawkesbury district – the first ex-convict to be appointed to the judiciary.⁹ Although emancipists greatly outnumbered freemen in the colony and several already sat on the civil court bench, none had until now the authority to fine, flog or incarcerate an offender. The appointment of worthy men was overdue in the colony, but no previous governor had risked refuting the widely held belief that ex-convicts were incapable of fairly administering a court that had treated them so harshly. Even though Chief Constable Thompson was by a long stretch the best man for the magistrate role, his unprecedented promotion shocked many in Sydney. This, and the later appointment of Simeon Lord and D'Arcy Wentworth as magistrates, astounded the British Colonial Office and the Tory government. They still considered New South Wales a penal colony, and Macquarie's actions were viewed more as anarchy than a much-needed step towards a society in which all inhabitants were equal under the law.

On 17 January 1810 William Bligh returned to Sydney on HMS *Porpoise*. On entering Port Jackson and seeing the two naval ships HMS *Dromedary* and HMS *Hindostan* anchored at the Cove, Bligh assumed they were there to return him to power. Indeed, military relief had arrived to remove the rebels but not to reinstate him as governor. As soon as HMS *Porpoise* dropped anchor Lieutenant Governor O'Connell came on board to inform him that Lachlan Macquarie was now governor. This undoubtedly shocked Bligh, and, although he understood the circumstances, he would have been angry. He was also dismayed to hear that his previous gaoler, Joseph Foveaux, now advised the governor. Bligh and his daughter were quickly housed in a residence on Bridge Street beside the Tank Stream, where he began compiling documentary evidence for the upcoming court martial of George Johnston in England.[10]

On 21 January 1810 'Mr. Redfern' announced in *The Sydney Gazette* that parents wishing to give their children the 'incalculable advantages' of being vaccinated for cowpox should register at the general hospital.[11] Redfern was so busy with vaccinations that he almost missed the deadline to revoke his land grant as required by Macquarie's edict to cancel all rebel grants. On 29 January he surrendered his deed, pointing out that he had received the land and fifteen cows as compensation for property owned on Norfolk Island and for his health services to the military on the island. He attached a letter from Foveaux that he had recommended Redfern for a grant of 500 acres as compensation for his unpaid 7-year service as assistant surgeon to the military on Norfolk Island and for property lost when forced to evacuate the island. Macquarie reviewed his grant and offered him land elsewhere.[12] It took another year before this was finalised.

Eight years had passed since William Redfern was transported to New South Wales and he was keen to return to Britain to see his family. And so was his homesick partner, Sarah McHenry. Joseph Foveaux had already obtained permission from Macquarie to return to England so that he could be examined for his conduct during the rebellion, and he was expected to depart on the first available ship.[13] Because of Lieutenant Governor David Collins' dispute with Bligh during the Hobart blockade, Macquarie predicted that Collins would soon be recalled. He recommended to the Colonial Office that Joseph Foveaux be made the next Lieutenant Governor of that settlement.[14]

On 19 February 1810 Redfern applied for leave to return to England for up to 18 months. In the same letter he requested that his appointment as assistant surgeon at the hospital be confirmed. A day later Redfern received the reply from the administration that his application for leave had been denied because there was no one to fill his position.[15] However, on 24 February, Macquarie announced in *The Sydney Gazette* that:

> Mr. William Redfern shall continue to act as Assistant Surgeon on the Civil Medical Establishment of this Colony, until His Majesty's Pleasure shall be known, it being His Excellency's Intention to recommend that Mr. Redfern may be confirmed in that Situation.[16]

A week later Macquarie wrote to the Colonial Office Secretary Castlereagh recommending William Redfern receive a commission from His Majesty as assistant surgeon and, if surgeon Thomas Jamison did not return to the colony, that D'Arcy Wentworth be appointed principal surgeon.[17]

Lachlan Macquarie was dismayed at the 'extraordinary and illiberal' stance taken by past governors towards emancipists.[18] Admittedly, this was at a time when high achievement could not expunge the stigma of low birth or having committed a crime. For this reason, prominent emancipists such as Redfern, Thompson and Lord were shunned socially. Despite good connections, even the wellborn D'Arcy Wentworth was treated coolly by "better society" because of his court appearances and close association with emancipists.

Macquarie saw the discrimination against ex-convicts as a significant obstacle to creating a cohesive community and he was determined to stamp it out. In April 1810 Macquarie wrote to Colonial Secretary Castlereagh that former convicts had 'by long habits of industry and total reformation of manners, had not only become respectable but by many degrees the most useful members of the community'. He pointed out that emancipation, combined with rectitude and established good behaviour, should enable a man to rise in society.[19] Macquarie prioritised criminal reform over punishment and believed that the biggest incentive for personal repatriation was acceptance into the society of freemen.

To show his commitment to egalitarianism, Macquarie invited all walks of life to dine with him at Government House. Such recognition was welcomed by emancipists, but it alarmed the

Sydney elite. They claimed that the social reputation of the colony and the Governor was irreversibly damaged when past criminals were invited to sit at the seat of power. Macquarie informed the Colonial Office that:

> The number of persons of this description whom I have yet admitted to my table consist of only four, namely, Mr. D'Arcy Wentworth, Principal Surgeon; Mr. William Redfern, Assistant Surgeon; Mr. Andrew Thompson, an opulent farmer and proprietor of land; and Mr. Simeon Lord, an opulent merchant.[20]

Thereafter D'Arcy Wentworth, Andrew Thompson, Simeon Lord and William Redfern became regular guests at Government House. Outraged letters about these scandalous gatherings were soon being sent to the British Colonial Office. Redfern also met regularly with Captain Henry Antill, Macquarie's Aide-de-Camp, and they formed a lifelong friendship and later became brothers-in-law. Antill was born in New York where his father fought in the British army during the American War of Independence. After the war the family moved to Canada where Antill spent his youth. In 1796 he joined the British army and served in India with Lachlan Macquarie in the 73rd Regiment of Foot.

During the rebel administration, NSW Corps officers had been at the forefront of excluding emancipists from society, no matter their official status or wealth. Corps Lieutenant Archibald Bell 'considered them as having been once tainted, unfit for associating with afterwards'.[21] He observed that 'I know that Mr. Redfern has been admitted as a professional man to many families but within the circle of my acquaintance I have not known of his being invited as a friend or a member of society'. Bell was then inferring that Lachlan and Elizabeth Macquarie preferred the company of ex-convicts to 'free persons' in the colony. On one occasion at Government House, Lieutenant Bell had been slighted when 'Mrs. Macquarie has passed me by without notice & has held out her hand to persons who had been Convicts & who were present'.[22]

Many Exclusives shared Bell's indignation. The naval surgeon Joseph Arnold had arrived with Macquarie on HMS *Hindostan* and regularly mixed in the society of free merchants and military officers. He was astounded at the success and wealth of the ex-convicts Andrew Thompson and Simeon Lord considering the lowness of their class and observed that 'free men' would never sit at their table. Arnold was also disparaging of D'Arcy Wentworth being 'a highwayman, [who] is now Surgeon General of the colony and is said to be worth £30,000 ready cash'.[23]

It was at this time that Joseph Foveaux recommended Doctor Redfern to the chronically ill Judge Advocate Ellis Bent. He had arrived sick from England and was being treated by the regimental surgeon John Carter. But Bent thought Carter 'did not understand my case, nor take pains to understand it' and on Foveaux's advice he consulted Redfern. After some treatment he partially recovered and praised Redfern as 'by far the cleverest professional man in this Colony'. Carter was very angry at being replaced by an ex-convict surgeon and thereafter refused to talk to Bent. However, the medical remedies available then were of no use to the 'infirm and lame' Ellis Bent, and a year later he was unable to walk.[24]

On 18 March 1810 Joseph Foveaux and Ann Sherwin departed for England on the brig *Experiment*.[25] Although William Redfern was denied leave because he was needed at the hospital, his companion Sarah McHenry was under no such constraint. There is no record of her whereabouts after returning to Sydney in 1808, but it seems likely she sailed to England at the same time as Foveaux. She was a close friend of Ann Sherwin and probably accompanied her on the *Experiment*. It is impossible to speculate on Redfern's reaction to Sarah leaving; the two had been together for nine years, so it was probably difficult for both. The demands of Redfern's work at the hospital and his medical practice are likely to have tested their relationship – perhaps Sarah decided that she no longer wanted to play second fiddle to William's passion for medicine.

With Macquarie's support, Joseph Foveaux planned to return to the colony in one year and replace David Collins in Hobart. But the Colonial Office had other ideas. Although a court martial cleared Foveaux of any serious illegalities in New South Wales, his role in the rebel leadership had prejudiced future governmental roles. Unfazed, Foveaux re-joined the British Army and, with his well-honed leadership skills, rose to be a Lieutenant General in 1831. Foveaux and Redfern would soon meet again.

At the end of April 1810, William Bligh was ready to sail for England with the fourteen men he had selected to give damning evidence at the court martial of George Johnston. On 12 May 1810 Bligh and his witnesses departed on HMS *Hindostan*, part of a three ship squadron with HMS *Dromedary* and HMS *Porpoise*. The ships also transported men of the disbanded NSW Corps, which included Sarah's husband James McHenry and Colonel Paterson.

Macquarie was certain that the promotion of capable emancipists greatly benefited the colony, especially with a shortage of educated men in the colony willing to work hard and take on new challenges. Many of his top officials had left for England with Bligh, and important public posts now had to be filled. On 31 March he appointed D'Arcy Wentworth as Treasurer of the Police Fund, which in effect made him the Colonial Treasurer. Revenues from duty and custom payments, road tolls and liquor licence fees were paid into the Police Fund. This financed all police and gaol expenses, road works, building repairs and the salaries of some civil officers.[26] The Police Fund would later finance some of Lachlan Macquarie's most ambitious building projects.

For some of the Sydney elites, particularly Reverend Samuel Marsden, the invitation for ex-convicts to dine with Macquarie was an inexcusable breach of social etiquette. A serious confrontation occurred between the two men after Marsden refused to join with emancipists Andrew Thompson and Simeon Lord on a Turnpike Trust overseeing the building of a toll road between Parramatta and Windsor. Marsden declared that, not only were these men ex-convicts they were also living in immoral *de facto* relationships. Marsden's bigotry infuriated Macquarie and he replaced him on the Trust with the ex-highwayman D'Arcy Wentworth, and, to annoy him further, appointed the emancipist Simeon Lord as a new magistrate.[27]

With D'Arcy Wentworth holding medical, treasury and trustee posts, most medical duties at the hospital fell to Redfern, who was at the same time running a large Sydney and rural private practice. Private patients ranging from the governor to poor families sought his attention. Government employees incurred no charges, but other private patients had to pay a fee; five shillings in Sydney and 1 to 5 pounds for a rural visit. Attending a childbirth was free for the poor and cost £5 for the rest.[28] Many poor patients paid for medical treatments with goods and services.

Overall, the health standards in New South Wales were good. The diseases prevalent in England such as scarlet fever, smallpox, measles, whooping cough, croup and influenza were rare in the colony. Typhus from ships was reduced by strict quarantine measures. Dysentery was the most common fatal sickness in the colony, mainly among newly arrived convicts and poorer residents.

Redfern commenced his daily hospital rounds as early as 6 am, examining outpatients at 8 am and finishing at noon. He then attended to his private patients. Hospital in-patients received free treatment independent of status, as did outpatients. Most were convicts working for, and victualled by, the government. Ex-convicts, ticket of leave convicts and poorer residents were only admitted to the hospital after a doctor received governmental approval. Assigned convict servants, whose masters wanted them returned after recovery, had to provide their food rations. If they did not, convict servants were returned to the government after hospital discharge. Doctors treated civil officers in their houses and provided them with free medicine from the hospital. Seamen were only admitted to the hospital if paid for by their employer.[29]

The government provided most of the medical supplies in the colony. Since 1788 it had been 'the general Practice of all the Medical Officers to administer the Hospital Medicines to all persons whatever, whether connected with the Government or not'.[30] In later years William Redfern justified dispensing hospital medical supplies to his private patients, explaining that:

> In a Country where there was neither a Public Dispensary, a Private Medicine shop, nor any means of procuring regular supplies of Medicines, being in fact regarded as a sort of General Colonial Dispensary from which all persons were considered as having a right to obtain Medicine, & without which the people must have been destitute of all Medicine whatever.[31]

He administered 'Medicine in the same way to the people in & out of the Hospital, connected & unconnected with the Government and amongst the rest to those persons whom he did charge for his services'.[32] Medication was given gratis to the poor patients, but charges may be applied to those who could pay.[33]

Governor Macquarie had ambitious visions for improving Sydney, both architecturally and economically. One of the most serious obstacles to commercial growth in the colony was the absence of large financial institutions. Macquarie's greatest desire was to establish a bank in the colony that would mitigate the current use of promissory notes for most transactions. These handwritten notes were liable to forgery and fraud, and they caused much of the litigation that flooded the courts. In March 1810 Macquarie recommended to the Colonial Office that a banking system be created with the power to issue a stable currency similar to that available in Cape Town.[34] He asked for £5,000 in copper coins to be circulated among the 'lower Branches of Trade' to relieve the need to accept depreciated promissory notes.[35] Colonial Secretary Liverpool rejected both requests, claiming that the establishment of a bank was premature and dangerous.[36] Macquarie was furious at the refusal, as he was certain a bank would benefit the colony. It would take another four years before this became reality.

In 1810 the colony had a population of 10,452 people, 6156 of whom lived in Sydney where medical care was provided at either a military or a civilian general hospital. The military hospital catered to 1853 soldiers and their families and was served by two surgeons and two assistant surgeons. The Sydney general hospital, headed by Principal Surgeon D'Arcy Wentworth and Assistant Surgeon William Redfern, was available to 4303 non-military residents, including 792 male and 63 female convicts. Evidently staff and facilities at the general hospital were struggling to cope with the ever-expanding patient numbers.[37]

Lachlan Macquarie was particularly dissatisfied with the overall quality of buildings in Sydney and elsewhere, just as William Bligh had been. One of his highest priorities was to establish a town plan and building codes. The street layout of modern Sydney is still largely based on the plans he drew up. The colony's most prestigious buildings were to be built on Macquarie Street – Lachlan, like most Governors, was not reticent to give his own name to prominent infrastructure. However, in 1810 no public works budget existed because the British government still saw the colony as a place for criminals who had no need of fine buildings or good roads. Macquarie scoffed at such nonsense and promoted an ambitious brick-and-mortar plan to populate Sydney with large official buildings in the Georgian style currently in vogue.

One of the most vital government buildings in Sydney, the general hospital on George Street, was close to collapse and Macquarie was determined to replace it, no matter the cost. On 8 March 1810 he told Lord Castlereagh in the Colonial Office that it was necessary for the Crown to fund the construction of new military barracks and other public buildings, which included a new hospital. He wrote:

> There will be an absolute necessity for building a New General Hospital as soon as possible, the present one being in a most ruinous state, and very unfit for the reception of the Sick that must necessarily be sent to it, of which there are on an average seldom less in it than between Seventy and Eighty Men, women, and Children.[38]

Macquarie considered the replacement of the hospital critical and urgent and did not wait for a response. On 19 May D'Arcy Wentworth called for tenders to construct a new Sydney hospital. Redfern undoubtedly contributed to the facilities planning of the hospital but was not involved in the architectural design.[39] Seven acres land facing Macquarie Street was set aside for a hospital that would accommodate 200 patients. It would be an 'elegant and commodious' three-winged two-storey building with colonnaded verandas on both levels, 287 ft (87.5 m) long and 28 ft (8.5 m) wide.[40] Today, two wings of this building remain – the southern wing is now 'The Mint' and the northern wing is the New South Wales Parliament House. The designer of the hospital is unknown, but it was widely rumoured that the general concepts originated from a book of "home designs" belonging to Elizabeth Macquarie.

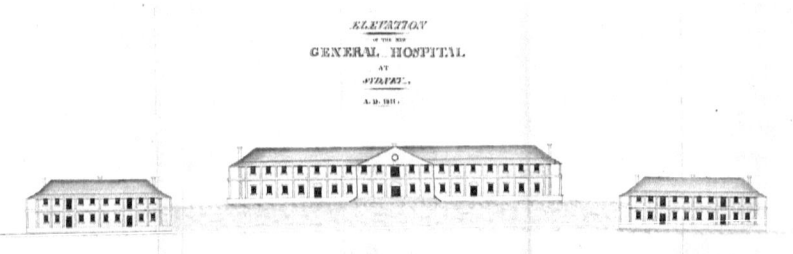

An 1811 architectural drawing of the three wings of the new General Hospital on Macquarie Street Sydney.

As had other governors, Macquarie wanted to halt the trade in alcohol but soon realised that his existing measures for regulating spirits were ineffective. If it was impossible to suppress the rum trade, he wondered if it could be harnessed to benefit the colony. In March 1810 Macquarie *doubled* the alcohol import duty from 1s 6d to 3s per gallon and allowed a less restricted ingress.[41] Rum importing now became easier, but at a much higher price.

THE RUM HOSPITAL

Macquarie saw the construction of a new general hospital as the start of his ambitious building program, so it had to be a success. In July 1810 the merchants Garnham Blaxcell and Alexander Riley submitted the first building tender. Their quote required that they be granted a monopoly on the rum trade and the right to import 45,000 gallons of spirit. Macquarie initially rejected the proposal. But when no further tenders came forward, he reconsidered their submission.[42] On 6 November 1810, he agreed that Riley and Blaxcell, in partnership with D'Arcy Wentworth, could build the hospital, provided it was completed in three years at no cost to the government. In return, the consortium was given a licence to import 45,000 gallons of rum for commercial sale. Moreover, they would be assigned 20 bullocks and 20 convict labourers to assist in the build.[43] When the extraordinary conditions of the building contract were revealed to the public, the new Sydney hospital quickly became known as 'the Rum Hospital'.

As principal surgeon, treasurer and hospital contractor, D'Arcy Wentworth now had his finger in almost every colonial pie. D'Arcy's private life was equally complicated. His eldest son William, aged 20, had returned from England in March 1810 and about this time his father had formed a close relationship with Ann Lawes, who had left her husband James Mackneal and a young child. On 28 April 1810, *The Sydney Gazette* printed a notice by James declaring Mary Ann had, without provocation, left his house and abandoned her son. It warned anyone sheltering her that they risked prosecution and would be liable for debts incurred in her name.[44] Mary Ann had arrived in Sydney in 1806 as the 13-year-old free servant of Provost Marshall William Gore. She married James Mackneal two years later and was only 17 when she left him for the 48-year-old D'Arcy. The liaison caused friction in the Wentworth family. His sons greatly admired their father's previous partner Maria Ainslie and insisted that she be cared for. At the children's urging, Maria was moved to Wentworth's Home Bush estate in Parramatta as housekeeper, while Mary Ann resided at D'Arcy's house in Sydney. To minimise colonial chatter Wentworth never discussed his family and he always attended public functions alone.[45] The first of his eight children with Mary Ann, George, was born in November 1810.

By June 1810, Andrew Thompson, William Redfern's friend and patient, was told he did not have long to live. Redfern regularly treated Thompson for respiratory disease when he visited Sydney, but now such trips from Green Hills were impossible. More often surgeon James Mileham visited Thompson's farm and occasionally Redfern was asked to come and assist. The journey to Thompson's Red House in the Hawkesbury district took several hours on horseback or by carriage. The close-knit community in Green Hills made sure Thompson received the best possible care; as did Lachlan and Elizabeth Macquarie, who were his close friends. Thompson's illness had resulted from days of cold wet exposure during his rescue of many settlers in the devastating 1809 Hawkesbury floods. As most lung diseases were untreatable then, everyone in the district realised Thompson's days were numbered. In early August 1810 Redfern treated him again but it was purely palliative.[46] By September his health had deteriorated further and on 22 October 1810 he died at the age of 37.[47]

Many distinguished officers and gentlemen, both Exclusives and emancipists, were among the large congregation at Andrew Thompson's funeral service in Green Hills. Among them was William Redfern 'who had attended the deceased during the long and painful illness that brought to a conclusion an existence that had been well applied'.[48]

Shortly after Thompson's funeral, Redfern was invited to join the Governor on a tour of the colony's farming districts. It would be Macquarie's first inspection of the colony's western farming areas. The Blue Mountains, 40 miles west of Sydney, remained a barrier to expansion – its forested gullies and sheer cliffs had so far prevented colonialists from crossing to the lands beyond. Macquarie had already advised settlers that many of the existing farms close to rivers were prone to flooding and needed to be relocated. He also wanted to improve roads in rural districts to provide better access to farm communities. It was expected that the Governor's visit to the estates of prominent settlers would take seven weeks. This was too long for Redfern to be absent from his patients, and he planned to return to Sydney after three weeks when the touring group reached Green Hills.

On 6 November 1810, on the evening of the day that the contract for the new hospital was signed, Lachlan and Elizabeth

Macquarie, Captain Antill, Captain Cleaveland, surgeon Redfern, surveyor Meehan, Macquarie's cousin Ensign John Maclaine, their servants and wagons full of camping gear, set off towards Parramatta.[49] On 7 November they reached an area on the Georges River prone to flooding and surveyed the site for a town to be named 'Liverpool' after the Earl of Liverpool, the current Colonial Office Secretary.

The next day Macquarie, Moore, Redfern, Antill and Meehan set out on horseback to the southern Minto district and, after visiting several large farms including 'Mr. Thompson's Farm called St Andrews'. On 12 November the touring party returned to Parramatta where the Governor, accompanied by Dr Redfern and contractor James Harrex, inspected the construction of the new toll road between Parramatta and Green Hills. That afternoon they visited farms near Parramatta, including that of Dr Wentworth. The whole day Macquarie felt 'bilious' and Redfern administered some medicine before the Governor retired to his camp bed.[50]

After two days Macquarie had recovered sufficiently to visit other farms north of Parramatta. On 16 November the tour group set out for the Cowpastures property on the west side of the Nepean River, where wild cattle grazed. They camped under the stars and were joined by John Warlby, Gregory Blaxland and four soldiers. The country between Parramatta and the Nepean River was mainly open forest with passable tracks, and the river was so shallow that their carts could cross easily. They set up camp near a lagoon at the foot of Mount Taurus and that night heard the wild cattle 'bellowing in the woods'. Early next morning Blaxland and Warlby shot a bull for the servant's meals. Guided by Warlby, the tour group were riding out after breakfast for another hunt when an accident occurred. Macquarie recorded in his diary that 'Mr. Meehan in hunting the wild cattle had the misfortune to be thrown from his horse and dislocated his arm; but Doctor Redfern having come shortly after to his assistance, immediately set his arm again, so as to secure his still preserving and recovering the use of it'.[51]

On 20 November the tour group recrossed the Nepean River and returned to St Andrews farm where they stayed for two days admiring the fertility of the area. In the following days the party travelled through undeveloped country, Macquarie judged to be the 'best and fittest' for farming. Here he planned to create a new farming district called 'Airds' in honour of his wife's Scottish estate.

Plans were also drawn up for the village of Campbelltown, in recognition of Elizabeth's family name.[52] In years to come William Redfern would be granted land in this district.

On 1 December the party rode along the Hawkesbury River to Green Hills. The Governor was 'quite delighted with the beauty of this part of the country, its great fertility, and its picturesque appearance'. Buildings, once the property of Andrew Thompson, covered much of the Green Hills government precinct, and dominated the vista from Government House. The touring party dined there soon after arrival, and Macquarie noted in his journal: 'after dinner our friend & family physician Doctor Redfern took his departure for Sydney'.[53]

The governor's tour of rural districts continued for another month. On 6 December 1810 Macquarie gazetted five new towns to be established in areas that were less susceptible to flooding: Windsor (formerly Green Hills), Richmond, Wilberforce, Pitt Town and Castlereagh. To honour Andrew Thompson's development of the Green Hills district, Macquarie named the central park in Windsor to be 'Thompson Square'.[54]

William Redfern would have been pleased that his deceased friend Andrew Thompson had been so recognised – it was particularly satisfying that the efforts of emancipists in the colony were starting to be officially rewarded. This was especially important to Redfern who hoped to be the future principal surgeon of the colony.

Chapter 10

MISS SARAH WILLS

> Redfern: *I am sorry, my dearest! But you know you are marrying a – doctor!*
> Sara: *I know, William. I am also marrying one of the kindest and most generous men in the world! And – I will come along with you – as far as you will allow me. Always!*
> John Antill et al., a play entitled The Emancipist, 1936[1]

As soon as William Redfern returned from the governor's tour, D'Arcy Wentworth, who had been his locum over the three weeks, updated him on hospital matters. This would have been a hectic period for Wentworth though he may have enjoyed practicing medicine for a change – civic responsibilities took up most of his time and these were about to get even more onerous. Concern about lawlessness in Sydney had soared recently, and nightly riots and assaults were common. In an attempt to eradicate the 'Midnight Ruffian and Thief', Macquarie had promulgated new police regulations and on 29 December 1810 he appointed D'Arcy Wentworth as the Superintendent of Police.[2]

D'Arcy and his family moved some distance from the hospital to a new residence on George Street and from here he pursued his innumerable official duties, which now included law enforcement. He had no opportunity to regularly practice medicine these days, but quite willingly replaced Redfern when he was absent from the hospital – he may well have found these duties therapeutic.[3] No such locum arrangement existed for Redfern's private patients, and they would have missed their doctor during his recent absence. One of these patients was Edward Wills, an emancipist merchant living close to the hospital. Redfern had become friends with the Wills family and their beautiful daughter Sarah.

Edward Wills, a London letterpress printer, was arrested for highway robbery in January 1797 and his sentence to be hanged was later commuted to transportation for life. In December 1798 he sailed from Portsmouth on the transport *Hillsborough* with his wife Sarah, their three-year-old daughter and 300 other convicts.

Because of the dreadful conditions on board many convicts, who were allowed little exercise, contracted typhus. The Wills family survived but a third of the convicts on the *Hillsborough* did not.

On arrival in Sydney, Sarah Wills requested that her convict husband Edward be assigned to her as a servant. By law, a married woman could not buy or own property, make contracts or incur debts, without her husband's approval. However, these restrictions did not apply to a free woman married to a convict. In such cases a wife had the rights of a single female until her husband completed his sentence.[4] With financial help from her family in England, Sarah began trading from a warehouse and opened a retail shop and tavern on George Street. She was a good businesswoman and would eventually own several farms. When her husband Edward received a conditional pardon in 1803, they became prosperous shop owners and traders.[5] In 1805 Thomas Reibey and Edward Wills became partners in the seal trade and built the sealer ship *Mary and Sally*. The increasing wealthy Wills family also bought the two trading sloops *Raven* and *Eliza*.[6]

During William Bligh's governorship, Sarah and Edward Wills opposed his reforms to curb alcohol trading, as it threatened their tavern business. Like many Sydney merchants, they supported the arrest of the governor and signed John Macarthur's petition.[7] In May 1808 Sarah wrote to her mother in England:

> But at last the Officers and Gentlemen in general found themselves so much imposed on that they could put up with it no longer - and for the good of the people in general Major Johnson took up the cause - and on the 26th January quite unexpected and to our great surprise the Drum beat to arms, the soldiers marched to Government House, put the Governor under arrest and Major Johnson took the command. The Major is a good man and I hope what he has done will be approved of.[8]

The Wills family planned a return to Britain after Edward had gained an absolute pardon. Their daughter Sarah, nicknamed Sally, had been well educated locally but she was to finish her schooling in England.[9] These plans never came to fruition. Edward was never well and when he finally gained an absolute pardon in late 1810 it was evident, he would not survive the voyage to England. By then, there were four more Wills children: Thomas born in 1800, Eliza in 1802, Edward in 1805 and Elizabeth in 1807.

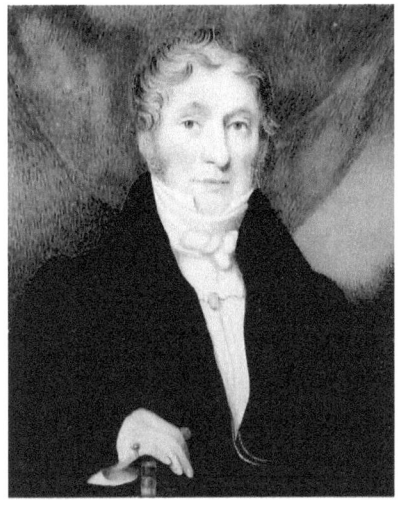 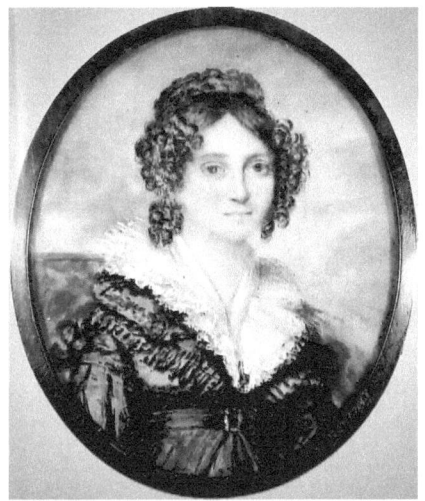

1832 portrait of William Redfern.   c. 1815 portrait of Sarah Redfern.

William Redfern regularly treated the invalided Edward Wills and shopped at their store. He probably also imbibed at their tavern just metres away from the hospital. With the decline in Edward's health, Redfern advised his 35-year-old patient in May 1810 to settle his affairs. Edward was especially concerned about the future of his 14-year-old daughter Sally, who was by now a young lady regularly working in the store and tavern, as well as caring for her younger siblings. In a colony with so few young females, Sally was practiced in fending off amorous approaches. Even so, her parents agonised about her future as she reached marriageable age – it was common then for girls to wed at 14. This was evident in Edward's will, which stated: 'should my Daughter Sarah Wills marry contrary to the Wish or Consent of her Mother Sarah Wills that the Mother shall cease to give her any further assistance whatever'.[10]

In early 1811, Redfern also treated the Wills' chronically ill baby Elizabeth, who died aged three. The death occurred just as Sally was about to sail on the *Indian* for England and this, coupled with her father's terminal illness, led her to cancel her passage and stay to help her mother. It was then that she also became friends with the 36-year-old Dr Redfern. How this romantic attachment started is unknown – quite possibly Sally set out to find a suitable partner before her father died. Despite the age disparity, William Redfern was probably one of the few promising bachelors she knew, and her parents approved of. Large age differences between couples were common then. All of this is pure speculation, of course, but with few marriage prospects for educated females in the colony, the reason for such a tryst seems logical.

On 2 March 1811, William Redfern drew up a prenuptial contract that provided £1000 to his future wife Sally on his death. It was witnessed by Reverend William Cowper as Executor and Captain Henry Antill. His wife-to-be Sarah (Sally) Wills, who was almost 15, would receive a 30-acre farm as a dowry settlement from her mother.[11] The farm, just south of central Sydney on Botany Bay Road, had 150 sheep and 11 cattle.[12] In later years, this land was added to, and it would eventually become part of the future Sydney suburb of Redfern.

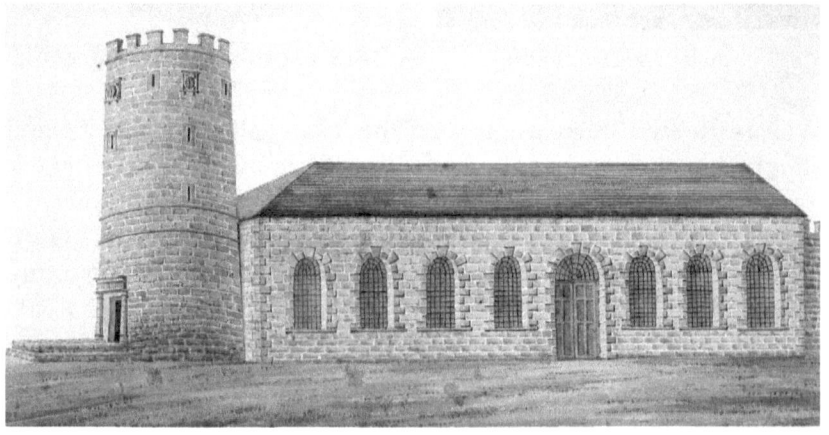

1809 painting of St Philip's Church where Sarah and William were married.

On Monday, 4 March 1811, the bells of St Philip's Church of England heralded the wedding of 'William Redfern, Gentleman, of this parish, Bachelor' and 'Sarah Wills, Spinster', who were married under 'Especial Licence' by Reverend William Cowper. Edward Wills, and William's friend, Captain Antill, acted as witnesses.[13] The passage of time would prove that Sarah and William were temperamentally and intellectually well matched, and they would have a mostly harmonious marriage. Being married to a doctor who practiced long hours was not easy, but the industrious Sarah would stand by William during his many challenges.

Mrs Sarah Redfern – she had dropped her childhood nickname – now resided in the assistant surgeon's house just down the road from her parents. Every day she visited the Wills store to assist her mother, and William continued to care for her father until he died just two months after their wedding, aged 33.[14] It was a highly emotional time for the Wills family. Not only had Edward passed away, but his 35-year-old widow Sarah was pregnant again. On 5 October 1811, baby Horatio Wills would be born.

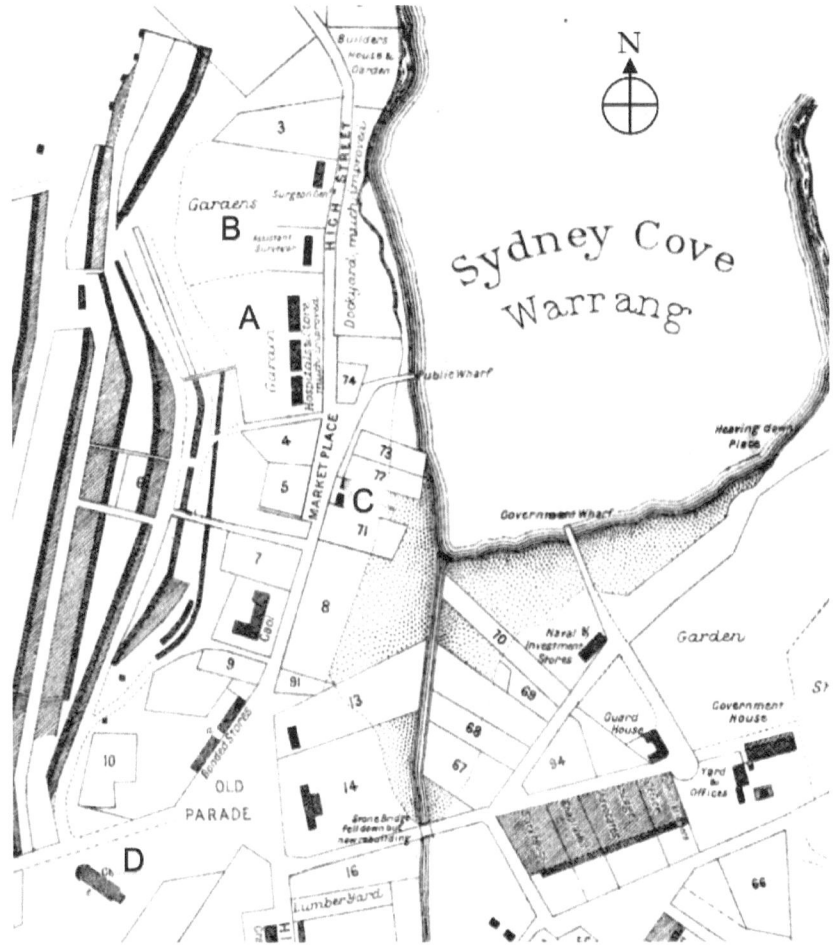

Part of surveyor James Meehan's 1807 plan of Sydney showing the hospital (A) and surgeon's houses (B) on High Street (later named George Street). The Wills family owned property (C) on Market Place. In 1811 Sarah and William Redfern were married at St Philip's Church (D).

The year 1811 proved challenging for William Redfern. There had been a serious outbreak of dysentery in Sydney between January and March, and thirteen men, eight of whom were convicts, died in the hospital. It is not known how Redfern treated dysentery, but the hospital records list the morbidity of the 41 patients who died. In addition to *dysentery*, the cause of death was *dropsy* (oedema, swelling of soft tissue), *venereal* (sexually transmitted disease), *paralytic* (paralysis), *haemorrhage* (loss of blood), *fever* and *asthma*.[15] The patients were convicts and others who could not be cared for at home. For most colonists the hospital was *a refuge of last resort*, a place where convicts, accident victims and poor people went for emergency care. Those with money stayed at home for treatment and relied on family or servants to look after their needs.

Some hospitalised patients suffered mentally. Convicts who left behind beloved partners and children in Britain when transported to the "ends of the earth" were susceptible to depression. But serious mental disorders were uncommon and most convicts adapted easily to colonial living conditions, which were often better than those they experienced in Britain. However, there were no facilities to support orphaned children, the incapacitated or the mentally ill. Medical services in the colony focused on physical ailments and anyone with emotional problems depended on aid from the church, friends or family. As the colony grew, those suffering psychologically were usually committed to the Parramatta gaol, as there was no other institution to care for them.

William Redfern was officially responsible for mental health aboard visiting ships. One such instance involved Alexander Bodie, the captain of the whaler *Frederick*, who was declared 'mad' on a voyage from London. On docking in Sydney in April 1811 Bodie had to be restrained and his possessions were handed to trustees. Redfern and Wentworth assessed Bodie's 'Health and Mental Faculties' to ascertain if he was fit to resume command of his ship. They found him 'perfectly recovered from his late Malady as to Warrant the removal of all Restraints'.[16] Governor Macquarie agreed, but it was another six months before Captain Bodie resumed command of the *Frederick*.

A more severe mental case was that of Jonathan McHugo, a merchant based in Calcutta. When arriving in Hobart Town on his ship *Active*, he claimed to be an incognito member of the British Royal Family who had the power to overrule colonial governors. McHugo convinced Lieutenant Colonel Gordon of this authority and was given command of the settlement. But other officers were less gullible; they intervened and arrested the deranged McHugo.[17] He was so violent on the passage back to Sydney that he was strapped to his cot to prevent injury to himself and others. After interviewing McHugo, Wentworth and Redfern informed Macquarie that he had a 'severe Mental Derangement rendering him totally incapable of attending to any business'.[18] This appears to be the first certificate of lunacy issued in the colony.[19] After a court inquiry Judge Advocate Bent declared McHugo a lunatic and appointed wardens to sell the contents of his ship. McHugo's 'unhappy condition' continued for nine weeks before he was sent back to Calcutta.[20]

The McHugo case, and a visit to the Parramatta gaol, alerted Governor Macquarie to the lack of facilities for treating mental illness in the colony. In May 1811 a Lunatic Asylum was built at Castle Hill, the first official institution dedicated to mental health in Australia. A two-storey stone structure was erected seven miles north of Parramatta and it was also used as a military barracks.[21]

As an assistant surgeon at the Sydney hospital, William Redfern was also in charge of inspecting the health and hygiene standards aboard incoming convict ships. These inspections were to prevent diseases entering the colony and also to ensure arriving convicts were fit and healthy. The latter was critical to ensure an active workforce in the colony and overburdening the crowded hospital. At Macquarie's urging, Redfern drew up a new inspection regime for vetting incoming convicts. Henceforth, medical inspectors had to be the first to board incoming convict transport ships. After this inspection convicts disembarked and were interviewed by Macquarie on their treatment by the ship's surgeon and master. This was a tense time for the ship's crew because their pay depended on Macquarie's approval. Secretary John Campbell and the Commissary William Broughton then mustered the convicts by trade and assigned duties: civil officials had first pick, followed by merchants and landowners seeking assigned convict servants.[22]

On 2 July 1811 Redfern inspected the transport *Providence* that docked with 174 convicts from Ireland. Six convicts had died on the voyage, and Redfern noted this was a 'lenient bill of mortality, compared with many former'. Disembarking convicts were in good health and Captain Barclay was praised for his humane 'liberal and indulgent' treatment of the convicts.[23] At that time

Redfern needed to replace a recently absconded convict servant of his own. After the muster and assembly was complete, he chose the 20-year-old John Grant, a ploughman from Tipperary transported for life for attempted murder.[24] It was a good choice, and he eventually became the overseer at his farm Campbellfield.

Macquarie praised Redfern's inspection regime and sent details of it to England. The new arrival requirements forced ship owners to improve the hygiene and food aboard transport ships. By October 1811 Macquarie reported that 'The Male Convicts arrived in those Ships proved a very Seasonable and acceptable Supply for the Colony'.[25] Redfern's inspection duties, coupled undoubtedly his own incarceration on a convict ship, instilled a lifelong interest in improving the health of transported felons. Having suffered the long passage to the colony himself and seen the health benefits Sir Jeremiah Fitzpatrick had enforced on ship captains and surgeons, Redfern was determined to further improve conditions on convict ships and make transportation as humane as possible.

In mid 1811 the building contractors of Sydney's new hospital were busy procuring a workforce and arranging for bricks, timber and stonework. The site on Macquarie Street had been levelled and a surrounding security wall erected. On 30 October Macquarie laid, with much pomp and ceremony, the foundation stone for the main building, witnessed by the 'principal Officers and Ladies of the Colony' who included William Redfern and his wife.[26] At the base of the foundation stone was a casket of gold and silver coins encased in a lead box. Five days later, the Macquaries sailed to inspect the settlements on Van Diemen's Land, accompanied by Captain Antill, Surveyor Meehan and Lieutenant Maclaine. This time Dr Redfern did not join them, but he went to the farewell breakfast on the *Lady Nelson* and returned to the hospital.[27]

In addition to William Redfern's successful medical pursuits, he renewed his interest in agriculture. In May he received a grant of 800 acres to replace Paterson's cancelled grant of 500 acres. This land was in the district of Airds on the Bow Bowing Creek, 35 miles southwest of Sydney. Redfern had seen the land when he visited the area with Macquarie, and he called the farm *Campbellfield* after Elizabeth Macquarie's maiden name. A month later he bought eight cows from the government herd for £224.[28]

In January 1812 King George III appointed 'William Redfern, Gentleman, to be Assistant Surgeon on the Civil Medical Establishment' and D'Arcy Wentworth as Principal Surgeon.[29] As an emancipist, the stamp of Royal approval for the government surgeon post at the hospital was of the utmost importance, and Redfern would have been relieved to have it in writing.

In April Lachlan Macquarie sought Dr Redfern's opinion on the health of Elizabeth. He informed the governor that he believed his wife was with child, but it was too early 'to pronounce decidedly whether Mrs. M. is Pregnant or not'. He advised against her taking further trips by carriage or horseback; in her present state she should 'keep herself as quiet and as free from any fear or alarm as possible'. Redfern's diagnosis was correct, but within three weeks Elizabeth had her fifth miscarriage and became extremely ill. Over the next few weeks Redfern visited her regularly to reduce the fever.[30]

Patient numbers at the hospital had ballooned to an extent that additional medical help was urgently needed. An overseer, clerk, gatekeeper, matron and nurses assisted Redfern, but they were mostly unqualified convicts who only recompensed with rations and accommodation. In July 1812, Redfern took on the 19-year-old James Sheers as a medical apprentice and he became, in effect, Australia's first medical student and the first that Redfern trained. He had known the Sheers family on Norfolk Island, where James was born in 1793. Mr Sheers Snr was a butcher who most likely prepared Redfern's pigs for market and James' stepsister, Mary Ann, later married the Commandant of the island, John Piper. Usually, parents paid for a son's apprenticeship and lodgings, but this was waived if the family was poor. Instead, Redfern managed to arrange that James was paid an annual wage of £25 with food rations through the Police Fund.[31] He resided in the hospital complex and accompanied Redfern on his daily rounds.

Redfern was a strong advocate that education was the best path out of poverty and took a particular interest in helping orphans. In 1801 Governor King had built a female orphan school on George Street opposite St Philip's church. Here girls were taught mostly spinning and weaving. Providing little formal education, the school was basically a clothing factory and a source of domestic servants. Redfern became the official physician for the school, and he and Sarah helped with the girls' education. They would have discussed this interest with the Macquaries, and it may have led to the Governor's decision that a new school for female orphans was needed. With no funds to build a new orphanage, public donations were sought and the Redferns were the first to contribute towards the purchase of land at Parramatta.[32] The design of the new Female Orphan School at Parramatta appears to be based on Elizabeth Macquarie's childhood home in Scotland, Airds House.

Another educational project of interest to the Redferns was the building of a school close to their Campbellfield farm in Liverpool, a town founded by Macquarie in November 1810 only 11 miles from their farm. When public donations were called for to build a schoolhouse in Liverpool, William and Sarah donated £5.[33]

The editor of *The Sydney Gazette*, George Howe, had been a long-time acquaintance of Sarah's parents Edward and Sarah Wills. Howe had been a printer in the West Indies where his father ran the government press. In 1790, aged 21, George moved to London to work at several newspapers but in 1799 he was found guilty of shoplifting and sentenced to death. This was later commuted to transportation for life. Howe arrived in NSW in 1800 with his son Robert, his wife having died on the voyage. In Sydney he became the government printer and, after a conditional pardon in March 1803, established the colony's first newspaper, *The Sydney Gazette*.

In 1806 George Howe received an absolute pardon and by then had fathered five children with his *de facto* partner Elizabeth Easton. Because the *Gazette* made little money, Howe opened a stationery shop and gave tutoring lessons. Edward Wills, also with a printing background, knew Howe and, when his newspaper premises were damaged by a storm in December 1810, he offered him rental space in the Wills' George Street building.[34] But in 1812 George Howe became insolvent and after Edward's death, he began courting the wealthy widow Sarah Wills. George abandoned his *de facto* partner for an opportunity to marry Sarah. Since a female's property belonged to her husband on marriage, George Howe saw this union as the solution to all his money problems.

Because 19th century couverture laws considered a married woman's legal identity to be merged with that of her husband, Sarah Wills took the precaution of drawing up a pre-nuptial 'Deed of Trust'. The deed, counter-signed by George Howe, Reverend William Cowper and merchant David Bevan, declared that her children would inherit Sarah's wealth and property.[35] George Howe and Sarah Wills married on 5 October 1812, exactly one year after the birth of Horatio. Howe moved into the George Street house bringing with him his 17-year-old son Robert and five of his children with Elizabeth Easton. Also residing in the house were Sarah's children, Thomas, 12, Eliza, 10, Edward, 7 and toddler Horatio.

Despite Sarah's diligence, George was soon paying off his debts with her money. She had to discharge a £500 promissory note written by George and finance the substantial enlargements to the house required to accommodate George's children. Although Sarah's ship *Mary and Sally* was named in the Deed of Trust, Howe put a notice in *The Sydney Gazette* a year later offering it for sale.[36]

Since taking office Governor Macquarie had intended to treat all inhabitants in the colony equally and fairly. He firmly believed that convict rehabilitation gave emancipists the opportunity to integrate into colonial society and that this was the key to the future stability and commercial success of the settlement. Some in the colony, especially the business elite, ridiculed such controversial objectives. Reverend Samuel Marsden complained bitterly to the Colonial Office that Macquarie was favouring criminals over free men and hence destroying the natural order of society. The rehabilitation of convicts and the advancement of ex-convicts in New South Wales became a hotly debated topic in the British parliament. So much so that in 1812 a British Parliamentary Select Committee was set up to inquire into transportation and its efficacy as a punishment.

News of Prime Minister Perceval's assassination reached the colony in late 1812. His successor the Earl of Liverpool and the newly appointed Colonial Secretary Lord Bathurst were conservative Tory politicians who were concerned by Macquarie's rehabilitation efforts in the colony. Bathurst held diametrically opposite views on the purpose of transportation and the benefits of rehabilitation. He believed in the separation of social classes and had little faith that the lower classes of society could be rehabilitated.

Interestingly, Lachlan Macquarie did not see his rehabilitation efforts as being those of a reformer. He simply believed that all free men had equal rights and that convicts should be given the opportunity to regain that status through their labours. In the 19th century such ideals were enlightened for intellectuals, let alone for a soldier. It was little wonder that conservatives in the colony and in Britain saw him as a radical who had to be muzzled. Macquarie's resolve to give emancipists equal standing and opportunities in the colony remained an ambition for the rest of his governorship.

On 26 November 1812 HMS *Samarang* arrived from Madras carrying 40,000 Spanish silver dollars, worth £10,000. Macquarie was about to use these coins to create the colony's own currency.[37] In the past foreign traders only accepted payment in hard currency and this removed coins from the colony. To deter this practice, Macquarie over-stamped the Spanish silver dollars and punched a hole in the centre. The holed coins still had intrinsic value because of their silver content but they became less attractive for traders to use overseas. The rebadged 'holey dollars' were valued at 5s each and the centrepiece called the 'dump' was valued at 15d.

The close of 1812 marked the third anniversary of Macquarie's governorship. On 30 December prominent Sydney residents met in Market Place next to the George Street hospital to plan a dinner and address to commemorate the occasion. They also discussed ways for the British Parliament to allow increases in the export of colonial commodities. Such permissions had been stymied because of Britain's contract guarantees with the East India Company.

The meeting, chaired by Simeon Lord, selected a committee of thirteen men who included William Redfern, D'Arcy Wentworth, John Blaxland, Robert Jenkins and Samuel Terry.[38] It was the first occasion that William Redfern was directly involved in colonial politics. It would not be the last.

Chapter 11

MEDICAL PIONEER

With a View therefore of providing Skilful and Approved Medical Men for this Service, it might not perhaps be deemed improper to suggest that the Surgeons ought to be appointed by Government, selected from the Surgeons in the Navy – Men of Abilities, who have been Accustomed to Sea practice, who know what is due to themselves as Men, and as Officers with full power to exercise their Judgment, without being liable to the Control of the Masters of the Transports. Redfern to Macquarie, 1814[1]

The public holiday on New Year's Day 1813 celebrated the third anniversary of Lachlan Macquarie's governorship. He received a Congratulatory Address signed by 134 colonialists acclaiming his administration for the 'Beauty and Improvement of our Metropolis' and the increased agricultural productivity leading to self-sufficiency. They thanked him for the improved policing in Sydney that had reduced crime to such an extent robberies were now rare. Macquarie was also praised for his egalitarian policies and his 'liberal, humane, and philanthropic Exertions to banish the narrow, illiberal Policy of invidious Distinctions, so long the Bane of this Colony'. However, they expressed disappointment that the Colonial Office forbid the export of surplus produce overseas, and they humbly requested the governor to support future petitions for expanding colonial trade. Governor Macquarie thanked everyone for the Address, telling the deputation that he was always willing to receive and support petitions from the community.[2]

On the evening of his anniversary Macquarie entertained 48 dinner guests at Government House. They included civil and military officers with their families and the 'Gentlemen who were deputed to present the Addresses'.[3] As a signatory of the Address, William Redfern was among the guests, accompanied by his wife Sarah.

The Sydney Gazette announced on 9 January that 'respectable inhabitants' of the colony would host a special Commemorative Dinner to celebrate Macquarie's governorship. An organising committee of free men and emancipists was formed, with 'Wm. Redfern, Esq.' among them.⁴ The cost of the Commemorative Dinner, including wine, was 22s 6d – many wishing to attend the occasion would have been sent to the colony for stealing less. In any case, the tickets sold quickly and on 29 January 1813 150 men participated in a lavish dinner held in a decorated marquee erected in the front garden of Robert Jenkins. By 6 o'clock all were seated 'without respect to rank or difference of condition' while the band of the 73rd Regiment played. In the course of the long dinner 15 toasts were given. The one for Macquarie was a 'bumper', followed by 'three times three' cheers. The 12th toast to the 'Establishment of an Export Trade' received an equal number of cheers.

The 13th toast at the dinner was to 'The intended Library' and was accompanied by a call for 'every Inhabitant of our Colony to unite in promoting the general diffusion of useful Knowledge!'⁵ Despite enthusiastic support, it took ten years before the British government allowed a public library to be built in the colony. And, although expanding exports would have greatly benefited the colony, the British refused to let them compete with the East India Company, a quasi-government enterprise that provided massive income to Britain and to many shareholding parliamentarians.

At one o'clock in the morning, four days after the dinner, a seaman knocked loudly on Redfern's door. Urgent medical help was needed on a ship in the harbour for Macquarie's cousin, Lieutenant John Maclaine. He had climbed the ship's mast during a drunken party and fallen 35 ft (10 m) onto the deck. Redfern dressed quickly and was rowed out to the ship. He found that Maclaine had 'dislocated his left arm in a most shocking and dangerous manner'. By three o'clock he had set the bone and Maclaine was taken to Government House where he remained dangerously ill. Macquarie had no sympathy for such foolishness and commented 'such being the Consequence of low Drinking and intemperance, this unfortunate young man deserves little pity!'⁶

On 12 June 1813 the *Fortune* docked in Sydney conveying a letter from the Colonial Secretary Bathurst concerning the rank of medical officers. Edward Luttrell, assistant surgeon at Parramatta Hospital, had written to Bathurst claiming that he had seniority over William Redfern but was receiving a lower salary of £91 5s per year. Luttrell's complaint read:

But Your Memorialist [Luttrell] was placed subordinate to the Situation he before held, and a Mr. Redfern, formerly an Assistant Surgeon in the Navy and who came to this Colony for Mutiny at the Nore and who was at the time of his appointment by the Lt. Governor a single Man, was placed before your Memorialist, the date of his appointment being one day previous to that of Your Memorialist, viz. Feby. 23, 1809, by which Mr. Redfern is entitled to receive seven Shillings and sixpence per day, and Your Memorialist's appointment being of a day's later date is only entitled to receive five Shillings per day as subordinate to the appointment of Mr. Redfern.[7]

Bathurst's letter told Macquarie that as governor he had no authority to determine seniority in the medical service. Acceptance into the government medical establishment, and promotion, could only occur after a surgeon had 'received a regular Commission from home' and that seniority was determined by the commission date, not by the appointment date of the governor. The letter stated that colonial medical officers appointed in Britain 'should have some prospect of rising in their profession, and of attaining in course of time to higher Salaries'. Bathurst expressed no knowledge of Luttrell's or Redfern's medical abilities, but, since there was a vacancy for an assistant surgeon with a salary of £136 17s 6d, he asked whether Luttrell should advance provided 'he is competent to do the duty of the Situation'.[8] Bathurst instructed:

> ... take care that in future every Person within the Colony, who is appointed provisionally to the Medical Department should clearly understand that he will by no means have any claim to be considered on the permanent Establishment, or to be promoted in rotation, until he has received a regular Commission from home.[9]

Macquarie's reply on 28 June 1813 strongly defended Redfern's appointment and rank. He pointed out that since the foundation of the colony it had been accepted practice that medical officers 'should take Rank and Succeed by Rotation according to the Seniority of the Dates of their Commissions' and that no colonial appointment was permanent until confirmed in London. However, 'immediately on such Confirmation taking place, the Officer, thus Appointed and Subsequently Confirmed at Home, enjoys equal Rank and Privileges, as if he had been in the first Instance Appointed and had received his Commission at Home'.[10]

Macquarie told Bathurst that although Luttrell arrived in 1804 as assistant surgeon with a pay of 5s per day, he resigned in 1807 to accept a position on HMS *Porpoise* at 10s per day. He remained there until being replaced in November 1808. Luttrell was not employed as a civil medical officer again until February 1809 when Paterson made him assistant surgeon in Parramatta. Although Luttrell said 'that the Date of his Appointment was only one day Subsequent to Mr. Redfern's' this 'widely departed from the Truth, for Mr. Redfern was duly Appointed by Warrant by Colonel Foveaux on the first of August, 1808' when Luttrell was still attached to HMS *Porpoise*. Redfern had been awarded a warrant as assistant surgeon on HMS *Standard* 'having previously Undergone the Necessary Examination'. In order that there was no doubt regarding his professional ability, Redfern had been re-examined, at his own request, before a medical board appointed by Colonel Foveaux. Lord Liverpool confirmed his appointment in 1811. Macquarie then wrote:

> Mr. Redfern's Claims with regard to Services in this Colony are far superior to Mr. Luttrel's .... I Consider Mr. Redfern as a Professional Man, a very great Acquisition to this Colony, his Talents as a Surgeon being far superior to those of any other Person of that Description in this Country, and perhaps equal to those of the most Skilful Medical Men in any other Country. With such Talents and such Claims, Mr. Redfern unquestionably looks forward to filling the highest Situation in the Medical Department of New South Wales in the regular Rotation of Seniority, being Able to produce Satisfactory Proofs of his Eligibility both with respect to professional Abilities and Character.[11]

Macquarie had a low regard for Luttrell's medical abilities and did not hesitate to inform Bathurst. He wrote that it would violate his 'own Sense of Duty and Propriety' if he recommended Luttrell for any additional pay or rank, beyond what he presently had. With the bluntness of a veteran soldier, Macquarie said he considered Luttrell 'totally undeserving, and unworthy of any further Favor' and, while not deficient in professional skill, he totally lacked 'Humanity and in Attention to his Duty' for the unfortunate people under his medical care. Many complaints had been received about Luttrell's negligence and inhumanity: that he was 'sordid and Unfeeling' to his patients; gave no medical assistance to people unable to pay a fee and routinely left the poor untreated.

Macquarie told Bathurst that he had severely censured him and unless his conduct changed Luttrell might be suspended or removed from public duties.[12] Not surprisingly, there was no further correspondence with the Colonial Secretary on this matter.

In late June 1813 Macquarie finally received the 'Report of the Select Committee on Transportation' from Britain. Although the document criticised some of Macquarie's policies, it supported his strategy that 'long-tried good conduct should lead a man back to that rank in society which he had forfeited, and do away ... all retrospect of former bad conduct'. The Report also granted permission for a distillery to be built in the colony and for law courts to allow trial by jury, provided the jurists were free men. Most importantly for Macquarie, the Report concluded that the humanitarian principles of his convict policies were in general beneficial to the administration of the colony.[13]

Macquarie was particularly pleased that law courts could now be adjudicated with a jury but, in a letter to Bathurst about the involvement of emancipists, he strongly disagreed that 'Jury Men ought to be Free'. It had always been his opinion that:

> Once a Convict has become a Free Man, either by Servitude, Free Pardon, or Emancipation, he should in All Respects be Considered on a footing with every other Man in the Colony, according to his Rank in Life and Character. In Short, that no Retrospect Should in any Case be had to his having been a Convict.[14]

Macquarie did not waver in his advancement of emancipists in society and believed they must be able to take their turn in a jury along with any other free man in the colony. He wrote bluntly that settlers opposed to emancipists having equal social standing 'Should Consider that they are Coming to a Convict Country' and if too delicate to associate with them, they should go where 'their Prejudices in this Respect would meet with no Opposition'.[15]

To celebrate their sixth wedding anniversary Lachlan and Elizabeth Macquarie invited friends to a dinner at Government House on 3 November. They were also celebrating the news that Elizabeth was pregnant again. The guests included Mr & Mrs Riley, Dr & Mrs Redfern, Dr Wentworth, Dr Mileham, Major Cameron and members of the Macquarie family.[16] As usual, the Macquaries ignored any social taboos about inviting emancipists.

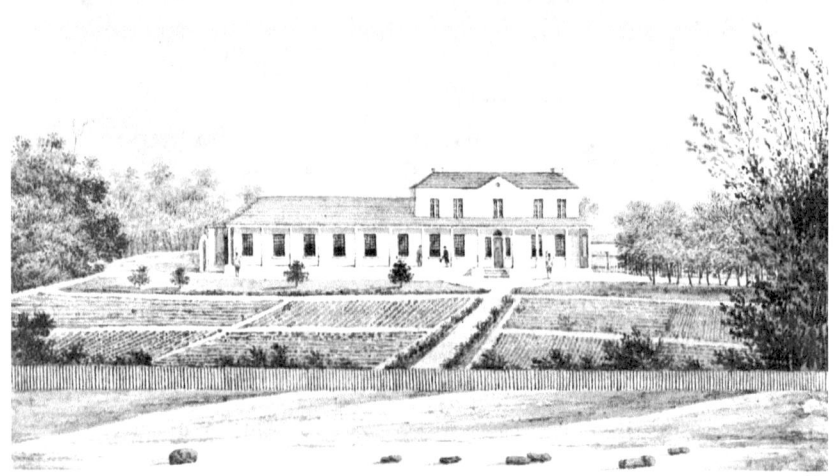

1809 watercolour of Sydney Government House. Redfern was Governor Macquarie's physician and close friend, and he frequently dined with him.

Governor Macquarie and Principal Surgeon Wentworth were considering what to do with Assistant Surgeon Luttrell. The arrival of Surgeon Henry St. John Younge in October 1813 opened up various options.[17] Initially, Younge was assigned to work at the Sydney general hospital, but his lack of training was soon apparent; instead of reducing Redfern's workload, he increased it. Wentworth now had two problem surgeons to deal with and they were too busy to train another "qualified" surgeon. It was decided that Luttrell and Younge should swap posts. On 17 December 1813 Redfern accompanied Governor Macquarie to the Parramatta hospital and offered Luttrell a position at the Sydney hospital with higher pay. Younge was then moved to the Parramatta hospital where Wentworth could closely monitor him.[18]

Younge's abilities as a government surgeon were eventually judged inadequate and Macquarie informed Bathurst in April 1814 that Mr Younge was not a 'desirable Acquisition in the Line of his Profession'. Macquarie did not mince his words and wrote that Younge was an ignorant doctor with little knowledge of medicine and 'very low and Vulgar in his Manners'. He was not suitable to fill a position of such responsibility. Macquarie asked for a more 'Minute Investigation of Medical Candidates' before they were sent to the colony and that they must be 'Certified as duly Qualified by the Army Medical Board' before appointment.[19]

William Redfern had a particular interest in preventive medicine. In 1814 he proposed sweeping reforms to the transportation of convicts after ships arrived in Sydney with major outbreaks of scurvy, typhus and dysentery. His work in health and patient care pioneered preventive medicine in Australia and Redfern is now recognised as the first 'public health' physician in Australia and honoured every year since 1994 by The Royal Australasian College of Physicians with the William Redfern Oration.[20]

On 7 February 1814 the transport *General Hewitt* entered Port Jackson with 70 men of the 46th Regiment and 266 male convicts. On board was the former naval surgeon John Harris returning as a settler and the former Corps officer John Piper, recently appointed Naval Officer and Collector of Duties, with his partner Mary Ann Sheers and their four children. The troops and ship's crew on the *General Hewitt* were healthy, but many convicts were very sick and 34 had died on the voyage.[21] Inspecting the vessel and the ship surgeon's report, Macquarie was disgusted at the health standards. Only six months earlier the report of the Select Committee had expressed satisfaction when the mortality rate aboard transports had fallen from 1 in 6 convicts in 1795-1801 to 1 in 46 thereafter.[22] The death of 1 in 11 prisoners on the *General Hewitt* had reversed these gains. Moreover, many disembarking convicts had to be hospitalised and two later died.[23]

On 14 March Macquarie instructed Wentworth, Redfern and Luttrell to hold a 'Medical Court of Enquiry' into conditions aboard the *General Hewitt*.[24] At the inquiry the ship surgeon Richard Hughes stated that on boarding the 300 convicts, 16 were 'in a state of debility' and three weeks into the voyage, ten had died of dysentery and four of typhus. The Medical Court asked Hughes why sick convicts were allowed to board so close to departure. Hughes asserted these men were not the main cause of sickness; it was due to bedding being saturated by bad weather on the passage to Rio and because convicts were not allowed sufficient exercise. He claimed that only after the bedding became wet did dysentery and typhus rage among the convicts. Redfern noted in the records:

> In Consequence of this Sickness, the Convicts were very properly allowed Access to the deck during the day for the remaining part of the Voyage. It was now, Alas! too late. No care, no exertion, however it might lessen, could now remedy the evil.[25]

The inquiry also revealed that convicts had washed and shaved only once or twice a week, six men sharing one piece of soap for a month. Proper ablutions were neglected in Rio and the convicts became 'exceedingly filthy'. Each man received only three pints (1.7 l) of water per day but no water for washing clothes. However, the inquiry concluded that the ship was regularly cleaned, fumigated and ventilated, and neither Surgeon Hughes nor Captain Earl had been intentionally negligent. Even so, the captain was criticised for offering to purchase the convict's salted meat ration, which some claimed caused scurvy, for coffee, sugar, tobacco and tea at 'most shamefully enormous prices'. This made a 700% profit for Earl when the surplus salted meat was later sold at visited ports.[26]

Late in the evening of 28 March 1814 Redfern was called urgently to Government House. Mrs Macquarie was in labour and the midwife Mrs Reynolds, who had attended all afternoon, needed the doctor's assistance. A formal dinner at Government House had just concluded when, two minutes before midnight, Redfern delivered a healthy baby boy. For Macquarie the news that mother and child were well was 'the most joyful sound I had ever heard'.[27]

Two weeks later the Macquaries were 'dreadfully alarmed' when their baby exhibited severe spasms and had difficulty in breathing. Late at night Macquarie 'immediately sent for Dr. Redfern, who administered some composing medicine to our dear Babe, and remained himself during the rest of the Night in the House, so as to be at hand when necessary'. The baby was ill for three days but recovered.[28] They had good reason to be alarmed; infant mortality then was very high, and they had already lost a baby daughter.

Because of this scare, the Macquaries decided to privately baptise their three-week old son as Lachlan Macquarie (Junior). On 18 April Reverend William Cowper held the service at Government House with Lieutenant Governor George Molle and his wife, Captain Antill, Mrs Cowper, Dr and Mrs Redfern, John Campbell and John Maclaine present. Macquarie wrote in his diary 'all of whom had previously dined with us in the Family way'.[29]

A more formal and less hurried public christening of Lachlan Jr took place on 1 May 1814 at the parish church of St Philip's. Again, Reverend Cowper performed the service and at the same ceremony, baptised the four-month old William Macquarie Molle, son of Lieutenant Governor Molle. Macquarie recorded that the friends present were Mrs Cowper, Mr & Mrs Riley, Mr & Mrs Redfern, Lieutenant Maclaine and Mr Campbell. A christening dinner followed for 23 guests, who included Dr & Mrs Redfern and Doctors Wentworth, Harris and Foster. At the dinner the 'new Christians' were toasted with 'overflowing bumpers'.[30]

Lachlan Jr was one of many babies William Redfern delivered. Of course, treating Mrs Macquarie was an official duty for Redfern but performing obstetrics for others incurred a fee of £5, except for poor patients.[31] Midwives usually attended childbirths if no complications were anticipated. However, Redfern's reputation for saving women's lives and charging only a small fee, generated a large demand for his services in the poorer parts of Sydney. It was a time when a caesarean section was a last resort to save the child – mothers usually did not survive the operation.

Although Redfern's separate private practise was successful, he found childbirths exhausting work, especially late at night. Even so he resolved to continue obstetrics until he 'had by patient industry acquired sufficient to enable me to lay the foundation of living comfortably in my old age whenever it shall arrive'.[32]

Improving the health conditions aboard convict ships was one of Redfern's greatest achievements. On 6 May 1814, the newly built transport ship *Three Bees* sailed into Sydney Cove with 210 male convicts on board. Nine convicts had died on the voyage and 55 were in 'a dreadful State' from scurvy and had to be hospitalised. Some convicts were lame and infirm from old age. Despite high morbidity among disembarking convicts, most expressed gratitude for the care of Captain John Wallis and Surgeon Thomas Andrews. An inquiry determined that prior to departure the convicts had been held for a month in an overcrowded ship in Dublin. It was here that illnesses broke out and was not detected when convicts boarded the *Three Bees* because screening by the harbour inspector was cursory. Even so, the inquiry determined that the main cause of illness on the journey was most likely due to the poor health conditions aboard the *Three Bees* during the voyage.[33]

The ship had left England at the height of the Napoleonic War and the two convict ships *Three Bees* and *Catherine* sailed in convoy under the protection of two armed frigates. Near the Cape of Verde, they encountered the French vessel *Ceres,* and after a brief battle, the *Ceres* was captured. The two convict ships continued onto Rio de Janeiro, but their cannons remained loaded in case of any further encounters. Shortly after departing Rio in February 1814, the *Three Bees* sighted a strange vessel believed to be an enemy, and convict's bedding was placed around the deck as a barricade. They evaded the ship, but the bedding was drenched by heavy waves and rain. All attempts to dry the covers failed. Although convicts were ordered not to use the bedding, many did; their clothing was just too thin for the freezing Southern Ocean weather. Scurvy and dysentery then became virulent below decks.

Redfern reported after the inquiry 'that the want of warm Clothing had a very considerable Share in the production of the inveterate degree of Scurvy, under which the Convicts in the *Three Bees* laboured, will require but little proof'. He also 'regretted that sufficient attention was not paid to the personal cleanliness of the Convicts on board the *Three Bees*, as those, who were landed ill of Scurvy before their Clothing was changed, were extremely dirty both in person and dress'.[34] Even so Macquarie told Bathurst that the circumstances by which convicts embarked 'in a diseased or feeble State' showed that inspectors must pay more attention to convict's health and treat them 'as Humanity demands'.[35]

The *Three Bees* saga did not end there. The ship was anchored at the government's wharf, not far from Government House, and was preparing to depart. At 4.30 pm on 21 May 1814 a fire broke out in the forward hold. That was dangerous in itself, but the ship had not unloaded its 14 cannons since the French encounter, and there were 30 kegs of gunpowder on board. These were expected to ignite, so the crew abandoned ship after cutting cables to set the *Three Bees* adrift.[36] The ship drifted just offshore from the Sydney hospital and orders were given to evacuate the wards. As a naval surgeon Redfern knew that if the gunpowder exploded it would destroy most of the wooden buildings in the cove and set off major fires, but he refused to desert the hospital or his patients.

As news of the floating firebomb spread, so did the panic. Residents fled into the country, Sarah was sent to their farm for safety and the Macquaries evacuated Government House. With the burning *Three Bees* drifting with the tides in Sydney Cove, other ships in Port Jackson weighed anchor and sailed out to sea. The first cannon exploded within two hours and was followed by the others, sending cannon balls whizzing into the streets near the harbour. Miraculously, no one was injured. The burning ship became snagged on rocks at Bennelong Point just as the fire reached the gunpowder kegs. Fortunately, most were now wet and failed to ignite; the fire quickly burnt the vessel to the waterline and the *Three Bees* sank the next morning. Its wreck was never salvaged and remains on the harbour floor beneath the modern and majestic Sydney Opera House.[37]

Just a month after the *Three Bees* drama there was another more sinister threat to Sydney residents. On 28 July 1814 the convict transport *Surry* limped into the harbour ravaged by disease. Of the 200 convicts on board, 36 died, along with the ship's captain, the first and second mates, the surgeon and four soldiers of the 46th Regiment guarding the convicts. Two days before reaching Port Jackson, the *Surry* almost foundered when the dangerously ill crew lost control. Fortunately, the transport *Broxbournebury*, also en route to Sydney, saw the distress flag on the *Surry* and a seaman, Samuel Nash, boarded the ship and took over the navigation.[38] The *Broxbournebury*, with 118 healthy female convicts on board, followed the *Surry* into Port Jackson.

The *Broxbournebury* carried Sir John Jamison who had come to the colony for his inheritance after the death of his father Surgeon Thomas Jamison, one of Redfern's examiners. Also, on the ship was the first Supreme Court Judge of the colony, Jeffery Bent, the older brother of the Judge Advocate, Ellis Bent. Jeffery was a proud man who expected to receive a welcome appropriate to the high rank he placed on his office. When Macquarie did not appear, he refused to disembark without an appropriate welcoming party. Macquarie eventually ordered a thirteen-gun salute and his Aide-de-Camp Lieutenant Maclaine received Jeffery Bent at the wharf.[39]

The convicts' health on the *Broxbournebury* was in stark contrast to that on the *Surry*, which was promptly quarantined. Wentworth, Redfern and Luttrell boarded the *Surry* on 30 July 1814 and found the prevalent sickness was ship fever (*typhus*).[40] Concerned that the fever would spread to the colony, Macquarie ordered all possible precautions to prevent transmission. On the advice of Wentworth and Redfern, all persons on the *Surry* were confined to the ship until the infection had subsided. No one, other than 'Medical Quarantine Officers and their Attendances', was allowed to contact those on board.[41]

Australia's first onshore quarantine camp was established on the north shore of the harbour opposite Dawes Point (today in the vicinity of Jeffreys Street, Kirribilli), with tents erected for the sick.[42] Wentworth and Redfern treated all infected sailors, soldiers and convicts sent to the camp. Those without symptoms remained on the *Surry* to be monitored.[43] Redfern told Macquarie on 18 September 1814 that 'Every plan was adopted and carried into effect, that had a tendency to cut short the progress of contagion. The Measures adopted proved so effectual, that but one Case of infection took place after the sick were landed'.[44]

In a later account of the *Surry* outbreak, Redfern reported that the first case of typhus occurred two weeks into the voyage and a week later the first convict died. Although the ship was routinely cleaned and fumigated, no attempt was made to ventilate the convict quarters. Redfern also criticised the inadequacy of the surgeon's journal:

> The Surgeon, altho' his journal is very uninteresting, containing no remarks of importance, or indicating much thought, seems to have paid All the Attention in his power to cleansing and fumigating the Prison up to the 2d of June, when his journal ceases. … neither his representations nor his efforts met with that Attention or Assistance from the Captain and his Officers, which it was their duty to have afforded him.[45]

The captain's log on the *Surry* was no better. Redfern noted that 'Nothing worthy of Notice' was recorded, not even the increase in deaths. *Surry* convicts had not lacked warm clothing, but 'from the wretchedly dirty and squalid appearance of their persons and dress' they were 'strangers to wholesome ablution'. Although there was enough soap on board, convicts received little for washing. When Redfern ordered all sick convicts be washed before entering the quarantine camp, the *Surry* purser claimed all soap on board had been used. A few days later a *Surry* crewmember offered five boxes of soap for sale in Sydney. A search of the ship found many more stacked away. 'This fact speaks for itself', Redfern censured.[46]

The danger of infecting the colony had eased by 13 August 1814 and the *Surry* was released from quarantine. However, typhus had not been eradicated in the quarantine camp and restrictions remained in force for another two weeks.[47] Macquarie later told Bathurst that 'these Unfortunate people recovered under the humane and Skilful Attention of those Gentlemen', referring to

Wentworth and Redfern. An inquiry into the *Surry* episode concluded that the outbreak of the disease had to a greater degree originated from the neglect of the master and surgeon.[48]

Recent illnesses on convict transports heightened concern among civic officials that the promulgated health regulations were not being adequately followed in England or at sea. In September 1814, Macquarie, Wentworth and Redfern reviewed the 'calamitous' state of health on the *General Hewitt*, *Three Bees* and *Surry*. Redfern had more knowledge of shipboard illnesses than Wentworth and had suffered firsthand from putrid conditions in English prisons, hulks and transport ships. He was asked to examine the most probable causes of these diseases and advise on the preventive measures needed to avert such incidences in future. Redfern sent a detailed report to Macquarie on 30 September 1814 that demonstrated the breadth of his experience as a physician and administrator. The document reviewed the health deficiencies on each transport ship. Redfern concluded that established regulations were being ignored or neglected, detailing their failure under the headings: *Clothing, Diet, Air* and *Medical Assistance*.[49]

Under *Clothing*, Redfern stressed that clothes were not just a body covering, but a means of personal cleanliness that had to suit the season and weather conditions. An extra blanket was needed to allow convicts to remove clothes at night 'since by confining the effluvia arising from the human body constantly about it, thus rendering it more virulent, it tends directly to supply the most effectual means of generating and diffusing Contagion'.[50] Redfern deemed personal cleanliness and ventilation essential. This often meant that extra water was needed for washing their body and clothing, as was an adequate supply of soap.

Diet was Redfern's next heading. He considered standard food rations to be adequate provided they were fully served. The substitution of convict's salted meat rations with anything but flour, suet or plums deserved the 'most serious reprehension'. The provision of wine to combat scurvy should be increased from two gallons per person per voyage to six gallons. The daily wine issue of a ¼ pint (0.142 l) per person would provide 'most beneficial consequences' and help 'maintain the Vigor of the System, Counteract debility arising from bad weather, confinement below, and despondency'. Wine should be diluted with water and a small amount of lime juice and sugar added. Like soap, salted meat and wine should not be withheld from convict's rations to gain profit.

Redfern's next addressed the topic of *Air*, the 'great Pabulum of Life'. He wrote that inattention to airflow in convict cells greatly contributed to ill health and mortality; poor air circulation and lack of exercise on the three transports was a major cause of convict illness. He advised: increasing convict access to upper decks; use of windsails; better bedding; routine fumigation and cleanliness below decks. Redfern pointed out that female convict ships rarely suffered contagious illnesses because women were not seen as a safety risk and were given freer access to upper decks and better air circulation in lower decks. Redfern concluded that 'On this principle, and on this alone, is the absence of Contagion to be Accounted for'.[51]

Redfern's final advice was under the heading *Medical Assistance*. He claimed most surgeons on convict ships were untrained. Men appointed to these posts are 'either Students from the lecture room, or men, who had failed in the respective lines of their profession'. If in the first category, they were 'ill qualified to take charge of the health of two or three hundred men about to undertake a long Voyage'. If in the second, 'the cause or Consequence of their failure, they totally devote themselves to inebriety'.[52] A serious deficiency was that surgeons were employed by shipowners and hence were overruled by the ships' captains who with few exceptions had 'little claim to education, refined feeling, or even common decency, generally treat their Surgeons as they do their Apprentices and men with rudeness and brutality'. These remarks reflected Redfern's own experiences as a surgeon's mate under Captain Parr on HMS *Standard*. He added that captains 'avail themselves of every opportunity to insult and Mortify their Surgeons', who then neglect their duty and 'the poor Convicts become the unhappy Victims of the Captain's brutality and the Surgeon's Weakness, want of Skill or drunkenness'.[53]

Redfern concluded his review of health problems aboard the *General Hewitt*, *Three Bees* and *Surry* by recommending that the British government only appoint 'Skilful and Approved Medical Men' with experience as a ship's surgeon, who were independent of the captain or shipowner. Aboard a convict transport this person should act as a medical doctor and a government official.

It was almost certainly true that, at that time, no one except William Redfern had the experience or knowledge to make such detailed medical recommendations on improving convict health. Both Governor Macquarie and D'Arcy Wentworth fully endorsed his report. On 1 October 1814 Macquarie forwarded Redfern's report to the Commissioners of the Transport Board in London and to the Colonial Secretary Lord Bathurst.[54] The British government adopted most of the recommendations. In June 1815 the naval surgeon Joseph Arnold was the first to sail on a convict transport in the capacity of a ship surgeon and an agent of transportation. This person, later called surgeon-superintendent, was not part of the ship's crew but an independent government agent, just as Redfern had proposed. The surgeon-superintendent had overriding powers in all matters relating to the health and welfare of convicts. This new system significantly reduced the mortality rate on convict transports sailing to New South Wales.

In early October 1814 Macquarie received instructions from Bathurst to reduce the costs of his administration. The families of civil officers would no longer receive free concessions, such as food rations, assigned convict servants or firewood.[55] This caused a flurry of complaints from civil and medical officers because these allowances formed a significant part of their salary. Macquarie wrote to Bathurst requesting that families of assistant chaplains, assistant surgeons, deputy surveyors and civil officers with salaries below £300, could receive government rations again.[56]

The medical officers Wentworth, Mileham, Redfern, Luttrell and Younge wrote a separate letter to Bathurst requesting that the service conditions of surgeons in the colony be improved. The style and content of the letter suggests that Redfern was the main author. The medicos pointed out that the provision of food, firewood and servants to their families had been stopped while those for army and commissariat officers had not. In fact, army surgeons, who had no patients beyond their stations, were assigned a horse while civil government surgeons with patients all over the country had no horses and often received no fee for their work. To perform these remote duties civil surgeons had to maintain a horse from an income that was inferior to other civil officers in the colony. This meant that a novice commissariat clerk writing official letters earned more than a qualified doctor with years of training who was saving the lives of the sick around the clock. Lastly, the letter pleaded that surgeon's wives be eligible for a widow's pension, similar to that for army widows.[57]

Over and above his arduous medical duties, Redfern had become more and more involved in farming his properties in Sydney and Campbellfield. The November 1814 muster (census) shows that he employed on his farms eleven assigned convicts, ten male and one female. Nine of the men came from Ireland. One convict received government rations while the others were clothed and fed by Redfern. A month earlier he had made a contract to supply the Sydney government food store with 4000 lb of meat (1814 kg).[58]

It is difficult to ascertain if Redfern's interest in farming was at Sarah's urging or if there had been a recent shift in his interests. The year 1814 had been a tough and exhausting one, and Redfern may well have needed a respite from medical matters. Certainly, Bathurst's cut in allowances and a surgeon salary incommensurate with his responsibilities would have annoyed him. Additionally, the persistent sniping by elites in the colony that emancipists were getting "too big for their boots" may have started to annoy him. It was not that William and Sarah were penurious – far from it, they were now among the wealthiest residents of Sydney. It was more likely that Redfern was frustrated at the lack of appreciation shown for the long hours he put into medicine, and, in particular, that he had not been assured he would be the Principal Surgeon after Wentworth retired. Redfern was not known for his stoicism, and it is possible he seriously considered quitting medicine and becoming a farmer. He could then spend more time with Sarah – after three years of marriage they still had no children, something they both wanted.

Redfern's mood would not have been helped by Luttrell's work at the hospital. Instead of reducing his patient load Redfern often needed to fix problems Luttrell had created. The work of both the surgeons, Edward Luttrell and Henry Younge, was disappointing. Redfern could still rely on the help of Wentworth and his assistant James Sheers but the performance of his latest apprentice, the 14-year-old Henry Cowper, was not promising and he would soon be in trouble. Cowper was the son of Reverend William Cowper who had for some time tried to find Henry a position that would make him a 'respectable Member of Society'. Because of a 'sincere friendship' with Cowper, who had married him and Sarah, Redfern agreed to give the boy a medical apprenticeship over four years, without a fee and without being bonded under an indenture.[59]

Tragedy struck the hospital on 8 November 1814 with the sudden death of Redfern's senior apprentice James Sheers. *The Sydney Gazette* recorded:

> DIED. - On Tuesday morning last, much lamented, Mr. JAMES SHEERS, Assistant in the General Hospital, aged 21. – He was a young man of an amiable disposition, with attainments that would have reflected honour to a more advanced age, and promised to have rendered him ornamental to his profession, and of general service to Society.[60]

The cause of death is unknown but, as Redfern knew well, treating contagious diseases with no known cure was usually futile and often personally dangerous. Not being able to prevent a young promising surgeon from dying was a distressing reality check for Redfern. It is likely to have rekindled his long-cherished ambition of learning the latest medical treatments in Britain and studying medicine at the University of Edinburgh.

Lachlan Macquarie was also going through a difficult period. His pursuit of gaining social acceptance for emancipists was now being strongly challenged by Judge Advocate Ellis Bent. Initially Bent cooperated with the government and in 1812 Macquarie built him a house with public and private offices to serve as a temporary courthouse. A major fundraising effort to build a new courthouse was launched, to which Redfern donated £21 and Wentworth £40, but the project failed because of lack of interest.[61] After that, the 31-year-old Judge Advocate became uncooperative and, in 1814 he had a major fight with Macquarie over allowing emancipist lawyers to practice in his court. Bent eventually permitted three qualified emancipists to practise in the Court of Civil Jurisdiction but only if attorneys without a criminal past were unavailable.

In July 1814 Ellis Bent's 33-year-old brother Jeffery arrived in the colony to be Supreme Court Judge. The two Bent brothers now often criticised Macquarie's efforts and supported Reverend Marsden's objection to emancipist advancement. Jeffery Bent also demanded a private house and a new courthouse. Macquarie offered him parts of the new hospital building as a courthouse, but the Bents insisted that the entire north wing of the hospital become their domain. Part of this wing was intended as the residence of the principal surgeon and the south wing had been earmarked for two hospital assistant surgeons.

The egotistical Jeffery Bent maintained that the principal surgeon should have no objections to this change, considering the much greater importance of the justice system to medical health.[62] By December 1814, six months after his arrival, Jeffery Bent was still refusing to open the Supreme Court until it was housed in a building befitting his status.[63] He also goaded his brother Ellis into refusing reforms to the port regulations controlling the flow of goods and people.

Chapter 12

MOUNTAIN CROSSING

I have taken the liberty to name ... the fine Valley ... "Redfern Valley".
Surveyor George Evans, 23 May 1815[1]

The medical supplies kept at the Sydney general hospital were a critical resource for the colony and had to be secured against theft. William Redfern, who was in charge of the medical dispensary, had cautioned his apprentice Henry Cowper about 'bad characters' in the hospital who might try to gain access to these supplies in his absence. If anything went missing from the dispensary, Redfern had to be informed immediately. Despite repeated warnings, Cowper fraternised with disreputable 'Underlings about the Hospital' and material was stolen. Only Redfern's concern for Reverend Cowper's reputation prevented him from dismissing Henry early in his apprenticeship. One of Henry's undesirable associates was the son of surgeon Edward Luttrell. This 'idle, profligate boy' had on one occasion enticed Henry to remove 'sulphur & nitre' from the store so he could make gunpowder. On discovering this, Redfern forbid his apprentice any further contact with the young Luttrell. This deeply offended Surgeon Luttrell and hampered Redfern's administration of the hospital staff.[2]

On 15 February 1815, Governor Macquarie reinstated food rations for the families of surgeons and other civil officers, but only for eighteen months.[3] Shortly after this announcement William Redfern resigned from the hospital. The precise reasons for this action are unknown, but on 18 February he wrote to Wentworth 'I have to beg you will have the goodness to tender my resignation to His Excellency The Governor, soliciting his acceptance of the same'.[4] Redfern told his friend that he was 'fully determined' on this course of action for numerous reasons, which he did not state. It was widely believed, however, that he was unhappy with staffing at the hospital and particularly with the recent behaviour of Surgeon Luttrell. Redfern had also expressed indignation at the proposed alterations to accommodation plans for the new hospital. Jeffery Bent's insistence that the north wing be a courthouse left no suitable accommodation for the assistant surgeons and he and Sarah were not about to remain in the old hospital because a pompous judge wanted new rooms! More importantly, if Bent's courthouse did occupy half of the new hospital building, then the space for wards would be inadequate. The recent decision to restore surgeon's families to the victualling list for only eighteen months may have been simply the last straw!

Macquarie contacted Wentworth about Redfern's resignation letter, and they agreed that the colony's best doctor must be kept on the hospital staff. They convened a meeting with Redfern and listened to his reasons for resigning. Macquarie made it clear that he had no intention of changing the new hospital building to place a courthouse in the north wing just because a petulant judge wanted it. They addressed Redfern's other concerns and convinced him that they were trying to fix them and, importantly, they stressed how indispensable he was to medicine in the colony. Redfern withdrew his resignation but made it clear that being a farmer was an increasingly attractive alternative to being a surgeon.

By March 1815 several rooms in the new building suitable as a temporary court were finished ahead of the hospital's opening. Even so, Jeffery Bent refused to open the Supreme Court on the grounds that an attorney due from England had not arrived and William Moore was the only free attorney in the colony. Macquarie requested the court convene with just one solicitor, but the judge refused even though his brother Ellis had allowed qualified emancipists serve in the lower court until free attorneys were available. Macquarie was furious and insisted the Supreme Court convene in May with the two emancipist attorneys, Edward Eagar and George Crossley.[5] Jeffery Bent reluctantly complied and agreed to open the Supreme Court on 1 May. Crossley had been a London solicitor for 24 years before being transported for seven years for forging a will. In the colony he had advised Governor Bligh in the John Macarthur convict escape trial, for which the rebels had sent him to the mines at Coal River for seven years. Edward Eagar was an Irish lawyer sentenced to transportation for life for forging a bill. After receiving an absolute pardon in 1813, he became a very successful law agent and attorney in Sydney.

When Macquarie met with Redfern to discuss his resignation letter, he invited him to join a touring party in April that planned to cross the Blue Mountains. Until recently, these mountains had been impenetrable to Europeans despite numerous attempts to traverse them. Sheer cliffs, deep gorges, dense forests and fast flowing rivers had thwarted early attempts but on 11 May 1813 Gregory Blaxland, William Wentworth (D'Arcy's 22-year-old son), Lieutenant William Lawson, a local guide and four convict servants succeeded by following the ridges rather than the river valleys.[6] In November 1813 Macquarie had surveyor George Evans follow the same route and survey a way for wagons to access the hinterland. William Cox was then contracted to build a thoroughfare suitable for carriages and stock along the surveyed route. In July 1814 the construction of a 101-mile (162 km) road across the mountains was undertaken with 30 convicts who were promised pardons after its completion. The Blue Mountain Road was completed on 14 Jan 1815 in only 27 weeks without any loss of life or serious accidents.

Macquarie was keen to examine both the road and the lush pastures reported beyond the mountains. His touring party would set out in April 1815 and take four weeks to cross the mountains and return. Macquarie could have used military surgeons to accompany this expedition but preferred Dr Redfern's company and medical support – quite possibly he also intended this trip to give William a break from the hospital and some time to reassess his medical future. D'Arcy Wentworth had already agreed to care for William's hospital patients and, as Elizabeth Macquarie would also join the tour, young Lachlan was to be minded by his nurse, under the watchful eye of Sarah Redfern.

On 25 April 1815 Major Henry Antill and William Redfern made the two-hour ride to Parramatta. Here, they had breakfast with the Macquaries who had arrived by carriage accompanied by Lieutenant John Watts, the new Aide-de-Camp. Several days earlier five baggage wagons with clothing, provisions and camping gear had been sent with a small team of horses to cross the Nepean River and wait at Emu Ford. Redfern's cart contained enough medical supplies to handle most emergencies for a month.[7]

At 1 pm, the tour group left Parramatta destined for Mrs Philip Gidley King's Farm on the South Creek, where Deputy Surveyor General James Meehan, the road builder William Cox and the manager of King's farm, Roland Hassall, were waiting for them.

They had dinner there and stayed overnight. Early next morning they left for the Nepean River and were met by Sir John Jamison, Secretary John Campbell, Surveyor John Oxley, painter John Lewin along with 40 servants and soldiers. The carriages and horses were driven over the Nepean River while senior tour members crossed by boat. They then assembled and proceeded in order of rank as an impressive procession of carriages, officials, servants, soldiers, carts, horses and cattle. At 3 pm they reached an area suitable for encampment near a spring of fresh water in an extensive forest of large stringy and iron bark trees. Dinner was laid out in the open and the touring party enjoyed their first meal in the mountains. Before Macquarie left the camp the next morning, he named the place 'Spring-Wood', a name still retained today by the second largest town in the Blue Mountains.[8]

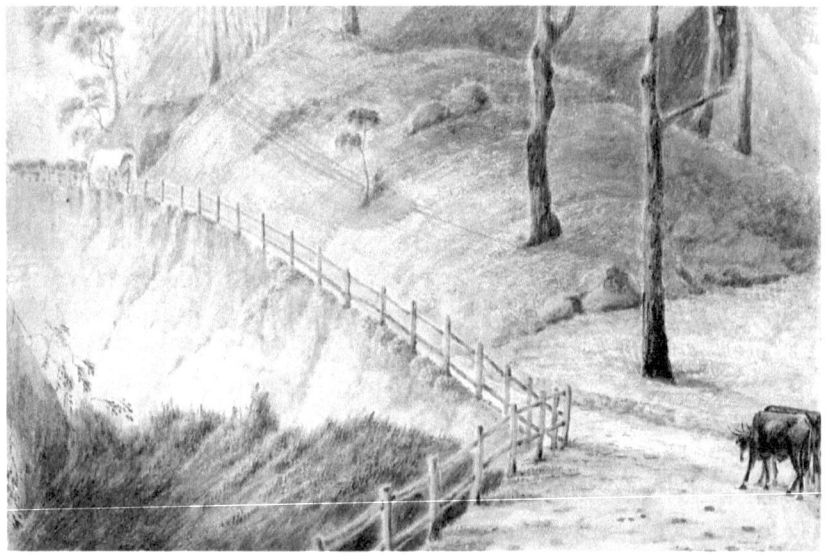

1815 watercolour of the track taken by Governor Macquarie's touring group to cross the Blue Mountains. Artist John Lewin was a member of the group.

On 27 April the touring party continued along the road recently constructed over stony terrain and up steep hills that were difficult for the carts and carriages to negotiate. They eventually arrived at an extensive plateau that offered a picturesque view of the deep valleys and forests below. Because of the 'majestic grandeur' of the area, Macquarie named it 'The King's Table-Land'. The main party reached the next campsite at 5 pm but it took another three hours before all of the baggage carts struggled up the rugged terrain.[9]

After two difficult days negotiating Cox's newly built track, they had traversed most of the Blue Mountains and faced 'a very abrupt descent almost perpendicular' to the countryside beyond. They stopped briefly to view a 'frightful tremendous Pass' and saw that the landscape below appeared to be suitable for fine grazing. The construction of the mile long pass had required a huge effort by Cox and his men, but it was far too steep and dangerous for the carriages and carts to be driven down by horses. With great difficulty these conveyances were brought down 'by fixing drag-ropes behind and holding on with the people'. During this ordeal Redfern would have hovered near his cart of medical supplies and been worried about injuries. After three hours of hard work, the carriages, people and animals safely traversed the pass. Macquarie was most impressed by the 'incredible labour and perseverance' William Cox and his men had undertaken to hack a road into the face of the mountain. In his honour he named it Cox's Pass for 'a most difficult and most arduous undertaking, and one which most people would have abandoned in despair as being impracticable'.[10] Today a large part of Cox's Road is encompassed in the modern Great Western Highway.

The touring party finally entered into a valley of open forest and good pasture and camped for two days by a river that Macquarie named Cox's River. On 1 May 1815, after crossing other hills and waterways, the tour group reached Fish River where a military post had been established during the road construction. Here, John Jamison went fishing and got lost in the woods for some hours. Gunshots were fired and eventually an exhausted Sir John found his way back to camp. The tour next crossed vast grasslands of fertile soil before reaching Bathurst Plains where surveyor George Evans was waiting for them. The route was now easier for carts and on 4 May the touring group arrived at the Grand Depot, a military outpost on the Macquarie River, and for three days they explored the area.[11]

On 7 May 1815, shortly after breakfast, Macquarie assembled everyone in front of his large tent with the British flag flying. After the soldiers saluted and fired three volleys, Macquarie declared the site for a new town, named Bathurst, in honour of the Colonial Secretary. On the same day Macquarie wrote in his diary 'Dr. Redfern having lost his two Caravan Horses, which had strayed away some days before, I had to furnish him with two of the Government Horses to carry Home his Caravan from Bathurst'.[12] Carriage horses cost between £10 and £40, so they were worth retrieving. Weeks later John Lee and several other men caught Redfern's horses and were rewarded £10 from the police fund.[13]

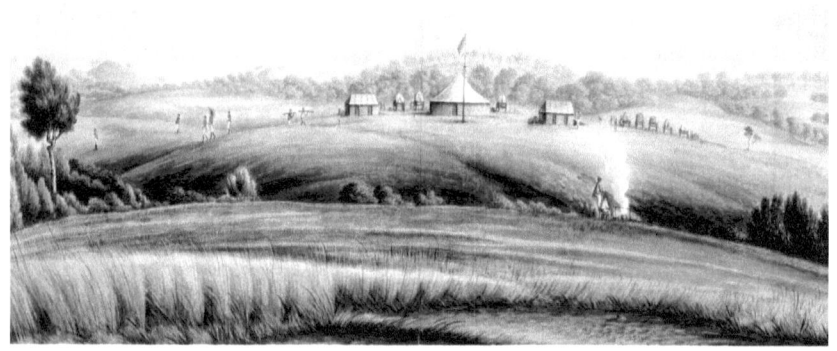

1815 watercolour by John Lewin of Governor Macquarie's camp on the Bathurst Plains after the touring group crossed the Blue Mountains.

Before departing on 11 May, Macquarie met with the soldiers remaining at the depot. They gave three loud cheers to the governor with such enthusiasm that many of the horses assembled for the departing party bolted with their carts. Mounted officers quickly retrieved them, but two carts rolled over and one broke a shaft. After they were repaired the tour finally departed.[14] Surveyor James Meehan remained at Bathurst to appraise land suitable for cultivation and George Evans set off to explore the region 200 km further west. A week later, Evans named various prominent hills he encountered Antill's Peak, Mount Lachlan, Mount Macquarie, Mount Molle and a 'Redfern Valley' along Coombing Creek. The name for this valley was unfortunately never registered.[15]

A day after leaving Bathurst Plains, a courier brought a letter from Sarah Redfern to Mrs Macquarie about her son Lachlan. Macquarie diarised that it gave 'us most pleasing and highly gratifying accounts of our beloved darling son's state of health and general improvement'.[16] On 15 May 1815 the tour group reached

Cox's Pass again and climbed slowly up the mountain. Three days later they had crossed the Nepean River where Jamison, Oxley, Cox and Campbell departed to their respective properties.

Henry Antill later wrote in his diary 'I cannot help mentioning with satisfaction, the unanimity and good understanding which subsisted between every individual composing our small society! Not a word of ill humour passed the whole time; on the contrary everyone appeared to use his endeavour to make the time pass as pleasantly as possible'.[17] Early in the morning on 19 May the Macquarie touring group set off for Parramatta en route to Sydney. At Parramatta Elizabeth Macquarie received a third letter from Sarah Redfern saying their son was in perfect health. On their arrival back in Sydney on 20 May 1815, they reunited with Lachlan Jr and everything was 'entirely to our satisfaction'.[18] In all respects, the mountain crossing had been a great success.

Returning to Sydney, Redfern immediately contacted Wentworth to check on the latest hospital news and the condition of his patients. He was no doubt pleased to hear that Edward Luttrell had been moved back to Parramatta. The Hobart surgeon Matthew Bowden had died, and Macquarie made assistant surgeon William Hopley his replacement. Henry Younge, who was due in Hobart in July, would be his assistant.[19]

William and Sarah spent as much time as possible at their Campbellfield farm at Airds. On Sunday 4 June 1815 they were returning to Sydney in a single-horse chaise when a serious accident threatened William's life. The chaise reins broke and their 'naturally fiery and spirited' horse galloped off at a ferocious pace with the chaise behind. Redfern tried to calm the horse, but when the chaise hit a tree stump, it was smashed to pieces and the two were thrown out. Sarah escaped unharmed but William was knocked unconscious. Alerted by the noise, servants ran to the crash and carried Redfern back to the house 'to all appearance past the hope of recovery'. Initial efforts to make him conscious failed but after 90 minutes he spoke, though it 'was a long time before he had any other than a confused recollection of objects'.

Sarah had a servant ride to Sydney and inform Macquarie of the accident. He immediately sent Wentworth in his carriage to Airds accompanied by Thomas Foster, the chief surgeon of the 46th Regiment. They reached Airds at 10 pm and found Redfern being treated by the Liverpool surgeon Charles Throsby, who 'had flown as soon as the information reached him'. The doctors concluded that 'As the head had received the chief injury, and no fracture could be discovered, the symptoms that ensued seemed to indicate a concussion of the brain'. The following day the patient was returned to Sydney in Macquarie's carriage and within a few days Redfern was back working at the hospital. *The Sydney Gazette* reported 'we are now happy to add, all dangerous symptoms have disappeared, and the health of Mr. Redfern mends daily'.[20]

Governor Macquarie found on his return from the Blue Mountain crossing that his legal officers were in a complete quandary. During the Supreme Court hearings from 5 to 11 May 1815, Justice Jeffery Bent had denied emancipist lawyers the right to address the court as attorneys. Bent maintained that he would not allow the court 'to be disgraced by the Practice of such Men. If they attempted it, he would Severely punish them'. Following bitter exchanges with the two magistrates William Broughton and Alexander Riley, the Justice refused to assemble the court until he had received instructions from England.[21] His behaviour and insulting attitude to emancipist lawyers outraged the magistrates. Broughton called it 'repugnant to the Benevolent principles' upon which the colony was founded. These gave 'a greater regard for the reformation of the People than the Punishment of the Criminal' and were supported by the British Select Committee.[22]

Macquarie was incensed at Jeffery Bent's conduct. Not only had he acted against his instructions, but his two best magistrates now wanted to resign. Although Broughton and Riley had asked to be replaced, they strongly advocated the judicial recognition of other emancipist lawyers. Jeffery Bent reacted by closing the Supreme Court and, to support his elder brother, Ellis Bent shut down the lower courts. When asked by Macquarie why all court proceeding had ceased, Jeffery Bent replied in five pages of utter rudeness that it was none of his business, as it was not his duty to report to the governor.[23] On 2 June 1815 Macquarie informed Bent his tone was 'highly disrespectful and offensive' and that he would have no further correspondence with him until his conduct improved. He would inform the Colonial Secretary Bathurst of his impropriety.[24]

On 18 June 1815 the convict transport *Northampton* arrived with

100 healthy female convicts on board. Only four women had died during the voyage. The first ever surgeon-superintendent on a convict ship, naval surgeon Joseph Arnold, had overseen conditions on the ship. Redfern would have been pleased that his recommendations had been acted on and were successful. He had previously met Arnold in 1810 when he came to Sydney as assistant surgeon on HMS *Hindostan*. Shortly after disembarking Arnold met with the Governor, who received him coolly. Arnold expected to have his lodging paid for and his passage back to England arranged but since there were no instructions from the Transport Board to do so, Arnold was told that Macquarie was currently preoccupied with public dispatches.[25] Indeed, at the time Arnold sought his attention, the governor was trying to have the courts opened and was writing to Bathurst about the intransigent Bent brothers. In any case, Macquarie had not forgotten that the 33-year-old Arnold had on an earlier visit made sneering remarks about emancipists being admitted to his 'shabby table'.[26] Macquarie would deal with this rude young surgeon when he had more time, but he first had to prevent the erosion of his administration and courts by prominent members of Sydney society.

A day later, Joseph Arnold called on William Redfern to deliver surplus medicine and instruments from the ship to the hospital as required by regulation. Arnold recorded in his diary: 'Mr. Redfern who is Surgeon General here, a little man who is a convict for life on account of the mutiny at the Nore'.[27] The 'little man' tag was a sneer at Redfern's "emancipist status" in society, not his physical height. It was typical of Arnold's scorn for anyone he considered socially inferior.

Joseph Arnold sought the company of establishment figures in Sydney society such as Sir John Jamison and the Bent brothers. He also paid his respects to Captain John Piper, Surveyor John Oxley, Lieutenant Governor Molle and officers of the 46th Regiment. Friends of the governor such as Captain Antill of the 73rd Regiment, refused to meet Arnold and Secretary John Campbell scarcely gave him notice. However, the socially conscience Sir Jamison even suggested Arnold set up a medical practise in the colony and, if Macquarie did not give him support, that he go back to England and return as an appointed surgeon.[28]

William Redfern was less interested in the class issues. Recently he had avoided making enemies in high places and was even willing to tolerate the company of men with anti-emancipist views. He was now the preferred physician of Ellis Bent and he certainly wanted to maintain good relations with Joseph Arnold. Redfern needed to demonstrate to surgeon-superintendent Arnold, and therefore to the Transport Board, his superior knowledge as a physician and surgeon as this might have a bearing on his future appointment as the principal surgeon. It was also important for him to hear how his reforms had worked on the *Northampton* voyage and Arnold may be able to update him on medical developments in Britain.

Recent events in the colony had accelerated William Redfern's determination to go to England to see his family and, if possible, to study the latest medical treatments in Edinburgh. In 1810 he had applied for leave but it had been declined by Macquarie. His desire for leave became even stronger after learning that his brother Thomas had died in October 1814 aged 51. They had always been close, and Thomas had helped him during the mutiny trial and imprisonment. Redfern had mourned his elder brother's death for months and most likely discussed this with Lachlan Macquarie when exploring the possibility of a leave of absence.

Joseph Arnold may have voiced his wish to avoid social contact with William Redfern, but he could not do so professionally. On 26 June, Redfern met with Arnold to discuss the health regulations on transports. He knew Arnold had gained a surgeon's diploma in Edinburgh and told him that 'he was going home with the Governor & that he was going to Edinburgh for Graduation'. Arnold later diarised that 'Mr. Redfern, principal surgeon in the place for abilities, paid me much court'. He added that Redfern apparently disliked private practice but made £2000 a year from it, even though he had been 'a partner with Parker in the Mutiny at the Nore; & was transported for life but has been emancipated'.[29]

The belief that as a naval surgeon, Redfern had cooperated with Richard Parker, President of Delegates during the 1797 mutiny, was rumoured widely in the colony and it distressed him greatly. Redfern had strongly refuted the charge at his mutiny trial and continued to do so all his life. Predictably, Arnold also sniped 'Mr. Wentworth, Surgeon General is principal magistrate, and was sent out on account of some highway robberies'.[30]

On 13 July Joseph Arnold departed on the *Indefatigable*. His diary entries on life in the colony reflect the opinions of the men he kept company with during his visit. He wrote of disillusionment with Macquarie's leadership and labelled the state of society in Sydney as 'very preposterous'. He noted that 'The Governor admits convicts to his table, & the officers of the 46th do not. The Governor appoints convicts to the highest offices; and seems to despise those persons who hold respectable situations not of his appointment'. He wrote, 'I myself was rather ashamed of being a guest at Mr. Redfern's table, although he is rich and a great friend of the Governor'.[31] In effect Arnold inferred that Macquarie never gave the "better members of society" the attention they deserved, himself included, and ex-convicts were favoured for appointment to the highest administrative offices. He made no mention that these men were fully pardoned and highly educated. Arnold was also astounded that Macquarie had made the emancipists Wentworth, Lord and Thompson magistrates, and wanted emancipist attorneys to serve in law court proceedings.

Arnold's diary entries also echo the views of the Bent brothers in observing that the new hospital resembles a 'magnificent villa' rather than a medical facility. Arnold censured the plan for the north wing to be a residence for the principal surgeon, whereas the Supreme Court had only two rooms as offices, and the south wing was for the residences of two assistant surgeons who could not decently furnish it for under £2000. He could not understand that an assistant surgeon, who could 'scarcely afford more than two chairs & a table', would do with 'large magnificent apartments'.[32] This insult was directed at Redfern, who Arnold knew made £2000 a year from his private practise. His diary is full of fatuous comments on the inferiority of Sydney and its residents – oddly, this was the settlement he desired to become a member of.

William Redfern certainly would not have relished the return of Joseph Arnold to Sydney as a government surgeon, for several reasons. First, he loathed the pomposity of the man and knew that his presence at the hospital would disrupt his established medical routine. And second, because of the obscure ranking of government surgeons Arnold might be placed above him as the next principal surgeon. Governor Macquarie detested Arnold and shared Redfern's concerns about his return as a government surgeon. On 30 June 1815 in a letter to the Colonial Office Macquarie verified that William Redfern had been made assistant surgeon in the civil medical establishment on 20 February 1810. He attached an extract of the dispatch from the Earl of Liverpool, Colonial Office Secretary, dated 26 July 1811, stating that 'Mr. Redfern will succeed to the Situation of Assistant Surgeon vacated by Mr. Wentworth'.[33] In a separate letter Macquarie informed Bathurst that he had lost patience with the concerted opposition to his policies by some government appointees, and offered his resignation. 'It now becomes absolutely necessary for the good of the Colony', he told Bathurst, that either the 'Messieurs Bent, or I, should be removed from it'.[34] Macquarie knew it would take at least a year before he received an answer, but he made clear that, unless his emancipist policies were adopted, he would go. Macquarie emphasised in his letter that he remained confident his policies were beneficial to the growth and prosperity of the colony and that this would eventually become self-evident to all.

The majority of patients in the Sydney hospital were convicts. Most were petty felons who had stolen in Britain to stay alive, but a few were more serious thieves who continued this practice in the colony. For this reason the windows of the hospital were bolted at night to prevent convicts from robbing nearby businesses. Even so, some managed to escape wards undetected and stealing from the dispensary became frequent. For this reason, Redfern kept the keys to the medical supplies, and only when he visited patients in remote districts was apprentice Henry Cowper given permission to issue the medicine and materials required in the hospital.

On one occasion Redfern returned from a midwifery case earlier than expected and found the dispenser John Tawell and the clerk James Frost leaving the store clutching bundles of towels and bed linen. When confronted, the men confessed they had received the items from Henry Cowper. Redfern immediately reported the matter to Principal Surgeon Wentworth. Convict Tawell was sentenced to labour at the Coal River and ex-convict Frost, who had worked at the hospital for six years, was dismissed.[35] To avoid disgracing his father, the Reverend Cowper, Henry was only reprimanded. This concession would have irritated Redfern, but he had no choice because Macquarie badly needed Reverend Cowper's ecclesiastical support to counter Samuel Marsden who was routinely lambasting him from the pulpit. Cowper's support might have been jeopardised if his son was incarcerated – justice sometimes had to be modified to meet political necessities.

Surgeon Edward Luttrell remained a persistent irritant to D'Arcy Wentworth. After Luttrell returned to the Parramatta hospital, the principal surgeon was inundated with complaints about his negligence and poor conduct. In August 1815 Wentworth instructed him to either take the medical post in remote Castlereagh or return to duties in Sydney. Luttrell protested to Macquarie but was told to obey orders or retire to his farm on a small pension.[36] Shortly after Surgeon Hopley died in Hobart and Luttrell was sent to replace him.[37] Complaints from Hobart soon followed, and in 1818 Luttrell was retired on half pay.

The colony was about to learn of one of the most dramatic voyages in the history of transportation. On 7 August 1815 the transport *Francis and Eliza* sailed into Port Jackson with 52 male and 65 female Irish convicts on board. This ship and the transport *Canada* had departed in convoy from Cork on 5 December 1814 but were separated in a storm near Madeira off the coast of Morocco. Defenceless, the small *Francis and Eliza* was captured by an American privateer, the *Warrior*, carrying 160 men and 22 guns. The Americans stole anything of value on the ship, including the property of Captain Harrison and that of Surgeon-superintendent Major West, who lost £1000 in cash and a chest full of medicine and surgical instruments. None of the passengers, who included the long-awaited free solicitor Frederick Garling, were robbed.[38]

Once the *Francis and Eliza* had been plundered of all its guns, ammunition, alcohol and valuable items, several of the crew agreed to join the Americans and they released the imprisoned convicts from their irons. After the *Warrior* sailed away, some of the remaining crew on the *Francis and Eliza* ignored Captain's orders and raided the rum supply. Wild behaviour reigned on board for hours before one of the more bizarre episodes in maritime history occurred. When several drunken crewmembers started to attack the female convicts the male convicts defended them and took control of the ship. Directed by the Captain, the convicts assumed all crew duties and set the sails. In Teneriffe the *Francis and Eliza* was again joined by the *Canada* and they made the rest of the long journey without incident. Despite the loss of his medicine chest, Surgeon West had dutifully cared for the convicts and only two males and four females died.[39] Solicitor Garling and Surgeon West reported that the Irish convicts had acted impeccably and because of their exceptional behaviour requested that they be pardoned.[40] Macquarie referred this to the Colonial Office, and a year later an unprecedented mass pardon was proclaimed for the *Francis and Eliza* transportees.

On 5 September 1815 William Redfern acquired a new staff member at his hospital. The surgeon-superintendent Major West on the *Francis and Eliza* had arrived with a recommendation from Bathurst to be an assistant surgeon in Van Diemen's Land. Since Henry Younge already filled this post, Macquarie appointed Surgeon West to work with Redfern at the Sydney hospital.[41]

For a long time Judge Advocate Ellis Bent had suffered from 'Dropsy in the Chest' (fluid on the lungs) but more recently his health had seriously deteriorated. Wentworth and Redfern treated him but could do nothing to stem the illness. As a last resort, it was proposed that the salt air of a sea voyage may help and in October 1815 Ellis Bent requested leave to sail for England.[42] Macquarie gladly approved the leave but refused his brother Jeffery Bent's offer to be the temporary Judge Advocate. Instead, that post went to the newly arrived attorney Frederick Garling.[43] On 11 November 1815, Ellis Bent died in Sydney aged 32.[44]

Jeffery Bent continued to block the opening of the Supreme Court and in early 1816 Macquarie announced that the new Judge Advocate Frederick Garling would occupy the two courtrooms in the new hospital building and that Jeffery Bent would soon leave the colony.[45]

Chapter 13

BANK DIRECTOR

The election of Directors by ballot was then proceeded on, and eleven Gentlemen being put in nomination by different Subscribers, lots were cast for the order in which they should be ballotted for, and the following seven were declared duly elected: D'Arcy Wentworth, Esq; John Harris, Esq; Robert Jenkins, Esq; Thomas Wylde, Esq; Alexander Riley, Esq; William Redfern, Esq; and John Thomas Campbell, Esq.

The Sydney Gazette, 8 Feb 1817[1]

Five years after laying the foundation stone for the new hospital on Macquarie Street, the spectacular two-storey brick and stone edifice neared completion. Overlooking Sydney Cove, the three separate wings of the hospital, each level surrounded by lofty colonnaded verandas, were an imposing addition to the townscape. However, the beauty of the building belied its difficult birth. Bankruptcy had threatened builders on more than one occasion and forced Macquarie to modify the signed contract by increasing the spirit importation limit from 45,000 to 60,000 gallons. Despite this and other concessions, the build was plagued by frequent interruptions arising from contract disagreements and a shortage of skilled tradesmen and suitable materials.

During these five years, the old hospital on George Street faced repeated demands for increased services, ward space and staff. In particular more surgeons were desperately needed and when William Bland applied to join their ranks in January 1816, Macquarie requested surgeons Redfern, Wentworth and West to form a medical board to examine his 'Medical and Surgical Knowledge and fitness for the situation of an Assistant Surgeon' and whether he was suitably qualified to hold a government post.[2] Bland had been a naval surgeon in Bombay and was sentenced to seven years transportation after killing someone in a duel. On arrival in Sydney in 1814 he was assigned to the Castle Hill lunatic asylum to care for inmates. Bland received a conditional pardon in October 1815 and moved to Sydney to start a private practice. He now wanted to be an assistant surgeon in government service but lacked any proof of his qualifications. The panel decided he could be appointed to a vacant post in Port Dalrymple if he passed a medical examination. Redfern was the first surgeon in the colony to be so examined, but Bland flatly refused, declaring he was already a naval surgeon and probably better qualified than the examiners.[3] That immediately closed his application, and he continued private practice in Sydney.

The "musical chair" approach to medical appointments in the colony persisted. Assistant Surgeon Major West was made head of the Parramatta hospital and this further short-staffed the old Sydney hospital. The new hospital building was not yet open, but the Governor decided to celebrate the birthday of Queen Charlotte there with a gala ball on the evening of 18 January 1816. The walls of the unoccupied wards were gaily decorated with floral arrangements and the floor painted with a scene of Wellington's victory over Napoleon at Waterloo. The ball was preceded by an elegant supper for 250 ladies and gentlemen. William and Sarah Redfern were there in their fineries and would have enjoyed every minute of it. A week later funds were raised for the widows and orphans of soldiers killed in the wars against France and William Redfern donated ten guineas (£10 10s).[4]

On 3 March 1816 contractors notified Macquarie that the new hospital was finished. The officials responsible for signing off the construction criticised aspects of the build and refused to approve final payments. The central block was 2 ft (61 cm) lower than planned and the front verandas did not extend to a large flight of steps in the middle of the hospital. It took another year to fix the reported problems. It was then revealed that the hospital building contract, with its liberal alcohol trading rights, had proved a tax bonanza for the government through increased receipts of alcohol duties. Conversely, the builders grumbled that the deal had sent them broke and financiers Alexander Riley and Garnham Blaxcell became political opponents of the Governor. D'Arcy Wentworth, who was also a contractor, continued to support Macquarie.[5]

The central block of the three-winged building, measuring 131 x 28 ft (40 x 8.5 m), contained the hospital wards. Each of the five wards on the two floors accommodated 20 patients. At least, that was the original plan. In the completed building the northern end of each floor was closed off for a courtroom and offices. The north wing remained Principal Surgeon Wentworth's quarters and the south wing was accommodation for the Assistant Surgeon Redfern and other staff.⁶ Remarkably, the original south and north wings remain intact today and are among the oldest public buildings in Australia. The wing William and Sarah Redfern lived is now 'The Mint' museum, with the same layout as 200 years ago.

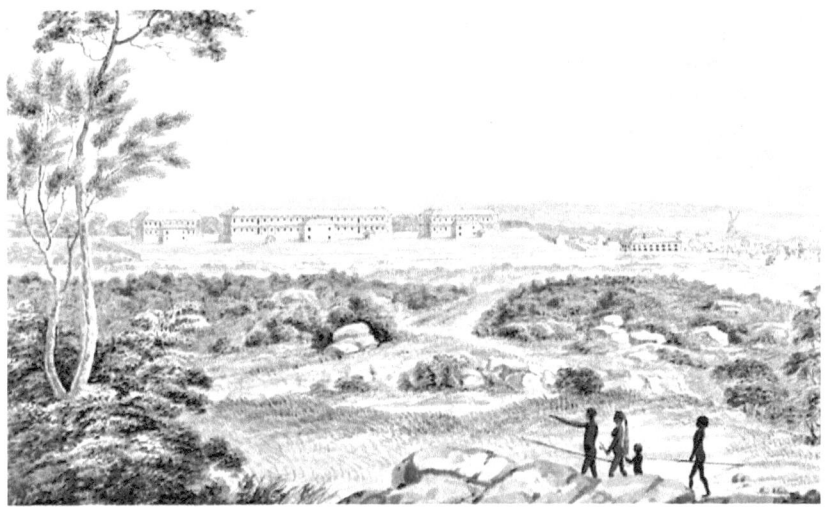

1818 watercolour of the new hospital looking west from Darlinghurst. The Redferns lived in the left wing and D'Arcy Wentworth in the right wing.

In late March 1816, just prior to the new hospital accepting patients in early April, William and Sarah Redfern took up residence in the south wing. D'Arcy Wentworth had already settled into the north wing. William Wentworth, D'Arcy's son, who had returned from schooling in England in 1810, was now a 23-year-old Provost Marshall. As a dashing young blade in Sydney, he rode in major horse races and had crossed the Blue Mountains in 1813 with Blaxland and Lawson. Although William was granted land for his part in the crossing, he had a grander ambition than being a farmer. He wanted to study law in England.

The youthful William Wentworth was an ardent defender of Macquarie's rehabilitation policies. In particular, he railed against the officers of the 46th Regiment who were openly hostile to emancipists holding official government posts. Lieutenant Colonel George Molle, Commandant of the 46th Regiment and also Lieutenant Governor of the colony, had declared that regimental officers would never admit emancipists into their company.[7] These men were often contemptuous of the governor's decisions and did not hesitate to openly mock him.[8] Unconcerned, Macquarie continued his policy of advancing emancipists he considered the most capable in the colony, no matter their social status or rank. In fact, criticism of these appointments from the elite and the military appeared to strengthen his resolve to promote social equity.

William Wentworth was disgusted at the constant vilification of the governor, and of D'Arcy and Dr Redfern. There would have been frequent discussions at dinners with his father and Redfern about the discrimination shown by officers and Exclusives. The indignation of Redfern on such occasions probably fuelled the young man's sense of injustice. On 6 March 1816 a pamphlet containing a 'pipe' (satirical verse) about Lieutenant Governor George Molle was sent to the military barracks and the hospital. The witty verse of 195 lines made fun of the Lieutenant Governor, ridiculing his hypocrisy and disloyalty to Governor Macquarie.

Molle was livid and particularly upset because he attributed the pipe to a fellow officer. He promptly offered £200 reward for the author's identity. Although Macquarie may have privately enjoyed the verse about his second-in-command, he expressed official outrage and offered to pardon any convict revealing the author's name.[9] Molle's anger raised public curiosity and the pipe was widely circulated but the author was never identified, and Lieutenant Governor Molle remained un-mollified!

On 25 March 1816 William Wentworth sailed for England to start a law degree at Middle Temple London. Although he never openly claimed authorship of the pipe, his father and Redfern suspected it and requested he confide in them. On reaching Cape Town in August 1816 William wrote to his father confessing it was his hand.[10] In the meantime, the lampooning of Molle had only served to harden the military's attitude towards Macquarie's emancipist policies, and officers of the 46th Regiment henceforth declined all invitations to Government House.

On 8 April 1816 the patients and medical stores were transferred from the general hospital on George Street to the new hospital on Macquarie Street. The patients were accommodated in three wards at the south end of the central building – two wards on the ground floor for male patients and one on the upper floor for females.

Extra beds had to be added to the wards for the 80 patients admitted and the hospital quickly exceeded its capacity.[11] Ten days later the hospital building on George Street was sold by auction. William Redfern and surveyor James Meehan bought most of the bricks, windows, doors, roofing and timber to renovate buildings on their farms.[12] Two weeks later the old hospital site was levelled.

Redfern enjoyed working in the new hospital wards but soon became aware of major deficiencies – there were no washrooms, storerooms, toilets or a morgue.[13] Also, the hospital failed to provide the better food and clothing promised to patients. Government rations were often not suitable for the sick and Redfern asked if the improved food aboard convict ships could also be served at hospitals, and he recommended the changes needed.[14] More immediate building alterations were also required. The walls enclosing the hospital were too low and convict patients scaled them at night to commit robberies. Macquarie agreed to raise the wall by 2 ft and top it with broken glass.[15] Thereafter thieving attributable to convict patients ceased.

Redfern's inspection of incoming ships continued. He was the first to board and inspect convict ships and was responsible for returning unused medicines to the hospital.[16] There were other maritime-related duties as well. When the Indian merchant ship *Lady Elliot* arrived on 23 June 1816, it gave a traditional cannon salute to the harbour battery. During one salvo a gun barrel exploded burning two sailors and seriously injuring another. One man was transferred to the hospital where Redfern removed three of his fingers and later amputated an arm.[17] The captain of the *Lady Elliot* was charged £30 for the sailor's treatment.[18]

By August 1816 Governor Macquarie had become exasperated at not hearing from Britain about his resignation letter. Surgeons Wentworth, Redfern and Foster were at the time treating the Governor for severe bowel pains. On 1 September Macquarie was totally incapacitated despite receiving 'every medicine and Surgical application they thought most likely to remove' his pain.[19] By 8 September Macquarie had recovered and that same day he granted Redfern 70 acres of land on the Botany Bay Road in Sydney, immediately adjacent to the 30 acres Sarah had received as a dowry from her parents.[20]

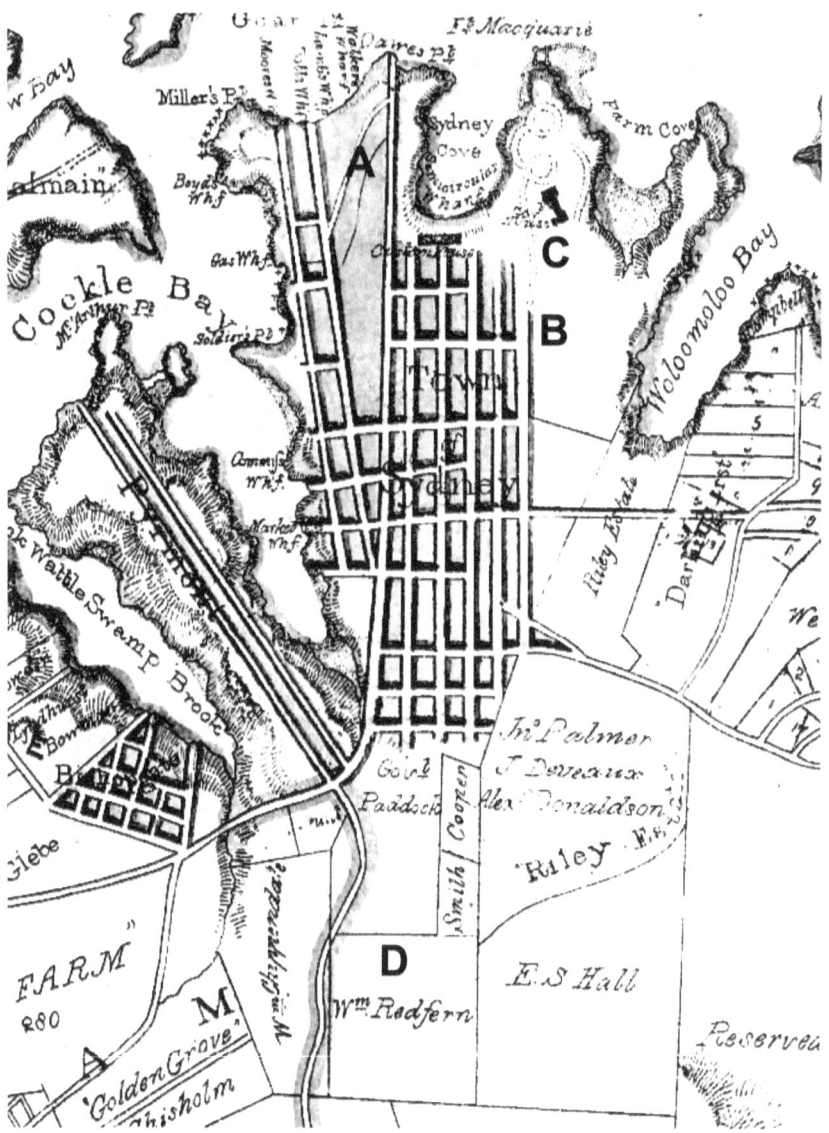

1840 map showing the Sydney Hospital (A) on George St., the new Hospital (B) on Macquarie St., Government House (C), Redfern's 100-acre farm (D).

Much of Governor Macquarie's time was taken up with the impressive building projects he had initiated across the colony. In central Macquarie Place he erected a large obelisk as the zero-point milestone for all roads leading to Sydney – it remains there today. Another of his surviving edifices is the barracks constructed at Hyde Park in 1817-19 to house up to 600 new convict arrivals.

The incidence of petty crimes had risen in England when soldiers discharged after the Napoleonic Wars could not find jobs. Despite a steady increase in convicts arriving in the colony Macquarie was optimistic about the future and maintained Sydney would one day 'be as fine and Opulent a Town' as any in the British Empire.[21]

On 5 October 1816 the transport *Elizabeth* docked with 153 healthy male convicts and the new Judge Advocate John Wylde on board. It also brought an official dispatch dismissing the Bent brothers from office and appointing Barron Field to replace Jeffery Bent as Supreme Court Judge.[22] Macquarie would certainly have celebrated that news with his close confidants. In the four months before Barron Field reached Sydney, Jeffery Bent had ignored his earlier dismissal and proclaimed the Supreme Court could now open because the arrival of Frederick Garling meant there were now enough "free" solicitors in the colony. Macquarie scoffed at the audacity of the fellow and issued an edict that, by order of His Majesty, Bent no longer had any authority. This prohibited him from practising law or from opening the court. Jeffery Bent would never forgive Lachlan Macquarie for enforcing the dismissal edict and, on returning to England, he denigrated the governor wherever possible in parliamentary circles.

In November 1816 the new Judge Advocate John Wylde told Macquarie of the financial chaos left by his predecessor Ellis Bent who had failed to apply Sterling currency regulations. The ensuing widespread use of promissory notes had swamped the courts with payment disputes, and this gave further impetus to Macquarie's ambition to establish a colonial bank. At Judge Advocate Wylde's urging, he met with magistrates, merchants and businessman on 22 November 1816 to discuss the establishment of *The Bank of New South Wales*. They agreed that a subscription bank should be created with a capital of £20,000, divided into £100 shares, each giving a shareholder a vote at bank meetings. After Wylde assured Macquarie of his legal powers as Governor, he approved the establishment of the first bank in Australia.[23]

By early December 1816, 104 shares for the new Bank of New South Wales were purchased. William Redfern bought two and the emancipist attorney Edward Eagar bought ten, believing it would secure him a bank directorship. A committee of 14 members was appointed to prepare regulations for the bank governance. It included George Molle, John Campbell, D'Arcy Wentworth, Simeon Lord and Edward Eagar.[24]

The first general meeting of the Bank of New South Wales was scheduled for 7 February 1817. Prior to this, committee members discussed whether ex-convicts would be allowed to own shares or become a bank director. Macquarie stressed that emancipists, who were among the wealthiest men in the colony, must be allowed to become bank directors. When the election of directors was called for, Redfern nominated Edward Eagar, a wealthy convict lawyer who had been *conditionally* pardoned. Whereupon four of the six nominated as directors declared they would withdraw if Eagar was elected. In the ensuing debate Redfern and Wentworth defended Eagar's right to be a director but they were outvoted.[25]

Following this debate, a rule was added to the bank charter that any person not absolutely and unconditionally free was ineligible to become a director. The members then elected John Harris, Robert Jenkins, Thomas Wylde, Alexander Riley, William Redfern, D'Arcy Wentworth as directors and John Campbell as president of the board. Macquarie was displeased with Eagar's exclusion and immediately gave him a full pardon. However, he accepted the election result and approved the printing of the first Australian bank notes with denominations 2s 6d, 5s, 10s, £1 and £5. The Bank of New South Wales opened on 8 April 1817 in the premises of emancipist Mary Reibey in Macquarie Place.[26] The first depositor was Sergeant Jeremiah Murphy of the 46th Regiment with £50, the second John Harris with £138 1s 4d, and the third William Redfern with £51 15s 7d.[27]

Macquarie's vision that Sydney would one day be as grand as any town in the British Empire came to fruition in 1817. Farming, trading and shipping in the colony flourished and new elegant buildings lining the streets gave Sydney an aura of prosperity. Paradoxically, Lachlan Macquarie, who was largely responsible for the growth that had occurred over his seven-year tenure, was routinely shunned by the Sydney elite because he appointed emancipists to official posts. Of the 155 guests invited to a dinner and ball at Government House to celebrate Queen Charlotte's birthday on 18 January 1817, 40 invitations were declined.[28]

Three months later, the Macquaries held a birthday party for their 3-year-old son. The celebrations began in the harbour with the launch of a small cutter given to Lachlan Jr as a birthday present. Captain Watts, Captain Gill, William and Ann Cowper, William and Sarah Redfern, and Sarah's 15-year-old sister Eliza Wills participated in this harbour occasion. They rowed around Garden Island with the little cutter in tow and breakfasted afterwards at Government House. Later 33 guests, including the Redferns and Eliza Wills, attended an evening birthday dinner party held for young Lachlan.[29]

Exclusives and emancipists in Sydney rarely, if ever, mixed socially but they regularly met on matters of civic and commercial importance. The Philanthropic Society, founded in January 1814, elected William Redfern to a committee of thirteen members headed by Reverend Marsden, who put aside his rigid policy of not associating with ex-convicts when it suited him. Redfern held a similar post at the Native Institution, which had been founded to care and educate Aboriginal children. In March 1817, he joined a large group of solicitors, chaplains, and civil and military officers to establish a Bible Society, responsible for reading the good book to poor children on Sundays. A year later he became a committee member and medical consultant for the Benevolent Society.[30] All of these charitable organisations were founded to assist the underprivileged in Sydney; people who Redfern encountered every day in his medical practice. He believed strongly in rehabilitation through education and was an active participant and generous contributor to many charitable institutions.

By 1817 the Macquarie Street hospital was a year old and surgeon Redfern's duties had expanded with the rising number of convicts landing in the colony. Previously about 1000 convicts a year came to Sydney but in 1817 over 2000 convicts landed, and by 1818 their number rose to 3350.[31] The medical needs of Sydney's civil population of 6700 were the responsibility of the general hospital and the two private practices run by William Redfern and William Bland. The seriously ill in rural areas were also brought to Sydney for treatment. Many were too poor to pay for private treatment and the Sydney general hospital was their last hope.

The increased demands on hospital services forced Redfern and Wentworth to trial different treatments and faster patient releases. These changes required additional funding and finding this money was the responsibility of the principal surgeon. At Redfern's urging

Wentworth proposed upgrades to patient diets, cleanliness and clothing. Hospital meals currently comprised raw grain rather than flour with some fresh meat. Wentworth advised that fresh meat, bread and vegetables be served every day to patients.

Another constant concern for surgeons was the appalling uncleanliness of patients and their clothing, as this seriously affected a patient's ability to recover. Often the convicts wore the tattered filthy outfits they were admitted in for their entire stay. It was proposed that, on entering the hospital, each patient be allocated new clothing. Wentworth also asked that the convict staff housed at the hospital be given a salary, so as to improve the quality of helpers and the level of patient care. He argued that paying clerks, overseers and matrons would attract and retain much better qualified people. Acknowledging that these changes would be expensive, Wentworth attached a full costing and argued that the expense would be offset by faster recoveries and reduced illness.[32] Macquarie agreed with these proposals, but he needed authorisation to make such major improvements and wrote to Bathurst seeking approval of increased hospital expenditures.[33]

In the meantime, the increase in sick convicts exceeded the hospital's capacity. In April 1817 Macquarie sought Bathurst's approval to move the courtrooms out of the hospital building to allow for more wards, and to provide funds for a new courthouse.[34] Money was also needed for an additional surgeon to assist Redfern with the surge in patients. Even Wentworth had to do occasional ward duties to assist with the influx. An opportunity to find an extra surgeon arose when the *Harriet* docked in Sydney. The 25-year-old ship surgeon Robert Wainwright Owen, who had a diploma from the Royal College in London, expressed an interest in joining the hospital. On 11 May 1817 Macquarie appointed Owen as assistant surgeon on a salary of 5s per day.[35]

The 46th Regiment's anger over the "Molle pipe" had not abated a year later, and D'Arcy Wentworth's clerk Robert Murray was accused of being the author. Judge Advocate Wylde summoned Murray to appear in court with D'Arcy as a witness. On 11 June 1817 Wentworth was forced in his defence of Murray to admit that his son William wrote the pipe. Initially Molle was relieved that the author was not a fellow officer and declined to prosecute further. But he changed his mind when regimental officers openly declared that men 'so much Our Inferiors in Rank and Situation among that promiscuous Class' had penned the libel. At their urging, Molle told Macquarie the next day that D'Arcy Wentworth was responsible for his son's actions and should be court martialed. Wentworth retaliated by releasing a list of potential charges that could be laid against Molle for his misbehaviour as Lieutenant Governor. After some bitter exchanges Judge Advocate Wylde ruled that Wentworth was not liable for a court martial trial, and the issue of responsibility and punishment was quietly dropped.[36]

The accusations against Wentworth annoyed Macquarie greatly. Friction between the civil and military officers had become so toxic that on 25 July he wrote to Bathurst that George Molle and his regiment should be recalled. He also suggested the abolition of the 'inefficient and altogether useless' office of Lieutenant Governor and stressed the importance of integrating emancipated convicts into colonial society.[37] He admitted that his rehabilitation efforts had not always succeeded, but many men with 'liberal Educations' had regained their original status in society and some of 'Superior order' sat at his table. The 46th Regiment officers had, by contrast, never accepted emancipist in any capacity.[38]

Macquarie's wishes were soon granted. On 7 August 1817, 200 soldiers of the 48th Regiment commanded by Lieutenant Colonel James Erskine arrived on the transport *Matilda* to relieve the 46th. The new Lieutenant Governor Erskine was given a 13-gun salute as his regiment marched to its barracks. That evening Erskine and thirteen officers of the 48th dined at Government House, together with the Judges Wylde and Field, and Doctor Redfern.[39] In Erskine, Macquarie had found an ally with similar social attitudes. A month later George Molle and the 46th Regiment left for India.

On 30 September 1817 the convict transport *Lord Eldon* sailed into Sydney harbour with John Macarthur on board. He returned from his eight-year banishment in England for provoking the coup against Governor Bligh and was allowed to return on the condition he avoided politics. Macarthur had agreed to this but was aware of the British Parliament's objections to Macquarie's policies and would exploit this knowledge where he could. Macarthur regularly communicated with his patron, a physician to the Prince of Wales, Sir Walter Farquhar, who promoted his business interests in British parliamentary circles.[40]

Also on board the *Lord Eldon* were 215 healthy male convicts overseen by Surgeon-superintendent James Bowman.[41] During the voyage, John Macarthur had befriended Bowman after receiving a letter from his wife about the 'continued ill health and suffering' of his daughter Elizabeth.[42] The early success of Redfern's treatment of Elizabeth had faded and the family was now searching for other remedies. Macarthur hoped that Surgeon Bowman would know of a treatment that Redfern did not.

It was James Bowman's second visit as surgeon-superintendent to the colony. On his first visit a year earlier Bowman had applied for the vacant assistant surgeon position at the Derwent. When this failed, he returned to England with a recommendation from Macquarie to Bathurst that he receive a future posting.[43] Bowman now claimed that the Colonial Office promised him the assistant surgeon post in Hobart to replace Edward Luttrell. However this contradicted earlier dispatches from Bathurst saying that Luttrell should remain assistant surgeon in Hobart. Bowman had no documents to support his claim and Macquarie was unable to act without them, even though he would have liked to have Luttrell replaced. Surgeon-superintendent Bowman had to return to England again and get written support from Lord Bathurst.[44]

In October 1817 Governor Macquarie and his family visited the town of Windsor on the Hawkesbury River to oversee the annual general muster (census). The hot weather distressed three-year-old Lachlan who developed spasms in his eyes. He was taken by carriage to Parramatta, where on 15 October Wentworth and Redfern came from Sydney to see him. They recommended the boy be blistered 'in the back of his Neck to relieve the Nervous affection in his Eyes' and that he should take a laxative the next day. Redfern remained to treat the boy for the next week while Wentworth returned to Sydney. Young Lachlan soon recovered.[45]

In November 1817 sections of the old hospital grounds in George Street, 'deemed one of the most attractive in Sydney', were put up for rent or building lease. Macquarie promised to grant the land to those leaseholders that would build a house on the land within two years. One of the lots was granted to William Redfern, another to his mother-in-law, Sarah Howe. In the next few years Redfern would buy two more plots of land in the area.[46]

William Redfern was now 42 years of age. This would have

been considered a good age at that time – life expectancy in England in 1820 was 41 – but the Doctor had not slowed down. In addition to his duties at the hospital, the bank and various charitable societies, he found farming an increasingly attractive pursuit. His Campbellfield estate had increased to 2050 acres after receiving another three land grants and purchasing four neighbouring farms.[47] Additionally, Redfern leased another 1300 acres of government farmland close to his estate.[48]

William and Sarah regularly drove their chaise from the Sydney hospital to their Campbellfield farm and discussed its management with their overseer John Grant. Part of this large property had been fenced to prevent cattle from straying, but this did not prevent stealing. In October 1817 William Redfern announced in *The Sydney Gazette* that cattle and calves had been stolen from his Airds farm and offered a £50 reward for the thieves' identities. In the same newspaper issue, Redfern sought a tender for the delivery of 40,000 bricks to build a homestead at Campbellfield.[49] Several timber houses already existed on their property, but it was time to build a larger brick house. Although he was wealthy, the new farmhouse was to be a modest single-storey building, similar in design to Redfern's houses on Norfolk Island. It had an attic, a large cellar made of sandstone that was accessible from the side, a stone-flagged veranda, and a detached kitchen and stables. Today, little remains of the original farmhouse because of a fire in 2014. The rebuilt cottage in Minto now houses a childcare centre.

Not all of the Campbellfield farmland was fertile, but Redfern applied an 'improved system of English husbandry' to increase the fecundity of the land. His employees cleared the tree stumps, rotated crops and grew clover and lucerne to enhance soil quality. From 1817 to 1820, the property sold 6000 lb of fresh meat every six months to the Sydney government store.[50]

Governor Macquarie was being kept well informed of the machinations in the British Parliament about the colonial administration. He knew that Members of Parliament, mostly with a conservative political leaning, were questioning whether convict transportation was the best solution to overcrowded gaols. He was also informed that some MPs claimed his "soft treatment" of convicts and emancipists was the main reason that transportation was no longer a deterrent to criminals. Adding fuel to British concerns were the many complaint letters from the colony about the promotion of emancipists to official positions. Some MPs even claimed that shipping villains offshore was illegal and unless the criminal classes feared transportation, British prisons were cheaper and more effective. It was apparent to Macquarie that many influential politicians in Britain now viewed his governance as far too liberal and his reputation in Tory circles had been irreversibly damaged. The abrasive tone of Bathurst's recent communications to Macquarie indicated he had also lost the support of the Colonial Office. On 1 December 1817 he tendered his resignation to the Colonial Secretary for the second time.[51]

Macquarie knew that it would take a year before he could hear back from the Colonial Office. In the meantime, he had a colony to govern and to nourish.

Chapter 14

CALM BEFORE THE STORM

> *In Succession to Mr. Wentworth, as Principal Surgeon in the Medical Establishment of this Territory, I beg most respectfully to recommend Mr. Assistant Surgeon William Redfern to be appointed Principal Surgeon, as in every respect perfectly competent and well qualified for executing the Duties of that important Office, being a man of very eminent talents, an excellent Scholar, and possessing universal knowledge.*
> Macquarie to Bathurst, 15 May 1818[1]

Much to Governor Macquarie's chagrin the social acceptance of emancipists in the colony did not improve markedly with the departure of the 46th Regiment. Officers in the newly arrived 48th Regiment adopted a similar prejudicial attitude and largely refused to admit this 'obnoxious class to their society'. In late 1817 Major Henry Antill wanted William Redfern to meet officers of the 48th and invited him to their regimental mess. To his mortification, they were denied entry. Such a blatant breach of etiquette angered several of the senior regimental officers, and Lieutenant Governor Erskine, Major Morisset and Major Druitt subsequently apologised to Redfern, making sure he was invited to private dinners. They became regular guests at the Redferns' house.[2]

On 6 January 1818 Lieutenant Governor Erskine invited Dr Redfern to dine with him at the regimental mess. As soon as the two were seated, Captain William Watkins left the table declaring he would not sit next to a convict. The next day Watkins was court martialed for not respecting another officer's guest and for writing an insubordinate letter to Erskine. This incident gave rise to a new regulation for the 48th Regiment that required officers to stay at their mess table until the 'first thirds' had been drunk.[3] An altogether more harmonious occasion occurred on 19 January 1818 when William and Sarah Redfern were among the 158 guests attending the annual Queen's birthday celebration at Government House. The supper and ball lasted until 4 am the next morning with 30 couples dancing through the night.[4]

A week later, on 26 January 1818, salvos from 30 guns on Dawes Point heralded the 30th anniversary of the establishment of the colony of New South Wales by Arthur Phillip. Later in the day Governor Macquarie inspected the 48th Regiment in Hyde Park. In his address to the troops, he cautioned officers to be respectful to all residents and avoid improper remarks about government policies. Macquarie later entertained these officers at Government House with William Redfern present as the guest of Lieutenant Governor Erskine.[5] Some officers still politely refused to fraternise with Redfern, but they now appreciated that he had very powerful allies. Not everybody had official supporters in high places and the majority of emancipists continued to be isolated socially. This situation was not helped by the increasing number of free immigrants arriving in the colony. Most brought with them the prevailing British class prejudices and they largely avoided integrating with ex-convicts except in remote rural areas.

Reverend Samuel Marsden was one of Governor Macquarie's severest critics about his rehabilitation of convicts and promotion of ex-convicts. Marsden was known in the colony as the 'Flogging Parson' because of his harsh treatment of convicts; he routinely sentenced them to hundreds of lashes when he was magistrate. In 1814 Macquarie forbid magistrates giving sentences of more than 50 lashes without official permission.[6] Disputes between the two came to a head in January 1818 when Macquarie summonsed Marsden to Government House and accused him, as 'Head of a Seditious low Cabal', of conspiracy and 'malicious attempts to injure' him. Macquarie never spoke to Marsden again except on public duty and dismissed him as magistrate three months later.[7]

In February 1818 William Redfern was re-elected to the board of the Bank of New South Wales. A month later the position of cashier became vacant at the bank. The person appointed as cashier had to be someone of undisputed honesty, who would reside in the bank building and not go out after dark. Applicants required the names of 'two opulent and respectable' nominees in Sydney who would commit to a security bond of £2000 (£133,000 today). On 28 March 1818 Thomas Wills, 18, applied for the cashier position supported by his brother-in-law William Redfern and stepfather George Howe – Sarah Howe most likely shared in the bond pledge. Redfern considered Thomas honest and competent, which was essential because his reputation as a director was at stake. On 21 July 1818 Thomas Wills was appointed to be the new cashier at the Bank of New South Wales.[8]

To provide Thomas with some financial experience prior to taking up the cashier position, Redfern sent him to Hobart to recoup money owed to him by Norfolk Island settlers who had resettled in Van Diemen's Land. Four months earlier Redfern advertised in *The Hobart Town Gazette* that all persons indebted to him should settle their accounts promptly to save him 'the painful necessity of having recourse to coercive Measures for the Recovery of the same'. Thomas was only partially successful in recovering these debts and when he returned to Sydney Redfern took legal action against several of the major defaulters.[9]

The embarrassment of Henry Antill's thwarted attempt to dine with William Redfern in the 48th Regimental mess did not in any way affect their friendship. In fact, it flourished and on 9 October 1818 Sarah's sister, 16-year-old Eliza, married 39-year-old Major Antill in St Philip's Church. The witnesses to the wedding were Sarah and William Redfern, and Thomas Wills.[10]

The health of 56-year-old D'Arcy Wentworth had been declining for some time and on 5 May 1818 he tendered his resignation as Principal Surgeon to the Governor. Macquarie informed Bathurst and recommended the appointment of Assistant Surgeon William Redfern as his replacement. Macquarie stated that Redfern was 'in every respect perfectly competent and well qualified for executing the Duties of that important Office, being a man of very eminent talents, an excellent Scholar, and possessing universal knowledge'. He informed Bathurst that, although James Mileham was the most senior assistant and 'a very worthy good man, [he] is very defective in medical knowledge; he is old and very much affected in his eyesight, which render him incompetent for the active and important Duties of Principal Surgeon'. For these reasons Macquarie strongly endorsed the next senior officer, William Redfern.[11] With this support Redfern felt confident that he was to be Wentworth's successor, especially as three Colonial Secretaries, the Lords Castlereagh, Liverpool and Bathurst had personally given him that assurance. Bathurst had also indicated this succession to William's brother Thomas and the local MP for Wiltshire.[12] It would take another year before the appointment was made and both Redfern and Wentworth continued their hospital duties.

William Redfern's daily rounds visiting hospital patients had a predictable pattern. Since Robert Owen had joined the hospital in May 1817, patient duties were shared; Owen was responsible for the outpatients visiting the hospital for medication or for a certificate if unfit to work.[13] Henry Cowper had completed his apprenticeship and was now an assistant at the hospital. Redfern discouraged Cowper's association with Owen, whom he considered 'low in his habits and vulgar in his manner' and 'grossly ignorant of his Profession'.

Prior to becoming a member of the Royal College of Surgeons in London, Owen had served on a slave ship to save money for medical studies. Redfern believed that Owen knew little besides 'Chalk diagrams' and how to grind medicine powders. He considered his training of Cowper to be superior 'in point of professional skill'. Owen and Cowper had been reprimanded several times for being drunk on 'spirituous cordial medicines' and Redfern was disgusted with Owen's treatment of convicts, particularly of females and 'His & Mr. Cowper's conduct towards the Nurse & others about the Hospital is too gross & filthy for me to soil my paper'.[14]

Despite Redfern's reprimands, Cowper continued to supply 'Underlings' with filched medicine. He had given hospital store clothing to a nurse with whom he had an affair. The nurse was dismissed and Wentworth admonished Cowper repeatedly for improper conduct; each time the young man 'shed tears & promised amendment' but his behaviour did not change.[15] If he had been an assigned convict, Henry would have been sent to the coalmines, but in order to protect his father Reverend Cowper, he was always put on probation. Some assigned convict staff in the hospital were just as corrupt and neglectful in their duties. Redfern dismissed overseer William Wakeman for 'Drunkenness, Incapacity, Corruption' and 'assisting in drinking the spirituous cordial Medicines'. Ward attendant Richard Prescott was found 'robbing the dead' by taking a shirt off a body in a coffin – an act 'so disgustingly horrid' that Redfern immediately sacked him.[16]

Addressing any questionable governance issues in remote New South Wales was a low priority for the Colonial Office during the

Napoleonic Wars. This changed after the Battle of Waterloo and peace was declared in Europe. Discharged soldiers quickly led to increased unemployment and petty crimes in Britain. It was then that Members of the Parliament started to take notice of Governor Macquarie's success in transitioning the New South Wales colony into a free and prosperous settlement. Most law-abiding people in Britain expected the colony to remain a penal settlement where criminals feared to be sent. The improvements Governors King and Macquarie made to the lives of convicts and ex-convicts had eroded this deterrent – the inmates of the colony were now better fed, dressed and employed than most poor in Britain.

Macquarie's egalitarian policies were criticised in the colony as well. Free settlers coming to New South Wales expected to live in a society where the lower classes were subservient, and cheap to employ. Their views matched those of British politicians who believed it unrealistic to try and reform illiterate felons – Britain was, after all, still the most committed nation to the slave trade. Few appreciated the extent the colony had matured into a law-abiding community, and the prejudicial views espoused by a bitter Jeffery Bent in London misled MP Henry Grey Bennet to vilify the leadership of Lachlan Macquarie in the British Parliament.[17]

In April 1817 Lord Bathurst alerted Home Secretary Viscount Sidmouth of the need to re-examine whether transportation had become 'neither an object of Apprehension here nor the means of Reformation in the Settlement itself'. He questioned whether it was the governor, or the system itself, at fault. Bathurst claimed transportation had worked initially because of the perceived remoteness and harshness of the penal colony. He observed that the colony had served its purpose for many years when populated by well-supervised productive convicts. But circumstances had recently changed and if transportation was no longer a deterrent to crime it should be made so or abandoned. Bathurst requested a Parliamentary Commission of Enquiry examine the administration of the colony.[18] This was approved, and for the next two years a suitable person was sought to lead the commission. This person was to instigate changes affecting the lives of most in the colony and would degrade convict rehabilitation for the next two decades.

On 5 January 1819 Lord Bathurst appointed John Thomas Bigge as the Commissioner of Enquiry to examine the functioning of the

New South Wales colony. Bigge had just returned from the slave colony of Trinidad where he had been the Chief Justice. He was instructed to sail to Sydney and report on all aspects of the government administration. The Commission of Enquiry should provide information to reappraise the nature of the settlement and to support a future decision on whether the New South Wales colony should be a penal or free settlement. Colonial Office officials briefed the Commissioner on their concerns that Lachlan Macquarie's liberal policies had caused serious doubts on whether transportation was still a cost-effective way of punishing convicts and deterring crime. Bathurst instructed Bigge to 'constantly bear in mind that Transportation' was intended as a 'severe Punishment' that must be 'rendered an Object of real Terror to all Classes of the Community'.[19] Where punishment was too lenient the commissioner was expected to recommend the establishment of harsher penal measures.

In effect, the prejudicial instructions given to Bigge largely pre-empted the inquiry findings. They assumed that the humanitarian policies of Macquarie and his 'ill considered Compassion for Convicts' had weakened the penal system and were preventing efforts to mitigate crime. Bathurst even suggested that free residents might be separated from convicts, and new penal settlements established where felons would be grouped according to their crimes, and that serious criminals should labour under more severe conditions.[20]

Bathurst also wanted Bigge to investigate another issue, but believed he had little chance of reconciling the divergent opinions in the colony. It was 'the Propriety of admitting into Society Persons, who originally came to the Settlement as Convicts'. Bigge was told that the Prince Regent supported Governor Macquarie's belief that emancipated convicts should be treated 'upon terms of perfect equality with the free settlers'. Bathurst informed Bigge that such beliefs were opposed within the colony by those 'who hold association with Convicts under any circumstances to be a degradation'. He suggested that the possibility of 'reconciling the conflicting opinions' made it a suitable topic to investigate.[21]

John Bigge was chosen to lead this inquiry at a fractious time in British politics. The Tory government was determined to stifle the large public demonstrations against poverty and unemployment that had followed the Napoleonic wars. Mounted cavalrymen had recently charged a crowd of 80,000 in St Peter's Field Manchester listening to a reformer advocating the universal right to vote. Nine were killed and 400 wounded. The so called 'Peterloo Massacre' epitomised the Tory government's disregard for the poor. D'Arcy Wentworth's patron Lord Fitzwilliam, a Whig, was dismissed as Lord Lieutenant of Yorkshire after speaking against the cavalry action.[22] Undoubtedly the severity of the government's actions would have instilled in John Bigge the importance of returning law and order to the wayward New South Wales colony.

Six weeks after John Bigge's appointment as Commissioner, Bathurst decided on D'Arcy Wentworth's successor as principal surgeon. Based on seniority and supported by strong testimonials William Redfern should have been the automatic choice. But he was passed over and on 27 February 1819 James Bowman was appointed the next principal surgeon.[23] When William Wentworth learnt of this decision in London, he wrote to his father D'Arcy expressing 'great pain that poor Redfern' who had 'set his heart' on this position had not been chosen. William believed the decision was strongly influenced by the illiberal hue and cry raised over Governor Macquarie's advancement of emancipists, such as William Redfern, to offices of trust and dignity.[24] It would be another six months before news of the appointment of John Bigge and James Bowman reached the colony.

On New Year's Day 1819 Governor Macquarie opened a new male orphan school on George Street. The renovated building had previously been for female orphans – they had been moved to a new school in Parramatta. Lieutenant Governor Erskine, Reverend Cowper, Secretary Campbell, Brigadier Major Antill and Dr Redfern escorted the Governor to inspect the 32 boys admitted to the institution for the first time. The orphan school accommodated young boys up to the age of ten and provided them with a basic education and some industrial training.[25]

The Queen's birthday on 18 January was a public holiday and in the evening the Governor hosted the colony's major social event of the year, a lavish ball and dinner at Government House. For the 200 invited guests it was an opportunity to display 'all the beauty and grace of the Colony'.[26] The Redferns would have had a good reason to enjoy the evening; they were expecting a baby.

A day later, landholders, merchants and other inhabitants met to form a committee to petition Governor Macquarie to apply for the removal of restrictions on agriculture, trade and shipping. They also pleaded to have routine trial by jury in the courts, the right to distil spirits from grain and the repeal of duties imposed in England on colonial imports. Freemen and emancipists proposed these resolutions jointly. At the close of the proceedings Edward Hall proposed, seconded by William Redfern, to thank Macquarie for the opportunity to meet and address important matters affecting their interests. Sir John Jamison was the most socially prominent in a committee of thirteen men that included the three emancipists Simeon Lord, Edward Eagar and William Redfern. Because emancipists were members, John Macarthur called it 'Sir John Jamieson's ragtag and bobtail' committee.[27]

The petition committee met regularly and 'transacted Business with the utmost harmony and union without objection to each other or any kind of jealousy'.[28] For some in the committee the proposed petition was the forerunner of changes to the political administration of New South Wales, in which Edward Eagar would play a leading role by introducing constitutional rights into the colony. Within two months the committee had finished writing a petition that purported to represent the aspirations of a colonist population of 25,000 diverse individuals. The chairman Sir John Jamison followed by William Redfern, committee members and 1250 residents and settlers, signed the petition. Macquarie sent the petition to Lord Bathurst for consideration by the Crown, describing the signatories as 'All the Men of Wealth, Rank or Intelligence throughout the Colony'.[29]

By May 1819, D'Arcy Wentworth and Governor Macquarie had still not heard back from Bathurst regarding their retirement and resignation. Without a replacement for Robert Owen at the Sydney hospital, Redfern and Wentworth were overburdened with medical duties. The number of convict transports arriving in Sydney had steadily increased to 18 ships landing 3140 convicts, most in the last three months of 1818. After a surge in illnesses among the poor between December 1818 and March 1819, the number of hospital patients rose to 105. This necessitated extra beds and the creation of two new male wards on the upper floor of the hospital by converting the storeroom and judicial offices.[30] In March 1819

Macquarie informed Bathurst that patient demands were so high that the courtrooms could no longer remain in the hospital, and a new courthouse was essential.[31]

Since the foundation of the colony, civil officials could receive personal medical care at any locality in the colony. This meant that Redfern often travelled long distances to treat them. For this he earned accolades from Alexander Riley who told the British Select Committee on Gaols in 1818 that the colony was 'very much indebted' to Mr Redfern 'for his unwearied and skilful attention to the private families in it, however distant, it was totally out of his power to meet the many calls for his services'.[32] One such rural callout came from a Windsor doctor, Thomas Parmeter, a surgeon transported for bigamy. His patient Laurence May had a 'mere speck upon his toe' inflicted during a flood and it now threatened his life. Redfern rode to Windsor, and he and Parmeter decided May's leg had to be amputated above the knee. The patient endured the amputation with such 'a degree of fortitude' that it surprised even the doctors. Laurence May quickly recovered and continued working on his farm with one leg.[33]

During Redfern's rural absences Wentworth treated his hospital patients in addition to administrative duties. One of Wentworth's most critical tasks was the procurement of pharmaceutical supplies for all hospitals in the colony. Redfern and Cowper compounded most of the common medicines for the Sydney Hospital. When Cowper proved incapable of doing this reliably, Wentworth had Redfern make these medicines after hours at his house, but when he was away Wentworth spent hours compounding the medicines himself.[34] The preparation of these materials was strenuous work for the overburdened surgeons.

In December 1818 Principal Surgeon Wentworth received news that the Colonial Office had agreed to improve hospital food. However, approval had not been given to upgrade patient clothing or to pay the convict staff currently recompensed with meals, clothing and accommodation. Because of difficulties in sourcing fresh vegetables, meat and bread the patient diets remained unchanged until mid 1819.[35]

After eight years of marriage Sarah Redfern, 23, gave birth to a boy on 27 June 1819, to the delight of his 44-year-old father. Four days later the boy was christened William Lachlan Macquarie Redfern at a ceremony in St Philip's Church.[36] Governor Macquarie, as the godfather of William Jr, gave the Redferns two miniature paintings of himself and Elizabeth as a christening gift.[37]

But the proud father's celebrations were short lived. The day after the christening, news of the principal surgeon appointment arrived on the transport *Canada*. When Redfern boarded the ship to inspect the convicts, Surgeon-superintendent Daniel McNamara informed him that James Bowman had been appointed to replace D'Arcy Wentworth. It was a bitter blow for William Redfern who had worked so hard to earn this promotion and been promised that he was next in line for the post. Angry and humiliated Redfern left the ship and immediately went to Government House to talk to Macquarie who was also baffled by the unofficial news. The Governor tried to console Redfern, but he was deeply hurt by his rejection and expressed 'Severe Mortification and Disappointment' for not gaining the office after almost 18 years of 'Meritorious Service' as assistant surgeon.[38] He felt the decision made no sense and must have involved 'secret and unjustifiable representations' by which Bowman had 'contrived to get himself nominated' contrary to the succession protocol and in contravention of the promises made to his supporters by the Colonial Office.[39]

Redfern immediately tendered his resignation as assistant surgeon at the hospital and declared he would cease treating patients in the hospital and at his private practise as soon as Bowman took office. Macquarie fully understood his anguish and granted him permission to resign under those conditions. Asked if he could 'serve him in any other way' Redfern replied that he would become a farmer and 'would feel highly gratified at being Appointed Magistrate in the District of Airds'.[40]

Macquarie was bitterly disappointed that his commendation of Redfern for the principal surgeon post had been ignored, and that Whitehall had not responded to his own resignation letter. He was more determined than ever to return to England soon and find out what was going on. In fact, Bathurst had already replied to his resignation request, but the letter had been lost in transit from England – seagoing mail was often misdirected and delayed. In the missing letter Bathurst had praised Macquarie's administrative efforts and asked him to postpone his retirement.

This hiatus in communications meant that the governor had no knowledge of James Bowman and John Bigge's appointment, or of the reasons for the parliamentary inquiry. On 21 September 1819, five days before John Bigge's arrival, Bathurst's letter reached Sydney informing Macquarie of an inquiry into the colony's governance and Commissioner Bigge would be in charge, but there was no mention of his own resignation request.

Quite unaware of the true intent of the upcoming inquiry – to ensure that New South Wales remained a much-feared destination for criminals – Macquarie expected, perhaps naively, a favourable assessment of his leadership of the prosperous colony.

Chapter 15

THE INQUISITOR

That memorable speech, conversation, & questions, so artfully calculated to wound & insult my feelings, have made too deep an impression on My Mind ever to be forgotten. The quiver of your lip, the curl of your nose, the expression of your eye – in short, your tout ensemble, revealed to me your very thoughts & intentions, as a Mirror exhibits the person of him who stands before it. I clearly perceived your intention was to alarm and intimidate and in the event of a failure in that object, to irritate me to a breach of good manners.

Redfern to Bigge, 5 Feb 1821[1]

The transport *John Barry* docked in Sydney on 26 September 1819 carrying 142 convicts, the principal surgeon appointee James Bowman and Commissioner John Bigge. Accompanying Bigge was Thomas Scott, his secretary and brother-in-law, who was also a clergyman and bankrupt wine merchant. On the day of their arrival Governor Macquarie was visiting Windsor, 37 miles from Sydney, for the annual muster but he had instructed the officer in charge of the Dawes Point battery that if Bigge's ship should appear, to welcome it with a 13-gun salute. The next day John Bigge took a carriage to Windsor to present to the governor his commission and papers explaining the purpose of the parliamentary inquiry. These surprised Macquarie, as they appeared to give Bigge authority over aspects of his administration. Having diligently led the colony for a decade, Macquarie believed he should have authority over a parliamentary appointee.[2] Macquarie initially gave Bigge his full support but as the true intent of the inquiry became embarrassingly clear – to denigrate his administration and malign him personally – he progressively refused to cooperate.

Lachlan Macquarie and John Bigge had quite different backgrounds and held contrasting views on social equality. Macquarie's father was a cousin of the last chieftain of the Macquarie clan, but his family was relatively poor and his upbringing down to earth. His father was a carpenter and miller on the Isle of Mull where he leased a small farm from the Duke of

Argyll. Lachlan joined the army with his uncle's help but his promotion in the military had been by merit and not privilege. As a combat-hardened soldier, Macquarie valued ability and courage over rank, and he sought the advice of clever men no matter their status. This meant that convicts and emancipists saw in Macquarie a natural champion for their fight to regain freedom. Such views were in stark contrast to those of the aristocratic lawyer and judge John Bigge, who espoused the values of a class system in which social status and breeding mattered much more than competence. Bigge was about to assess colonial activities by these standards and would never appreciate that his criteria for worthiness meant very little to most people he would encounter and interview.

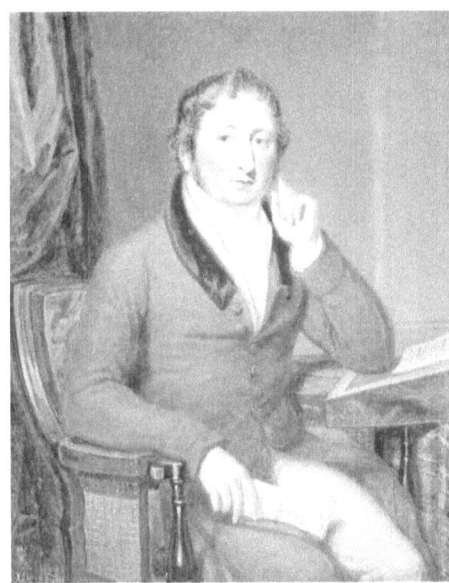

1819 portrait of the British Parliamentary Commissioner of Inquiry, John Bigge.

Shortly after disembarking from the *John Barry*, John Bigge and James Bowman were invited to dine in the 48th Regimental mess. It was later reported that Bowman, after an alcohol-fuelled dinner, declared 'that there would be no more Convict Magistrates in the Colony – the Commissioner would take care of that'. Bowman also boasted that he enjoyed Bigge's complete confidence.[3] The cosy relationship between the two had been apparent to William Wentworth in London who wrote about 'the means which he had resorted to, in order to defeat Mr. Redfern's just right and expectations' to the principal surgeon post. Bowman 'did all he could to undermine Mr. Redfern' and to influence Bigge during the voyage. Redfern's friends were disgusted when Bigge 'from the very hour of his landing in the Colony, treated Mr. Redfern with a marked superciliousness, for which no other reason is assignable'.[4]

Two days after landing James Bowman visited the hospital. When told that D'Arcy Wentworth was at the bank and William Redfern sick, he insisted that Henry Cowper show him around. This contravened the hospital regulation that no one was allowed into the wards without Wentworth or Redfern's permission. Cowper toured the wards with Bowman and answered questions on how Redfern's patients were treated. A hospital convict assistant rushed to Redfern's quarters and told him that a stranger was in the wards. Cowper was ordered to see Redfern immediately. He found him in bed exceedingly angry that Bowman had been admitted into the wards and had talked with his patients.[5] Redfern told Wentworth that Bowman's visit was a clandestine plot 'to discover something in his treatment of the sick, and general mode of management in the hospital, which Mr. Bowman might find fault with'.[6]

The next day, 29 September 1819, Redfern informed Bowman by letter that he was astonished by his visit without the incumbent principal surgeon being present, and annoyed that Bowman had questioned Cowper about his patients. Redfern asked that he be more diligent 'in his conduct' and reminded him that hospital patients were still in his care and that no other surgeon should visit them without his permission. He pointed out that in a few days Bowman would be well acquainted with the responsibilities of the principal surgeon post he had pursued with 'so gentlemanlike & honorable a cause'. Until then, he was not accountable to Bowman but hoped there would be no repeat of his intrusion.[7]

Soon after it was reported to Redfern that Bowman had said in Wentworth's presence 'that the Commissioner would completely turn his back on Mr. Redfern'. Redfern expressed disbelief that Commissioner Bigge would say such a thing.[8]

> Such assertion made in such manner impressed me with feelings of astonishment, commixed with indignation – Astonishment, that any Man would utter so unguardedly the predetermination of his friend, and with indignation that such predetermination had been formed, without the party, to whom such predetermination had been attributed, having known me, or having once seen me.[9]

A few days later, during Redfern's daily hospital rounds, several patients complained of not receiving their regular medicine. When Redfern queried his convict clerk William Johnstone on how this was possible and why the dispensary records were not up to date, he revealed that Cowper had failed to provide medications for the dispensary or to enter this into the records.[10] Johnstone was a well-educated and reliable clerk who did Redfern's paperwork so that he could concentrate on medical diagnoses and treatments. In England William Johnstone had been a skilled compositor in a London printing office before being sentenced to transportation for life, most likely for forgery. The notes of Johnstone that have survived exhibit an elegant copybook style of writing that is far more legible than either Redfern's or Macquarie's.

The disclosure of Cowper's latest dispensary antics was the last straw for Redfern, and he flew into a rage. He found Cowper and 'went so far in his anger as to box his ears'. After Redfern left the room Cowper and Owen were so enraged with Johnstone informing Redfern of their deceit, Owen beat him severely over the head with a large ruler. The commotion alerted Redfern who returned and warned Assistant Surgeon Owen that his conduct would be reported to the principal surgeon and the governor. Thereafter, William Johnstone, under constant threat from Owen and Cowper, delayed reporting other hospital misdemeanours to Dr Redfern until months later.[11]

Hoping to gain sympathy and parental support, Henry Cowper informed his father that Redfern had hit him. The pastor advised Henry to have the principal surgeon resolve the matter. On returning to the hospital Cowper reported the attack to Wentworth who told him that it was a difficult time for Redfern at the moment, and to let the matter rest.[12] Redfern later met with Henry in front of his parents and asked him whether he 'had ever manifested any anger or inflicted any chastisement upon him' except when his conduct called for it. Henry agreed that Redfern usually treated him fairly, and the matter was dropped.[13] Henry was well aware that if he pressed the assault charge further, many other instances would be revealed that were liable to criminal charges. In any case Cowper knew Redfern and Wentworth were leaving the hospital soon, and then James Bowman would be in charge.

After the ear-boxing incident Redfern put Johnstone in charge of dispensing medicines to the nurses.[14] This loss of responsibility infuriated Cowper, who 'scribbled upon and defaced' pages of the dispensary records. When Johnstone tried to stop him, Cowper threatened him, and two record books were found torn up. Owen saw the damaged records and commented, 'I don't know what will Redfern say, when he sees this'.[15] Quite unaware of Cowper's latest destructive rampage, Redfern instructed his clerk the next day to remove the hospital records to his own library. Johnstone was so worried about the state of the hospital records that he first took them to a bookbinder for repair.[16]

Commissioner Bigge was officially sworn in on 7 October 1819.[17] Three days later, Principal Surgeon James Bowman, accompanied by Wentworth and Redfern, met the hospital staff and examined the medical stores. Bowman's earlier prejudicial remarks about Redfern in the officer's mess apparently led to heated exchanges between the three men during this meeting. On 18 October William Redfern decided that he had had enough of the new hospital regime and requested Macquarie's permission to retire.

> I had every reasonable expectation from the strong recommendation of Your Excellency in my favor, from a long, laborious and I trust useful Service of Eighteen Years, and from the promise of Earl Bathurst to Viscount Castlereagh, and from His Lordship to my Brother, that I should succeed to the Vacancy occasioned by Mr. Wentworth's resignation, I cannot but feel deeply that those reasonable expectations have thus terminated in severe and mortifying disappointment, that my most sanguine hopes and best prospects in life are thus utterly blasted.[18]

Redfern requested that Macquarie forward his resignation letter to the King and to permit him to suspend duties as assistant surgeon until His Royal Highness's decision was known.[19]

On 23 October *The Sydney Gazette* announced the retirement of D'Arcy Wentworth as principal surgeon and that James Bowman would be his successor. The public were also informed of William Redfern's resignation and the Governor's sincere regret for the reasons leading to Redfern's departure from medical services to which 'he has been so great and valuable an Acquisition', praising him for 'his superior Professional Skill, steady Attention, and active zealous Performance'. With the strongest 'Sense of his superior Talents and Merits' Macquarie wished him all the best for his future 'Happiness and Prosperity'. On Principal Surgeon

Bowman's advice, the *John Barry* surgeon, Christopher Tattersall, was appointed to act as assistant surgeon at the Sydney hospital.[20]

On 24 October William Redfern visited his hospital patients for a last time – Bowman was to assume office the next day. Before departing he prepared a history of patients in his care. Redfern also provided detailed notes on the dietary system he and Wentworth strived to introduce. It stated 'I drew up the Memorial and its concomitant papers' on moving to the new hospital and that Wentworth may wish to provide Bowman with their detailed recommendations for patient clothing, the employment of better-qualified hospital workers and improved remuneration. Redfern pointed out that, because of a lack of funds, the Governor had been unable to authorise all changes to the 'dietic System and Economy of the Hospital' and had referred the matter to London for consideration. After a long delay, part of the scheme was approved, and new diets began in September.[21]

In his departing letter, Redfern also clarified the progress on improving and rebuilding of the hospital, stating that if Bowman had arrived a few weeks later this would have been implemented. To counter the criticisms Bowman had already levelled at the past hospital administration, Redfern wrote 'My conduct has been open and independent' and 'it will bear the effulgence of the noon day sun; the more it is scrutinized the more it will redound to my credit'. He ended the letter wishing Bowman, and 'the Gentlemen who may be carrying on the duty' under him, find the situation 'more conducive to your case, your comfort, and happiness than has been the case with Mr. Wentworth and myself'.[22]

This letter signalled the end of William Redfern's long and distinguished contributions to the Sydney hospital duties, and a halt to his Sydney private medical practise. The next day, William, Sarah and their little boy vacated the hospital quarters and moved to their Campbellfield farm at Airds. It is apparent that William Redfern was unsure of his future in the colony at that time and whether he and Sarah would soon return to England.

The Colonial Office officials had emphasised with Commissioner Bigge that Governor Macquarie's egalitarian policies eroded the Tory strategy of transportation being a strong deterrent to crime. The emphasis on punishing felons would have reinforced any beliefs John Bigge had nourished as chief justice in the slave colony of Trinidad, and shortly after arriving in the colony Bigge slammed Macquarie's rehabilitation efforts with a force that surprised even the Exclusives. Bigge would soon discover, however, that this veteran soldier was not about to surrender his liberal principles easily, and he had a battle on his hands.

The first direct confrontation between Macquarie and Bigge occurred when William Redfern was nominated as a magistrate. Redfern had been promised this post and on 26 October 1819, the day after Bowman replaced Wentworth, Judge Advocate Wylde was instructed to draw up Redfern's commission. Wylde advised Macquarie to 'pause' this decision because of the increasing opposition in England to appointing emancipists. But Macquarie insisted the nomination go ahead. Redfern's appointment must be treated identically to that of any free person in the colony.[23] Bigge learnt of this on 30 October at a meeting when Macquarie praised Redfern's credentials as a person and a surgeon. He also revealed, perhaps unwisely, that Redfern was being made a magistrate to compensate for not becoming the principal surgeon. Bigge protested that it had been 'striking & absurd' to make Simeon Lord a magistrate but 'placing a convicted Traitor on the Bench would be doing still greater violence to the rules of common sense & Decency'.[24] Bigge had no doubt that the British would oppose the appointment, especially after hearing that 'Mr. Redfern had become obnoxious to many Individuals in the Colony'. Here, of course, he referred to James Bowman.

Macquarie argued that Bathurst had not told him to exclude emancipists from judicial appointments and, based on his considerable experience in leading the colony, he was convinced of the right-mindedness of his approach to reform and rehabilitate convicts. Macquarie told Bigge that the view of any minister, parliament or individual would not alter his opinion and he refused to cancel Redfern's appointment, since this would bring triumph to those opposed to returning ex-convicts into society. Macquarie added that, rather than expose himself to the censure he would incur if these decisions were reversed, he would prefer Bigge take control of the government. Astonished by this level of resistance, Bigge warned him of the consequences, adding he would take no official notice of Dr Redfern outside of Government House and would not meet the doctor unless he chose to do so.[25]

Three weeks of heated letters between the two followed. On 6

November Macquarie wrote that he failed to comprehend how Bigge saw any danger or 'mischief' for the colony if Redfern, a talented man with irreproachable conduct and qualifications, was made a magistrate. Macquarie asserted that he was willing to make the personal sacrifice of bowing to the wishes of the Crown but after abandoning his authority, honour and principles he was then 'no longer worthy' of being Governor. He told Bigge that the men who the Commissioner considered 'first class' – the Exclusives – had overthrown the last government and caused the premature retirement of every other Governor. These 'factious, discontented and turbulent' men have sown 'Seeds of Discontent' in the community and only raised themselves in society through the free labour of the convicts they wished to suppress.[26]

The Governor told Bigge that he could not understand why William Redfern had been singled out for persecution; he was a man who had been 'One of the Most Loyal and Useful Subjects' to the government of this country. Macquarie confided that when he first arrived in the colony, he did not expect to interact much with convicts or emancipists. However, he quickly realised that the 'Most Capable and Most willing to Exert themselves in the Public Service, were Men who had been Convicts!' He then reminded Bigge that 90% of the colony's residents were convicts or ex-convicts and he should not be 'overwhelmed by an over Strained Delicacy, or too refined a Sense of Moral Feelings'.[27]

> Avert the Blow You appear to be too much inclined to Inflict on these unhappy Beings (if You make them so!); and let the Souls now in being as well as Millions yet unborn, bless the Day on which you landed on their Shores, and gave them (when they deserve it) what you so much admire Freedom![28]

Macquarie was astounded by the Commissioner's attitude. He had always believed that one of the most important functions of government was to rehabilitate and reform convicts, and he was appalled at Bigge's total opposition to this.

The battle lines between the two men were now entrenched. Bigge would not agree to support Redfern's appointment and was angry that Macquarie challenged his views on convicts. He would not accept that the faithful discharge of the duties of assistant surgeon should form any claim to the honours of a judicial post. Moreover, Bigge considered the crime of mutiny Redfern had been transported for to be 'the most foul and Unnatural Conspiracy that ever disgraced the Page of English History'. When asked by Macquarie why Redfern was singled out as 'the Victim of National Vengeance', Bigge replied that 'Mr. Redfern's Crime is unparalleled even amongst those of his unfortunate Brethren' and although 'his Crime may be forgiven by Englishmen, it Never Can be forgotten by them'. Bigge concluded by disclaiming all responsibility for Redfern's appointment as magistrate and protested at being forced when doing his duty to have made public contact with him.[29]

D'Arcy Wentworth and Henry Antill would have kept Redfern informed of progress on his judicial appointment. The intensity and rudeness of Bigge's opposition astonished them but they were heartened by the Governor's determination not to be 'degraded and dishonoured' by backing down on the issue.[30] Shortly before the official announcement of Redfern's appointment as magistrate appeared in *The Sydney Gazette* on 12 November, Commissioner Bigge received a notice from Governor Macquarie about his decision to appoint William Redfern as 'Justice of the Peace and Magistrate in the District of Airds and throughout the Territory of New South Wales'.[31] On the same day Macquarie wrote to Principal Surgeon James Bowman and denied him the use of a government carpenter to make alterations to the surgeon's wing, citing a shortage of labour.[32] That particular row would last for months. The Governor and his officer in charge of civil engineering, Major Druitt, were less willing to assist Bowman as they had been for Wentworth.

With the notice of Redfern's appointment in *The Sydney Gazette*, Bigge promptly wrote to Bathurst stating that Redfern's 'good education' made 'his guilt more inexcusable and his character more suspicious'. He added that it was widely believed in the colony that Redfern had 'Considerable Influence over the mind of the Governor' and was the only person with whom Macquarie 'maintained any Confidential Intercourse'. He recommended that all future emancipist candidates for official posts be blocked and disputed any inconsistency between his support of Wentworth and Lord as magistrates and his rejection of Redfern. Bigge told Bathurst that the whole system of emancipist magistrates should be quietly abandoned.[33]

Bigge's letter emphasised Macquarie's close relationship with his doctor. William Redfern was a man Lachlan Macquarie trusted and relied on – perhaps his only true confidant – and this letter revealed his determination to keep a promise to someone who had always supported him. As a military veteran, Macquarie knew the importance of allies who stuck by you in the heat of battle, and he pressed ahead with his far-reaching egalitarian policies.

News of Bigge's repeated clashes with Macquarie became common knowledge in the colony and many questioned why the inquiry interviews were being held in private without witnesses. There was particular concern that the interviewees were not sworn in and that evidence was not cross-examined. The legal obligations on those giving verbal evidence were being ignored. The inquiry procedures also provided no right of reply to charges being made by an unrepresentative group of civil officials, military officers, estate owners and merchants. These men were invited to give evidence, often repeatedly, but few settlers were interviewed.

Some of the inquiry formalities were also criticised. Why were those interviewed first asked: 'Have you any complaint to make against Governor Macquarie?'[34] This and similar questions meant that much of the evidence given and recorded verbatim was gossip, hearsay and opinions that, more often than not, reflected well known jealousies and prejudices. Because few knew details on how the colony was administered or understood the inner workings of government, responses were often useless and unlikely to identify real deficiencies in governance. They did, however, frequently criticise the governor and his supporters, and this certainly satisfied Commissioner Bigge's primary objective.

Of course, the Exclusives in the colony fully backed the inquiry processes and queued up to entertain the commissioner. John Macarthur, the bane of all colonial governors, dined regularly with Bigge and strongly berated the current administration. Macarthur was disgusted at the success of emancipists and was livid in 1810 when the successful Andrew Thompson became chief magistrate of the Hawkesbury district. Macarthur and fellow graziers espoused the view that the colony's future was in the export of wool, not in cereal crops or rehabilitating convicts. He firmly believed the cheap labour provided by convicts was much more important than Macquarie's grand building plans. Macarthur made sure that John Bigge received every comfort during his stay in the colony. He provided him with two of his best horses and a gig, and every morning sent him fresh eggs, butter, milk and mutton from

Parramatta. Bigge and his secretary Scott became regular guests for breakfast, dinner, and supper at John Macarthur and Justice Field's houses. Often James Bowman was also present. Years later the newspaper editor Edward Smith Hall remarked that Bigge was the 'creature and the spy of the faction' and 'his reports team [sic] with mis-statements'.[35]

Once Macarthur had gained the Commissioner's confidence, he asked him to recommend to the Colonial Office that the colony be made a bastion for the sheep industry and that farm productivity focus on large privately owned estates. Instead of raising such a blatantly commercial proposal with Macquarie, Bigge confined his discussions to major landholders and business leaders.

In an obvious challenge to William Redfern's medical capabilities, the inquiry delved into current hospital practices. Redfern's former apprentice, Henry Cowper, was interviewed over four days in November 1819. Cowper was queried on hospital administration, patient care, bookkeeping, the medicines prescribed, the hospital dispensary and whether Redfern removed medication or anything else from the hospital for his private patients. Cowper revealed that Redfern had assaulted him but declined to say why.[36]

Later evidence given to the inquiry by the hospital clerk William Johnstone contradicted much of what Cowper said. Johnstone was interviewed four times between December 1819 and January 1821. He had left the hospital after James Bowman instructed him to 'peaceably ... retire'.[37] Johnstone now worked for Redfern as a clerk, and in January 1820, after recommendations from Redfern and Wentworth, received an absolute pardon.[38] In the Bigge inquiry interviews, Johnstone consistently disputed the evidence given by Cowper and produced a signed affidavit denying accusations made against himself and Redfern. He told the inquiry of Cowper's false bookkeeping, theft, incorrect medication to patients and the destruction of record books. Johnstone admitted to the inquiry that, fearing punishment by Cowper and Owen, he had not always told Dr Redfern of their malpractices.[39]

At William Johnstone's fourth interview, Bigge asked Henry Cowper to be present so he could defend the accusations directly. Johnstone was told he had to countersign the record of his responses. On hearing the incredible nature of Cowper's charges, Johnstone refused to even acknowledge them, despite threats from

Bigge. He subsequently wrote to the Commissioner demanding that all charges made by Cowper be struck from the minutes as being totally 'untrue'. Cowper had accused him of making £1000 from illegal sales at a lumberyard and taking £20 from each settler he referred the fittest convict servants to. Cowper claimed that the clerk 'would hang his own father for liberty'. Johnstone said that all of Cowper's charges were utter lies, and he was ready to declare this under oath – after all, his father had been dead for 20 years.[40]

Of particular importance to Bigge was the supervision of the hospital stores. Prior to the interviews Cowper warned Johnstone he must swear under oath that he 'had knowledge of Mr. Redfern having appropriated certain Tin Ware & Spices severally to his private use'. Johnstone refused and told Bigge 'he had frequently seen Mr. Cowper take spices and convey them into his own pocket' and as these were not recorded in the dispensary logbook 'I consequently considered they were for his own private use'. Johnstone emphasised that Cowper's personal withdrawals from the store certainly did not 'occur with the approbation & by consent or knowledge by Mr. Redfern'.[41]

Johnstone informed the inquiry that Cowper had told him to 'acknowledge Mr. Redfern had used Government Medicine'. He had 'answered in the affirmative, that Mr. Redfern's dispensary was not to the Gentleman & alike [but] to the pauper in distress'. Johnstone rejected with 'high repugnance' the accusations made against Redfern, declaring that 'Morality, Christian Feelings, Veneration for the Dead, Respect to the Living & Religious Sentiments' were constantly abused by Cowper and Owen.

In a lengthy rebuttal letter to Bigge after seeing the transcripts of the interviews, William Johnstone related other malpractices of Cowper that he had seen in the hospital. In Redfern's absence he had attended the dissection of an executed man in which Cowper took out the heart and several large lumps of flesh. Cowper then enticed several hospital helpers into the theatre, threw the flesh at them and 'exposed the heart in a rough uncouth manner to the terror' of all present. But he did not stop there, Johnstone related:

> Mr Cowper cut away the Penis of from the said dead body, & conveyed into the dispensary, when he exhibited the said Penis very frequently to the Nurses on Duty, & to one particular Nurse he gave the said Penis wrapped in a sheet of paper, saying it was a present for her, who on opening it, threw it away.[42]

Johnstone also told Bigge that Robert Owen had taken an abortion foetus into the dispensary and immersed it in rum.

> Dr Owen & Mr Cowper, first consulting with each other, took the said Rum from around the said Foetus ... then gave by mutual Consent the said Rum ... to one Margaret Cuddie, a Nurse then on duty, desiring her to drink it, she took it into the ward among the patients.

Johnstone did not know if the nurse drank the rum, but he noted that no attempt was made by 'either Mr Owen or Mr Cowper to prevent her drinking it'. He repeated that he would swear on oath to the above evidence and could provide witnesses to verify these events. He added that there were other instances of depraved behaviour by Cowper and concluded sarcastically 'What a moral private Witness' you have listened to! Johnstone apologised for not coming forward sooner to inform the inquiry, but he was concerned for his personal safety and the reputation of Cowper's father. These were the reasons he had avoided telling Redfern until recently. Johnstone concluded his letter asking if Cowper should 'be considered a man on whom simple communication of "He said so & so" can be depended upon?'[43]

Despite William Johnstone's detailed and verifiable statements, Bigge decided that he much preferred Cowper's version of hospital behaviour. It better suited his need to damage Redfern's and therefore Macquarie's reputation. In fact, Bigge wrote in his 1822 *Report into the State of the Colony* that 'Mr. Henry Cowper ... whose testimony is confirmed rather than contradicted by that of a prevaricating convict, [who was] corrupted by the emancipation that he had received'.[44] In keeping with most of his report, Bigge was very selective about what he included and what he did not. As later inquiry reports reveal, Bigge totally changes his assessment of these witnesses in 1823, where he praises Johnstone and states that Cowper's evidence could not be relied on.[45]

William Redfern was now performing the duties of a Magistrate and Justice of Peace. The cases before him were mainly breaches of the peace, larcenies of a petty nature, complaints about convict servants and other minor matters. Much of his time was spent on convict administration: assignment of convict servants, convict discipline, granting of tickets of leave, administration of local and government orders and overseeing the general musters.

Since his retirement from the hospital, William Redfern had become a dedicated farmer and acquired a reputation as one of the best agriculturalists in the district. The November 1819 land and stock holding report shows his estate covered 2365 acres: 640 acres were cleared, of those 76 were in wheat, 26 in corn, 10 in oats, 10 in beans, 2½ in potatoes and 2 were garden and orchard. Redfern had 13 horses, 600 cattle, 2319 sheep and 50 pigs.[46]

Bigge's presence in Sydney was causing other problems. At the urging of the Exclusives, Bigge supported the exclusion of emancipists from a new 'Agricultural Society' being organised in the colony. Macquarie had initially agreed to be the patron of the society but when he heard of its exclusive membership he declined. Macquarie pointed out that such discrimination was nonsense since ex-convicts owned most of the land in the colony. The Exclusives countered Macquarie's criticism by contending that emancipists seldom lived on their large cereal farms and could not be 'considered as practical farmers'. Gentlemen farmers were 'graziers' who actually resided on and managed their estates.[47]

By December 1819 relations between Macquarie and Bigge had reached a simmering standoff. The stress of the inquiry had affected Macquarie's health and when he contracted dysentery, which was raging in Sydney at the time, he was confined to bed for four weeks. Redfern and Wentworth did their best to treat him during the critical stages of his illness. At one point Redfern advised Wentworth that their patient was so weak that he should come to Government House without spreading alarm.[48] The crisis passed but it was weeks before the governor returned to full strength.[49]

Dysentery devastated Sydney residents for another seven months and many poor, who did not have the benefit of the expert and dedicated medical attention the governor received, lost their lives.

Chapter 16

THE SLAUGHTER HOUSE

Mr. Bowman shall have full Credit given him, for the ample & steady employment he has furnished to the Coffin-Makers - the Grave-Digger, & the Chaplains - the cause of which I shall not fail to develope; whilst I shall only aspire to the honor of having the Hospital ... considered while under the charge of Mr. Wentworth & Myself the voluntary resort, the last mundane hope, of all the Maimed & Sick from the different parts of the Colony, and of those discharged, as incurable from all the Hospitals at the out stations - instead of being denominated, since we left it, the slaughter house of New South Wales. Redfern to Bigge, 5 Feb 1821[1]

Commissioner Bigge feared emancipist magistrates might try to disrupt his inquiry. These influential members of the community had gained the judicial post through achievement, and it was the promotion of these men that the inquiry sought to reverse. Bigge's resolve to preclude emancipist magistrates from his inquiry deliberations became apparent on 7 January 1820 when he sent a letter to all magistrates except William Redfern, Simeon Lord, Reverend Henry Fulton and D'Arcy Wentworth. His letter requested details of inhabitants in the magistrates' districts; the names of adult males with their own property; whether they were free, ex-convict or born in the colony, and if any might be eligible to serve as jurors. He later sent out another letter seeking information on the use of convict labour and views on the future of agriculture in the colony. This time Reverend Fulton was on the circulation list, but Redfern, Wentworth and Lord were not.[2]

Weeks later Redfern was contacted by Magistrate Robert Lowe and asked to contribute to Bigge's survey on land usage. Redfern replied that he would not participate in the survey unless requested officially. This required Bigge to write to him for his input, and he reluctantly did this.[3] A week later the Commissioner travelled to the Newcastle coal mines to collect evidence there. When his vessel sailed out of Port Jackson, Governor Macquarie and his guests William Redfern, Thomas Moore and Henry Antill toasted

Bigge's departure over breakfast.[4] It is likely that this gathering persuaded Governor Macquarie to later write to all magistrates requesting their views on the state of the colony and whether it had improved under his administration.[5]

On returning to Sydney Commissioner Bigge was informed by Secretary Scott of Macquarie's circular letter. Bigge promptly went to Government House and accused Macquarie of 'very improper Interference with the Objects of his Commission'. Because of his 'Violent Umbrage' at this action Bigge swore to never speak to Macquarie again and stormed out of their meeting. Mediation by Secretary Scott calmed matters, but Bigge asked Macquarie to defer publicising the magistrates' replies until he had left the colony.[6] Macquarie refused and told Bigge that he had every right to solicit views from residents and that delaying their publication might prove injurious to his own interests and the colony. The governor accused Bigge of treating him with indignity and a 'continued Spirit of Hostility and Insult', and he therefore saw no reason not to release the responses to questions he had asked *all* of his magistrates, *all* of whom had replied.[7]

Commissioner Bigge's determination to remove Redfern as a magistrate was made clear in a letter sent to Bathurst that quoted statements given by Henry Cowper and other hospital 'underlings' denigrating the doctor's abilities. Somehow Redfern learnt of this and was outraged at not being given an opportunity to defend himself against such slurs.[8] It was no consolation to learn that he was not the only magistrate in Bigge's sights – all four men who had dined with the Governor, Thompson, Redfern, Wentworth and Lord, had received similar treatment. During the actual interviews, Bigge had treated Simeon Lord and D'Arcy Wentworth decorously but not Macquarie's two closest friends, Redfern and Thompson. Although Thompson had been dead for ten years, the inquiry extracted as much fallacious gossip as possible about him. Fortunately, Macquarie and other friends easily refuted most of it.[9] However, Redfern was interrogated harshly and faced many accusations. But he was fully capable of defending himself against the charges and repudiating the scurrilous evidence submitted by others, and he would soon do so comprehensively in writing.

One of the most distasteful consequences of the inquiry was that it served to amplify social differences between convicts, emancipists, immigrants and Exclusives in the colony. Exclusives now openly opposed the progress of emancipists, especially if it competed with their own interests. They hoped that the rejection of Redfern as a magistrate would stop Macquarie's advancement of emancipists. Bigge wanted this as well and his secretary Thomas Scott told John Macarthur that the Commissioner saw his evidence to be 'the Key or Touchstone of the Truth of all they had heard'.[10]

Similar damaging evidence against Redfern was expected from James Bowman, who was on 'intimate terms and confidence' with Bigge. Macarthur claimed Bowman had 'performed miracles' at the hospital and yet to the Governor and his supporters, he remained 'an object of aversion which they take little pains to conceal'. Of course, Macarthur always exercised the belief that flattering a powerful person 'seldom does mischief'.[11] Judge Barron Field, who had joined Macarthur's cabal, increasingly gave legal advice to the Exclusives and actively fuelled social division in the colony.

By February 1820, Lachlan Macquarie had been governor for a decade and was weary of defending self-evident rights against an intrusive and rude Commissioner. Bigge had even started to interfere in his building projects. The construction of the large new courthouse was underway but before Bigge left on a four-month tour of Van Diemen's Land, he demanded that the building be converted to a church. The authority given to Bigge by Bathurst was such that Macquarie had little choice but to comply. The half-finished building on King Street was transformed into St James Church. Bigge claimed that this was necessary to save construction costs, but most knew otherwise. His secretary and clergy brother-in-law Thomas Scott would soon become the Archdeacon of New South Wales and needed a church to occupy. To calm judicial concern at the loss of court space, Bigge insisted that the principal surgeon's quarters in the hospital be converted into a courthouse.[12]

On 22 February 1820, Macquarie wrote to Bathurst supporting Redfern's appointment as magistrate and disputing Bigge's criticisms of his doctor. Macquarie had been dismayed when Bigge told him that Bathurst opposed promoting ex-convicts to posts of 'Trust and Confidence'. Macquarie told Bathurst this was 'highly prejudicial to the future Prosperity and Welfare of the Colony and tend greatly to excite a Spirit of Discontent and Party Animosity'.[13]

> It must never be forgot that this is, at present, a Convict Country, Originally established for their Punishment and Reformation; that

at least Nine-tenths of its present Population Consist either of Convicts, Persons who have been Convicts, or the Offspring of Convicts; and that the principal part of the property in the Colony at this day is possessed by the two latter Classes. Consequently some Consideration appears to be Justly due to so very large a Portion of the Population of the Country.[14]

Macquarie informed Bathurst that if he had 'kindly Condescended' to make his views known to him before Bigge arrived he would have 'bowed Submissively and respectfully to the Mandate'.[15] Two days later he wrote again to Bathurst entreating him to understand Redfern's disappointment at not being appointed as principal surgeon and grant him a 'Pension on Half Pay as a Reward for his past Services' (£68 per year).[16]

Defamations were also being levelled at Macquarie. A pamphlet produced by British MP Henry Bennet had just reached the colony condemning him and his administration. Bennet had been strongly influenced by the complaints of former Judge Jeffery Bent and Reverend Samuel Marsden. The pamphlet reinforced Macquarie's determination to go back to England soon and refute accusations made in the House of Commons based on 'the most polluted Sources and the false Communications of Unprincipled Individuals'. Two years had passed since Macquarie had submitted his resignation and there was still no reply. On 29 February 1820 he submitted another resignation and requested prompt action.[17]

Macquarie continued to communicate with all magistrates. His letter on 20 April concerned the transmission of governor's orders; the sentencing of men to do hard labour at Newcastle; the abuse of the ticket of leave system by magistrates; the appointment of constables; the withdrawal of tickets of leave, and a request for the names of suitable police constables and pound keepers. Four days later a detailed response from Magistrate Redfern endorsed the reappointment of two constables and recommended a new candidate as constable, a man who had been in Redfern's service for nine years, John Grant.[18]

In contrast to his repeated censure of Redfern, Bigge sent glowing reports to Bathurst on the progress of Principal Surgeon Bowman, praising the improvements he had made at the hospital. In reality, most of these advances had occurred before Bowman's arrival. The success of the new patient dietary scheme Bowman claimed credit for was mostly the 'borrowed plumes' of reforms Redfern and Wentworth instituted earlier. What Bigge did not reveal to Bathurst was that the standard of medical care across the colony had deteriorated under Bowman's watch, and the health of the poor was being severely neglected. In Wentworth and Redfern's tenure, the hospital was seen as a place of hope and recovery. Now many poor refused to be admitted to the hospital for fear of dying there.[19] The higher mortality rate and the overuse of bloodletting meant many avoided seeking medical attention until it was too late. And, since Redfern no longer had a private practise, there was a huge gap in medical care for the poor in Sydney, and beyond.

Between November 1819 and May 1820 contagious dysentery hit the colony causing 1060 to be hospitalised and 88 deaths. Hospital deaths doubled over the previous dysentery epidemic when Wentworth and Redfern were in charge. They 'did not bleed so much, unless there was a good deal of Inflammation' and Calomel (mercurous chloride) was not given in such large doses.[20] The use of bloodletting was now excessive, and convicts began to refer to the hospital as 'the Sidney Slaughter house'. A patient with 'fever of the brain' was bled by Henry Cowper 'Two Pounds in the morning & about Three in the evening' (about 2½ litres of blood – today's blood donors give below ½ litre). The patient was allowed to get out of bed and he immediately 'dropped down Dead'.[21]

Many other breaches of hospital care occurred. In one instance a male patient was declared dead, his body was sent for burial, but he woke up 'when the Clergyman was reading the valediction, he kicked off the lid of the Coffin, & walked home'. The man received a conditional pardon as compensation.[22] In another case a man delayed going to the hospital for fear of mistreatment, but a 'lump in his stomach' forced him to become an outpatient. He was given the 'blister' treatment and within hours of returning to his barracks, he suffered severe pain and died crying out 'Oh the Doctors have killed me'. After this incident Bowman introduced a 'broom stick discipline' at the hospital.[23] It is uncertain whether this meant that anyone guilty of unsafe practices was beaten, promptly dismissed, or that the matter "swept under the bed".

In April 1820 Macquarie appointed a medical board to inquire into the likely causes of the hospital's high mortality rate. The board comprised of Principal Surgeon Bowman, a military surgeon and three ship surgeons. They reported that the colony had suffered the most sicknesses ever recorded, and the high death rate was due to the hot summer, overcrowded hospital wards and patients' reluctance to seek hospital help until it was too late. The board also reported that hospital convict staff members were 'ignorant of every branch of the Medical profession', except for one man who acted as the apothecary. The board exonerated Principal Surgeon Bowman, declaring that he had adopted sufficient means to stop the disease and because of his 'unwearied attention' to the sick there was no need to enquire further.[24]

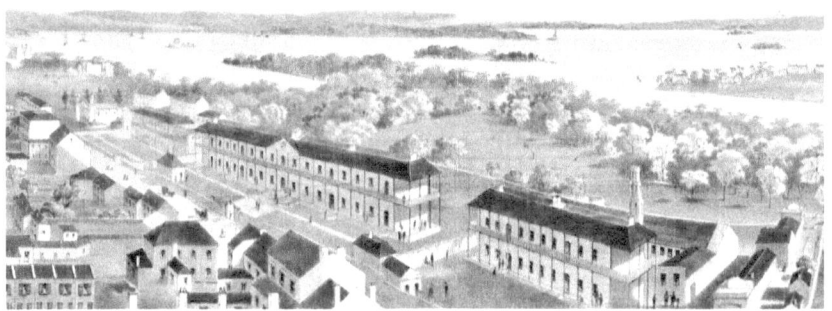

1860s lithograph of Macquarie Street showing the three wings of the new Sydney General Hospital.

On reading the report William Redfern held opposite views on Bowman's competence but initially kept them to himself. However, in February 1821, after much praise had been heaped on Bowman's work at the hospital, Redfern wrote to Bigge telling him that the principal surgeon was being given credit at the hospital for 'superior arrangements adopted in its management' long before he assumed office. Redfern asserted that 'Those arrangements ... are mine'. Redfern sarcastically gave Bowman full credit 'for the ample & steady employment he has furnished to the Coffin-Makers – the Grave-Digger, & the Chaplains – the cause of which I shall not fail to develope'. He reminded Bigge that despite its 'Augean' filth, the hospital under his and Wentworth's charge was 'the voluntary resort, the last mundane hope, of all the Maimed & Sick from the different parts of the Colony, and of those discharged, as incurable from all the Hospitals at the out stations – instead of being denominated'. He closed the letter to Bigge observing that since 'we left it' James Bowman had transformed the hospital into 'the slaughter house of New South Wales'.[25]

As this letter clearly showed, Redfern did not suffer fools gladly or let injustices go without comment. To close colleagues he was probably seen as a likeable but prickly know-it-all. He certainly would have considered Bigge as an arrogant pen pusher who had no authority or qualification to question his abilities. Conversely, Bigge expected ex-convicts to defer to his social superiority and breeding. This, Redfern would certainly never do.

Commissioner Bigge must have been fully aware of the problems at the hospital, but his *raison d'etre* for being in the colony was to discredit Macquarie's policies, so Bowman's inadequate response to the dysentery outbreak was never mentioned in his final reports. Quite the contrary; Bigge, who had no medical expertise, praised Bowman for his 'zealous exertions' in creating a new state of order and cleanliness in the hospital, while deriding the earlier reform efforts of Redfern and Wentworth.[26]

Conditions for Sydney hospital patients had not improved eight years later. An 1828 article in *The Monitor* reported a high mortality rate in the hospital and demanded authorities explain the rising number of convict deaths. The article sparked a contrary view in *The Sydney Gazette* claiming that convicts in the hospital were safe because of its 'cleanliness, attention, food, and medical ability, no hospital in the world can be better off'.[27] There is no indication that this assurance increased patient numbers or their health.

It is claimed that the 1822 Bigge Report on the inquiry provides historians with insights into the workings of the Sydney Hospital. In 1911, based on the Report Frederick Watson wrote in *The History of the Sydney Hospital* that 'The appointment of James Bowman ... was a fortunate one for the welfare of the Sydney Hospital itself'.[28] Similar sentiments are expressed in the 2003 book *A History of Medical Administration in NSW* by Cyril Cummins. He claims William Redfern gave preference to his private patients and was 'dilatory and careless in his hospital practise', while James Bowman was 'a vigorous and dynamic leader who had at heart the interests of the Colonial Medical Service and the Colony'.[29] Analogous conclusions, based solely on the Bigge Reports, appear in other historical accounts.

In her 2017 article *The Sidney Slaughter House: Convict Experience of Medical Care at the General Rum Hospital*, Fiona Starr doubts that the credits given to James Bowman in the Bigge Report for improving the Sydney hospital are true. She writes, 'If these new standards were actually put in practice, conditions may have improved somewhat, although no evidence for change is available'. She wrote 'By curing the incurables sent from other colonial hospitals, Redfern and the Rum Hospital perhaps should have been better acknowledged in their own time as providing the best medical care available in the colony'. Furthermore, Starr claims that health care at the Sydney General Hospital under Redfern was probably superior to that available to the working class in Britain.[30]

In his 1824 publication *Statistical Account of the British Settlements in Australasia*, William Wentworth denounced the Bigge Report as a piece of 'nauseous trash'. 'Instead of confining his report to public objects, and public interests', Bigge polluted almost every page with 'private scandal and vituperation'. Wentworth claimed that, without scruples, Bigge broadcast to the world evidence from 'whores, and rogues, and vagabonds in Sydney' and like a public scavenger had 'raked together all the dirt and filth, all the scandal, calumnies, and lies, that were ever circulated in the Colony'.[31]

Malcolm Ellis observes in his book *Lachlan Macquarie: His Life, Adventures and Times* that some of the phrasing in the Bigge Report resembles that of John Macarthur, and he was not the only witness whose words 'were embodied as accepted fact'. Ellis concludes:

> Both in the recording of "evidence" and of findings there is slovenliness. The reports teem with error from end to end. Often where the Commissioner has gone to endless trouble to elucidate the details of some old scandal with an array of damning facts, the "facts" prove to be mere gossip. He was not even accurate in stating the crimes for which many of the victims of his comments were sent to the Colony.[32]

Since the foundation of the colony in 1788, convicts believed that their civil rights would be fully restored when they completed their sentence or earned a pardon for good behaviour. Between 1810 and 1819 Governor Macquarie had granted 352 absolute and 1164 conditional pardons.[33] The first colonial civil court in New South Wales was based on the same principles as English courts but with statutes added by Judge Advocate David Collins to allow for the predominant convict population. The statutes enabled the convicts Henry and Susannah Kable to sue Captain Sinclair for the loss of property in his charge during their transportation were awarded £12 compensation. This set a legal precedent in the colony that overruled the English law forbidding a felon to sue anyone. An absolute pardon or the completion of a sentence restored full civil rights to a convict and gave an emancipist unfettered property rights in the colony.

In April 1820 a ruling in a Sydney court challenged the right of ex-convict Edward Eagar to be a legally entitled plaintiff seeking a debt repayment. This threatened to turn the emancipists' legal world upside down. The origins of this challenge began in late 1819 when the London case *Bullock vs Dodd* disputed if someone with a *colonial* pardon had legal rights. The emancipist Bullock had sued Dodd for the repayment of a debt and the defendant challenged the legitimacy of Bullock's pardon, asserting that it did not give him the right to initiate a court action. The King's Bench ruled that since Bullock's pardon had not been stamped with the Great Seal of Britain, his civil status was that of a serving convict, who had no right to sue. This 1819 ruling was cataclysmic for all ex-convicts, but the Colonial Office had failed to inform Macquarie, even though John Bigge was in London when the verdict was given and would have understood its ramifications.[34]

Prior to the 1819 English court ruling, the rights of emancipists had never been questioned. When Edward Eagar sued Justice Barron Field for defamation in 1820, Judge Advocate Wylde was confronted with a challenge to Eagar's pardon. Wylde adjourned the case until details of his conviction could be obtained from Ireland.[35] The decision to consider the defence's challenge to Eagar's legal rights caused an absolute furore in the colony, as it had ramifications for property transactions across the colony. This issue was particularly perplexing because the Colonial Office had never instructed the governors to have pardons ratified under the Great Seal of Britain.

Commissioner Bigge returned from Van Diemen's Land on 4 June 1820. Among the many witnesses he had questioned during his tour were former staff members at Sydney hospital. Redfern later labelled those interviewed 'the sober & pious Mr. Luttrell - the elegant & graceful Mr. Owen - and One Frost of no less notoriety - and in short every person, however mean & contemptible' who could be relied upon to give falsehoods injurious to his character.[36] Wentworth was also a target in these interviews. The surgeons Mileham, Harris, Evans and West told Bigge of problems at the Sydney hospital during the tenure of Principal Surgeon D'Arcy Wentworth. They cited poor supervision and record keeping in hospitals because Wentworth always delegated responsibilities to other staff and did not check their performance.

At 9 pm on the cold winter's night of 26 June 1820, William Redfern was summoned to Commissioner Bigge's residence for his first interview. The confrontation would not be easy for either man. Redfern was questioned about his appointment, his promotion to assistant surgeon, his medical studies, his 'Nore trial' and his sentence for transportation. Bigge queried him on every aspect of his work since arriving in the colony, and in particular on the Sydney hospital patient records, his access to the stores and the removal of medicine.[37] Redfern was to discover months later when reading a draft of his recorded inquiry answers that they bore little resemblance to what he had said during the interview, and a lot of his important answers and comments had been omitted.

The session was paused when Redfern vigorously protested at Bigge's personal and rancorous hostility. The accusation that Redfern had forgotten his crime and his 'correct place in society' put the so-called interview onto a dangerous footing. Redfern, who was accustomed to respect from officials such as Macquarie, Foveaux, Erskine and Antill, would not have tolerated Bigge's arrogance and was capable of fierce retaliation. Months later when reviewing draft minutes of the interview, Redfern refuted Bigge's claim that he had been uncooperative and reminded him of his disrespectful line of questioning. He wrote that Bigge's sarcastic sneers and threats would have fitted a 'Spanish Inquisitor'.[38] He later wrote to Bigge:

> The appearance of the Room, – the Piles of Books, the dress of yourself & Secretary, the gravity of your countenance, the awful Solemnity with which you made your opening speech – the threatenings you denounced, the dreadful charges you had to exhibit against me, not forgetting the stale trick in imitation of Banquo's Ghost, forcibly impressed on my mind the introduction of some unhappy victim, Clothed in his Santo Venito, with his

own picture portrayed thereon, surrounded with the figures of flames & Devils, to the inquisitorial Hall at Madrid, preparatory to the Auto Da Fe.[39]

Redfern accused Bigge of intentionally trying to 'alarm and intimidate' him and when that failed, he tried to irritate him to commit a 'breach of good manners'. Only his high respect for His Majesty's Commission induced Redfern to 'listen for a Moment to such insulting language'.[40]

> That memorable speech, conversation, & questions, so artfully calculated to wound & insult my feelings, have made too deep an impression on My Mind ever to be forgotten. The quiver of your lip, the curl of your nose, the expression of your eye-in short, your tout-ensemble, revealed to me your very thoughts & intentions, as a Mirror exhibits the person of him who stands before it.[41]

Many of Redfern's responses to questions were not recorded in the inquiry reports. These included his answers on the arrest of Governor Bligh, his role in the Nore mutiny and the accusation that he was the author of the pipe lampooning George Molle. Bigge also accused him of causing the rift between Governor Macquarie and the officers of the 46th Regiment. Redfern was queried on his hospital appointments, his early medical training, his farm, his business connections with Edward Eagar and his views on the transportation of convicts to the colony. At one point in the interrogation Bigge threatened to charge Redfern with the misappropriation of Crown property and for an insulting letter that accused James Bowman of clandestinely visiting the hospital when it was still under his control. Redfern demanded to have these charges put down in writing. It took some 'very unpleasant correspondence' before he was able to extract them from Bigge.[42]

In his 1824 publication *The Statistical Account of the British Settlement* William Wentworth detailed the 'personal and rancorous hostility' Redfern had endured during Bigge's interrogation that were intended to wantonly damage his feelings. Wentworth wrote that this 'was inflicted under the shelter of a high commission' and the wound all the more 'dastardly' because it was intended solely for public purposes, 'a species of political sacrilege, to make the vehicle of private revenge'. He had long wondered why 'Mr. Redfern did not on the instant apply some degrading chastisement to the nose or breech of this cowardly inquisitor'. In not doing so,

Redfern exhibited a restraint that Wentworth greatly admired.[43]

On 18 July 1820 Bigge provided Redfern with details of the six charges laid against him and the next day he responded. Redfern denied the first charge: that he had ever been absent from hospital duties without approval. All his leave had been approved by Macquarie, and Wentworth had attended to the hospital duties during his absence. He also denied the charge that Cowper had administered medicine without his authority; he had only been permitted to administer prescribed medicine during Redfern's absence or after consultation with Wentworth. Redfern refuted the third charge that he had misappropriated medicine, tinware and spices from the hospital for his own personal use. He had used those medicines when attending civil officers and their families, as was his duty, but had not kept an account for it. However, all medicines prescribed in his private practice were recorded. He said that the tinware and spices taken from the hospital were of little value. The storage and preparation of medicines at his house was necessary and was known to Wentworth and other officers in the colony; nor had it been prohibited or disapproved of.[44]

Redfern emphasised that since the foundation of the colony, it had been the common practise for the hospital dispensary to be regarded as a resource 'from which all persons were considered as having a right to obtain Medicine'. Under these circumstances, Redfern wrote, he had never conceived that he could or would be called upon to pay for the medicine used for private patients. He had not been asked for payment, but if the British government thought that he ought to pay for the medicine used in his private practise, he was willing to do so. Redfern refused to answer the last three charges about writing an insulting letter to Bowman and his conduct towards his former apprentice Cowper, as these were private matters and had no bearing on his professional conduct.[45]

A serious legal crisis regarding the civil rights of pardoned convicts now threatened the colony. In the court case *Eagar vs de Mestre* in September 1820, Judge Field declared that convicts pardoned without the Great Seal of Britain, remained 'Convicts attaint, incapable of taking by Grant or Purchase, holding or conveying any property, real or Personal, of suing in a Court of Justice, or of giving Evidence therein'.[46] In effect, this ruling invalidated all assets and transactions of pardoned convicts in the colony. Eagar's two court actions were not altruistic, but they highlighted a serious gap in the colony's legal system and the need to retrospectively validate all granted pardons under the Great Seal of Britain.

The wealthiest emancipists were the first to fully understand the ramifications of the court decision and they forecast heavy losses of property and official positions. The rest of the colony, both emancipists and freemen, quickly appreciated that this judgement affected everyone. Many business and financial dealings involved pardoned emancipists, who were the wealthiest farmers and merchants in the colony. Now their land grants, businesses, shops, shipyards, farms, properties and shares appeared to be at risk. If a free person had bought land belonging to an emancipist, the new owner had no right to hold it and no right to pass on the title.

Uncertainty surrounding the fundamental rights of ownership in the colony cast a gloom over the entire community. How had such a basic legal matter been overlooked and why had the Colonial Office never objected to a pardon-granting process that had been used by every Governor since 1788? Why did it take 33 years to discover this? Judge Field's decision appeared to invalidate the purchase of the largest estates in the colony, including those sold to free emigrants. Questioning the legitimacy of pardons dramatically raised the political temperature in the colony and influential people demanded the matter be immediately resolved in Britain. Edward Eagar and William Redfern sought Governor Macquarie's permission to hold a public meeting to petition the Crown for legislative relief of the emancipists' predicament.

Since his retirement from the hospital Redfern had become totally immersed in farming. In July 1820 this commitment led him to resign his directorship at the Bank of New South Wales – a post he had held for three years.[47] The Campbellfield farm of 2360 acres now had a work force of 40 men and women; free servants, assigned convicts and ticket of leave men and it grazed 547 cattle, 2159 sheep and 51 pigs. The leased farmland at Bathurst grazed 400 cattle and 2113 sheep.[48] Redfern continued his judicial duties, as he found being a magistrate interesting work that kept him informed about district matters. While no records have survived of his verdicts and sentencing as magistrate, there are details of his servant assignments, of absconding prisoners, recommending land grants and positions as constables, and rain damage of crops.[49]

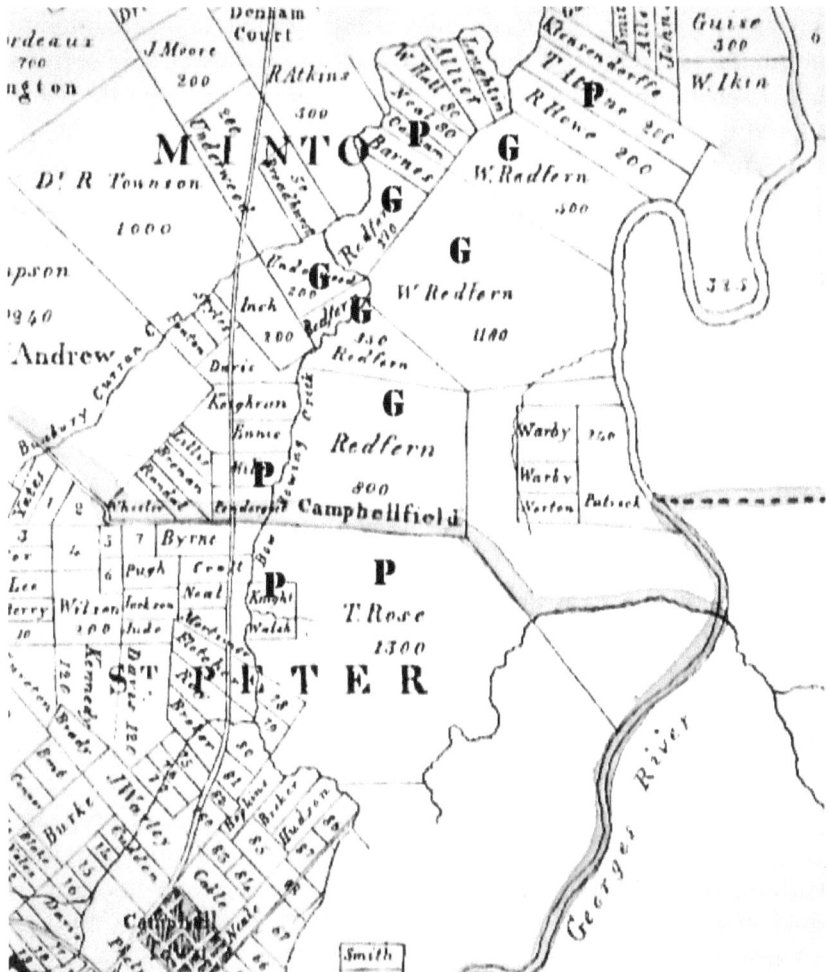

1840 map showing Redfern's Campbellfield estate composed of land grants (G) and land purchases (P). It is on the George's River and close to Campbelltown. His house and vineyard were on 800 acres granted in 1811.

Regardless of his commitment to farming, Redfern always kept an interest in medicine and a caring for the sick. Although he no longer ran a private practise, he remained the Macquarie family's physician and treated the farm's servants and labourers. It is also unlikely that he ignored local requests for medical assistance.

In the first three decades of the colony's existence, the overall health of its inhabitants had been excellent by Britain's standards. Its remoteness and strict maritime regulations had largely shielded the population from many infectious diseases that were endemic in

Europe. However, the recent increases in convict and free migrant numbers had removed the isolation barrier. Convict ship arrivals had risen dramatically, and the population of New South Wales soared to 26,000 people. In June 1820 influenza swept the colony. On 5 July Governor Macquarie was among the first to be infected after interviewing colonists applying for land grants.[50] The flu virus spread quickly into the remote settlements and by late August few families in the colony had escaped its impact. Those most at risk of severe morbidity were the young, the old, and Aboriginal people. *The Sydney Gazette* editor noted on 19 August that although influenza had been rampant in Sydney for a month, nothing had been heard from the 'medical gentlemen of the Colony'.[51] The deaths peaked in September and dropped off a month later. This epidemic barely rated a line in the Bigge Reports, and then only mentioned that 'several instances proved fatal'.[52]

In the early 19th century, influenza, known then as epidemic catarrh and *grippe*, was almost indistinguishable from the common cold or other respiratory infections. It was not known that flu is a transmissible virus; the belief then was that it was due to sudden changing winds or the level of humidity. Residents at Airds caught the epidemic catarrh in late August and William Redfern became infected with 'a severe visitation of the malady, and his lady being on the verge of suffering under the like disaster'. Most Europeans carried flu antibodies, but Aboriginal people did not, and they suffered badly. This concerned Redfern and he wrote about it to the newspaper. On 16 December 1820 *The Sydney Gazette* published a letter from a 'Medical Gentleman of Bunbury Curran' reporting on 'the mortal efficacy of the late influenza' affecting the colony 'with increased violence, and particularly among the scattered tribes of natives'.[53] The article was anonymous but it was clearly written by Redfern; he was the only medical resident in that area. The article reported that 'the natives of the interior had suffered excessively' and 'many young stout and robust people' became flu victims. It noted that the Aboriginal people had responded to the disease by retreating into the thinly wooded interior and the coast, where there were quantities of honey. Redfern understood how social dislocation and dietary stress exacerbated the impact of influenza's spread and had spoken to various tribes about this.

> Thirty years ago a prodigious mortality was spread among them by a contagious distemper resembling the small pox, of which the

indented marks remained on many till very lately; and which, had it continued to rage any longer, would probably have left but few alive in our vicinity. The natives of Broken Bay, and other tribes, not very distant from Sydney, reported that the calamity had proved fatal to many of them; and one, who was considerably intelligent, being enquired of the cause, gave it as his firm and unalterable opinion, that it was owing to the putrescence of a whale that had gone on shore to expire on a neighbouring part of the coast. ... Its [influenza] spreading throughout whole and many families would appear to denote that it was communicative from person to person, and that if contracted by any one, the whole in the same close connexion were liable to receive the contagion. Many have witnessed the effects, but we have not heard that its causes have been as yet defined.[54]

Despite their relative isolation on Campbellfield, William and Sarah kept up their friendship with Lachlan and Elizabeth Macquarie. On 1 December 1820 they visited the farm with Thomas and Racheal Moore, Miss Broughton, the Reverends Cartwright and Reddall, Surveyor James Meehan and Charles Whalan. After being served a handsome 'Cold Collation', the Macquaries, Redferns and their guests set off in carriages to an official naming of a new town, three miles to the southwest where the Governor set the boundaries of *Campbelltown* and marked the future sites of a chapel, school and burial ground. The day was attended by 60 settlers of the Airds district and by the magistrates of Liverpool and Airds, Thomas Moore and William Redfern.[55]

On the last day of the year 1820 the convict transport *Hebe* sailed into Sydney harbour with dispatches from Bathurst. Macquarie would later write in his diary, the dispatches were 'all of a very unpleasant and mortifying nature'. However, he did find one dispatch that was welcome. His resignation had been accepted and he would be relieved as soon as a successor had been selected.[56]

One of the most unpleasant letters aboard the *Hebe*, dated 10 July 1820, ordered the removal of William Redfern as magistrate. The reason given for his dismissal was that Commissioner John Bigge objected to his appointment. Bathurst expressed regret at the decision but ordered William Redfern's name be struck off the renewal of commissions list.[57]

Chapter 17

RIGHTS ACTIVIST

That your Petitioners ... are to be considered as Convicts attaint, without personal Liberty, without Property, without Character or Credit, without any one Right or Privilege belonging to free Subjects. ... Your Petitioners do therefore with the most profound humility approach Your Majesty, and ... Most Humbly pray that your Majesty will be graciously pleased to take, into your royal Consideration, the Condition in which we your Majesty's Petitioners are placed in by this State of the Law, as interpreted and acted upon by the Courts of Civil Judicature in this Territory, and afford your Petitioners such relief as our Situation and Circumstances in Your Majesty's Royal Wisdom shall seem to deserve.
WM. REDFERN, *Chairman, &c.*
HENRY FULTON.
F. H. GREENWAY.
and 1,363 others.   Petition to the Crown, 22 Oct 1821[1]

In early January 1821 Edward Eagar, William Redfern, Simeon Lord and six other emancipists sought permission from Governor Macquarie to hold a public meeting on the legal and civil rights of emancipists. Judges Field and Wylde opposed the meeting and tried to convince Macquarie that the emancipists' concerns about reduced legal status were baseless. Justice Field even went so far as to recommend that Eagar be banished from the colony to prevent further discontent and sedition among the convicts. He maintained that if Eagar were expelled most concerns about legal rights would fade away. Notwithstanding this council, Macquarie permitted the meeting to go ahead.[2]

Colonists were most troubled about the legitimacy of colonial pardons, but they were also seeking other legal concessions. One was the right to distil spirits. Rather than allowing overseas traders to profit from imported alcohol, local production would benefit both grain growers and local merchants. Bigge supported the granting of this concession on the grounds that distilling was an industry that could employ convicts at no cost to the Crown. On 9

January, with his departure to England only a month away, Bigge invited respectable residents wishing to engage in distillation to come to Government House and hear his opinion on the subject.[3] William Redfern was among the small group of attendees. Bigge spoke at length on the regulations and dangers of spirit production and various colonists commented. He warned that the cheapness of locally distilled alcohol might induce excessive consumption. Someone pointed out that this did not happen in other countries distilling alcohol and, in any case, this could be controlled by taxes.

Bigge shifted his ground and argued that the arable land in the colony was only suitable for growing grain to make flour. Redfern disputed this describing the farming practises in Flanders where gin was produced. Bigge interrupted him, saying that local farmers were less advanced than the Flemish in agriculture. Redfern agreed and added 'the sooner we begin to approximate towards their perfection, the better. We were only just beginning to develop our powers'. He said that it was important to place colonial farmers 'on the right end of the road; when once there, we could then steadily pursue our course & own object' but, if inhibited, they would risk 'breaking their necks' leaping over unnecessary hurdles.[4] A duty of 5s per gallon for local spirits was suggested by current importers but this was opposed by Redfern and others who haggled it down to 2s 5d. A month later, Macquarie announced that distillation would be permitted from 1 August 1823 and the present duty of 10s per gallon for imported spirits would remain.[5]

On 23 January 1821 Chairman William Redfern opened the much-anticipated meeting of 'Emancipated Colonists' and every seat in the room was occupied. Edward Eagar spoke in detail about the petition to be presented to the Crown and British Parliament. The draft of the petition was unanimously approved. Clauses in the petition emphasised the emancipists' interests were 'exposed to infinite prejudice and danger' and that this affected 'their personal liberty, their property, their civil rights as citizens, the rights and properties of their children, and the properties of their fellow Colonists'. After considerable debate, a committee was formed to lead a campaign for the restitution of emancipist legal rights. It was also decided that a delegation would need to be sent to England to advocate these causes, and that funds should be raised to cover their expenses. A drafting committee comprising William Redfern,

Simeon Lord, Reverend Henry Fulton, James Meehan, James Underwood, Daniel Cooper and William Hutchinson was formed, with Samuel Terry as treasurer and Edward Eagar as secretary. At the conclusion of the proceedings Redfern was thanked for 'his able, upright, and impartial conduct in the chair' of a meeting, where debates were as 'orderly, and well-conducted' as had never previously been 'witnessed in the Colony'.[6]

The meeting elected Edward Eagar and William Redfern as the delegates who should go to England and present the petition to the King and the Parliament. A petition-writing committee would meet every Tuesday and Friday evening at Edward Eagar's house to finalise details. Redfern clearly valued his involvement in the delegation and travelled from his farm to Sydney twice a week for this task. His election to the delegation would prove important, both because of his skill at explaining things clearly and his ability to calm the impetuous Edward Eagar, who was easily angered.

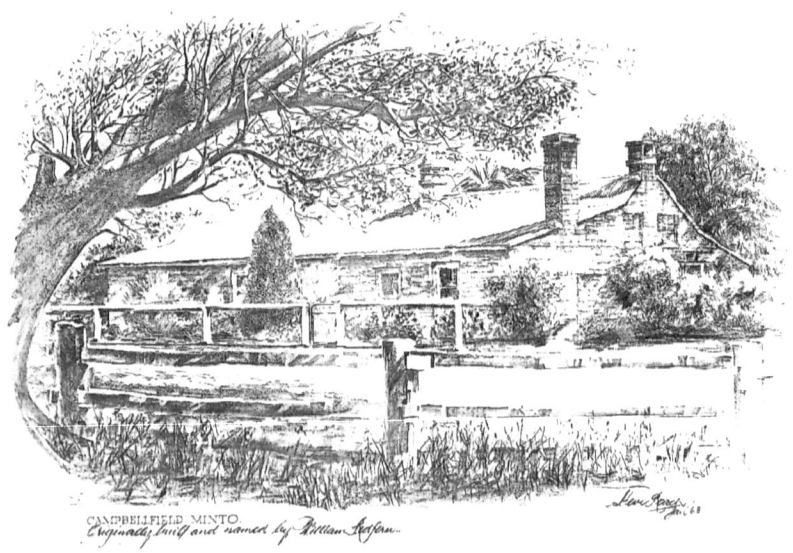

1963 pencil drawing of William and Sarah Redfern's house at Campbellfield.

William Redfern was also the president of a committee responsible for celebrating the foundation of the colony. At the anniversary dinner held at Hyde Park on 26 January 1821, more than 100 men sat down to sumptuous food and wine with President William Redfern at one end of a large table and Vice President Simeon

Lord at the other, with Governor Macquarie and Commissioner Bigge seated in the middle. After an excellent repast the President rose and offered a toast to 'Mr. Commissioner Bigge, May we have cause to transmit his name with veneration to Posterity'.[7] Most present, except perhaps Bigge himself, would have understood the irony of Redfern's toast; they were the same words he had used in his toast a year earlier before he knew how prejudiced the inquiry and the inquisitor would be.

Redfern continued his duties as Magistrate and Justice of the Peace until the end of January. His name had not appeared on the list of reappointed magistrates and neither had that of Simeon Lord, who resigned the post earlier claiming poor health and increased business commitments.[8] Most likely Lord was tired of the sniping by Exclusives and decided that being a magistrate was not good for business. For Redfern the judicial post was far more important and, following his rejection as principal surgeon, he would have been embarrassed and hurt at losing the position. Not only was this injunction ridiculous considering his long service to the colony, but Redfern could not reconcile why he had been singled out for such treatment. He suspected that Bowman was behind these attempts to diminish his standing in the community. This belief was later confirmed in the Bigge inquiry minutes.

In late January 1821 Macquarie received a 64-page preliminary report from Bigge summarising the accusations against him and his administration. Staggered at the number and nature of charges, Macquarie quickly wrote a 55-page response. The full extent of James Bowman's influence on the inquiry was evident in the allegations; a quarter referred to hospital matters and Macquarie's relationship with William Redfern. Other charges concerned the preferential treatment the Governor and his wife had given to emancipists. This particularly enraged Macquarie and he responded that all people in the colony were treated equally, but he was most willing to favour the individuals possessing 'conspicuous merit'.[9] He rejected the implication that his wife had given 'undue ascendency' to former convicts.

> It has ever been her wish to bestow the greatest share of her regard where she finds the greatest share of Merit. A Man having once been a Convict is not considered by her as a bar to his being treated in the same manner as if he never had been one, and she

considers it her duty during her residence in this Colony to show as much kindness towards those Persons as their good conduct can justify.[10]

Another accusation in the draft report was that Macquarie had forced regimental officers to associate with ex-convicts by having Major Antill take Mr Redfern to the officer's mess. Macquarie replied, 'If Major Antill chose to accompany his friend Doctor Redfern on such occasion, he most assuredly had a right so to do, and is therefore, a most absurd charge to be brought against the Governor'. Macquarie was also accused of ignoring Mr Redfern's insolent letter to Mr Bowman, and that he approved a medical board to investigate the high number of deaths at the hospital so as to damage Bowman's reputation. Macquarie called this a charge of 'bespeaking frivolity & Malice'. He also denied treating Bowman unfairly or having refused assistance when 'such Indulgencies' had been previously granted to 'favoured Individuals, among whom was Mr. Redfern'.[11]

With regard to the draft report criticisms of the new hospital, Macquarie admitted that some facilities had escaped consideration in the planning, but this was unintentional. He pointed out that, as Governor, he could not be expected to know about such matters in detail and took no responsibility for the oversights. Macquarie also refuted allegations that the colonial hospitals were dirty and dilapidated; pointing out that it was not the Governor's duty to make daily, weekly or even monthly visits to hospitals. In any case, he did not believe the hospitals were in a poor state; they had appeared satisfactory on occasional visits, and he had not observed any negligence. Macquarie emphasised that hospital patients 'were treated with a degree of Skill and Humanity which could not be exceeded'. Regarding the charge of unjustified use of medicine and hospital stores by Assistant Surgeon Redfern, he asserted that at no time had charges of that kind been made to his administration, or he would have immediately acted to censure 'the conduct of an Officer in whose integrity I had full confidence'.[12]

On 3 February 1821, while Redfern and his family resided in Airds, a draft record of his fiery interview with Bigge was delivered to his Sydney residence. It included a request that Redfern forward copies of his medical qualifications and respond to the interview draft immediately. When Redfern reached Sydney two days later, he carefully read the inquiry minutes and also the latest issue of *The Sydney Gazette*. A *Gazette* article had reviewed the progress of the inquiry and included a claim by Commissioner Bigge that there had been only one instance when cooperation with the inquiry was 'positively resisted' and had involved disrespect to his office. Redfern realised that could only have been himself, and with undisguised vengeance immediately wrote to Bigge, 'Now, Sir, as I am, I presume the Person to whom you allude as having positively resisted that Authority'. He reminded Bigge of the circumstances in June 1820 that had induced him 'to adopt the line of conduct' when 'you went so far as to tell me that I had appropriated large quantities of Medicines'. Bigge had also insinuated that his letter to James Bowman was 'heresy & treason not to be forgiven' and when questioned regarding the chastising of 'my apprentice ... you told me that if there were an Attorney General in the Colony, you would proceed against me in a different way'. Redfern reminded Bigge that at this point it became 'high time to resist - and I then determined no longer to submit to such a course of proceeding'.[13]

> The only regret I now feel on the subject, a regret I shall feel to the last Moment of my existence, is, that, when you, Sir, in my estimation, descended from the dignity becoming His Majesty's Commissioner of Enquiry, to a mode of examination by Menaces of heavy charges to be preferred against me, in order to confuse, perplex, & intimidate me, in a Manner More becoming a Spanish Inquisitor, I did submit to it for a Single Moment; – that I did not make you a low bow, and instantly retire from your presence.[14]

Redfern also informed Bigge that when Bowman arrived in the colony, he claimed the Commissioner would 'turn his back on Mr. Redfern' and ensure no more convict magistrates were appointed. These sentiments had been expressed repeatedly. At Bowman's request the hospital junior assistant Henry Cowper had been interviewed six times in order to extract as many accusations as possible against him. Redfern accused Bigge of seeking scurrilous input from all the 'underlings' in the hospital, some of whom had been dismissed by Redfern, and having interviewed even 'common strumpets in the streets of Sydney respecting the Character of Mr. Wentworth & myself'.[15]

Redfern's letter condemned Bigge's pernicious and malicious intent, asking why he had advised against paying Wentworth a half pension and ignored Wentworth's commendation that Dr Redfern was 'the only Man in the Colony in whom he would Confide' if dangerously ill. Why had Wentworth's testimony been deliberately omitted from the inquiry evidence? Did Bigge consider he was 'a Man of Much less responsibility' or of much less importance 'than to that of the confidential Mr. Henry Cowper?'[16]

Redfern then pointed out that the inquiry minutes also omitted his replies to Bigge's accusation that he was the 'Secretary to the Mutineers at the Nore, & even to Parker'. He wrote heatedly, 'I told you then, Sir, as I tell you now, that I never wrote a line for any Mutineer nor for any person connected with the Mutiny; nor did I ever see Parker'.

Another matter omitted from the minutes was Redfern's report proposing reforms to 'the Transportation of Convicts to this Colony'. Redfern added that because of this document 'your Protege, Mr. Bowman, and the other Naval Medical officers are indebted for their introduction into this Colony'. He reminded Bigge that 'you carped at my having stated that the present mode of conveying Convicts to this Country was nearly as perfect as possible' and dismissed my transportation report because others had written about it prior to this. Redfern responded:

> I, on the contrary, was placed at nearly the distance of half the circumference of the Globe I wrote my letter before those publications made their appearance – was no otherwise connected with the Subject, than a wish to prevent the dreadful Mortality among the Convicts on their passage to this Country – otherwise, I, without the vain presumption of aspiring to emulate your ability – and imitate your industry, in acquiring information – would have humbly endeavored to make myself Master of My Subject.[17]

Redfern closed the letter wryly wishing him a good voyage and hoping they would meet in London in a few months where 'the Press will be equally open to both – & where, if necessary, I shall defend myself in the face of the British Public'.[18]

Throughout his administration of the colony Governor Macquarie had consistently maintained that a government had a moral duty to act in the interest of all citizens, not just the privileged few. John Macarthur and the British Tories considered such views as almost anarchy and deemed these attempts at democracy in Australia as dangerously radical. Before Bigge departed, Macarthur continued to lobby the Commissioner on this point, writing:

... this democratic feeling has already taken deep root in the Colony, in consequence of the absurd and mischievous policy, pursued by Governor Macquarie and as there is already a strong combination amongst that class of persons, it cannot be too soon opposed with vigour.[19]

At their numerous private meetings Macarthur had also imbued Bigge with his grand visions of the colony's future: convicts should be assigned mostly to large landholders and punishments should be harsher. Macarthur advocated that farming estates should have a minimum of 10,000 acres and that new land grants should only go to 'men of character' who had the necessary skills and capital.[20] John Macarthur's views closely paralleled those of the landed aristocracy in rural England, who, ironically, had caused most convicts to be sent to New South Wales. Macarthur had long argued that emancipists should be kept in a state of 'degradation, Vassalage and Bondage' and should not reach a higher status than that of labourers, or tenants of gentlemen.[21] These ideas appealed to the class conscious Bigge and he gladly took them on board.

On 9 February, the day after Bigge embarked the *Dromedary* ready to sail, Redfern had his responses to the inquiry minutes delivered to the ship. An accompanying note stated that at such short notice he had been unable to fully examine all accusations but, in a few months, he would be in London and provide full explanations to Bigge.[22] Redfern had responded to only five of the forty questions.

The first response concerned his examination before the Court of Examiners of the Company of Surgeons in London. His answer to this query, which had been omitted from the minutes, explained the history of the Barber Surgeons Company founded in 1301, the formation of Company of Surgeons in 1745 and the renaming in 1800 to the Royal College of Surgeons.

During the interview Bigge had told Redfern that charges on his conduct would be exposed in his report and insinuated he ought to know about 'Murder and Treason'. Redfern demanded to see the charges in writing and on reading them now, he scornfully replied that the Commissioner was 'pleased to rate my Professional Abilities in examination, very low, & that my expectations in the way of My Profession were raised more than they ought to have been'. To the claim that his qualifications were insufficient for him to judge the suitability of someone for an assistant surgeon post,

Redfern responded 'I must now say, Sir, that, in the Judgement of any thinking Man, this is as unfair, illiberal an attack on My Medical character as the Most predetermined Malice could invent'.

Redfern admitted he was not a member of a medical society but pointed out that few men embarking on a naval career were, and not one of the surgeons Thomas Jamison, John Harris and William Bohan who validated Redfern's medical qualifications in 1808 was a member of a medical society. All had entered the navy and army with the same qualifications as Redfern. He reminded Bigge that he had welcomed an examination by a medical board, unlike William Bland who refused such scrutiny but whose qualifications Bigge apparently accepted. Since Bland had had the same medical training in England, Redfern wrote 'I do therefore consider this a most invidious attack'.[23]

Redfern next addressed Bigge's charges regarding the validity of his posting as a surgeon's mate on HMS *Standard*. In an obvious attempt to devalue Redfern's medical abilities, Bigge had noted the lowness of the surgeon's mate rank. Redfern pointed out that when he joined the navy the title of 'assistant surgeon' was not used and it was not until 1805 that it replaced 'surgeon's mate'. Redfern concluded his response to Bigge demanding that the numerous omissions in the interview record be corrected, as he considered them essential to his 'reputation'. He would provide more corrections now if Bigge delayed his departure, otherwise they would be delivered to him in London in a few months.[24] The *Dromedary* with John Bigge on board departed Port Jackson on 14 February 1821.[25]

Sarah Redfern would accompany William and his co-delegate, Edward Eagar, to England and she now busied herself for the trip. On 10 February 1821 Sarah placed an advertisement in *The Sydney Gazette* seeking a 'steady middle-aged' woman of 'good character' to accompany a family to England and care for an infant. All responses to the advertisement should be sent to the residence of Major Antill on Castlereagh Street where the Redferns stayed these days when visiting Sydney.[26]

Governor Macquarie was greatly relieved to be rid of Bigge and could now depart on his long-planned inspection of the Van Diemen's Land settlements. He asked his physician and close friend Dr Redfern to accompany him and although the departure of the 'rights' delegation to England was not far off, Redfern accepted the invitation because it provided an opportunity to talk to emancipists there about the petition. During his absence Sarah would stay with her sister Eliza Antill.

For the past few years the Wills siblings had been concerned about their mother and her unhappy marriage to George Howe. Sarah and George Howe had a daughter Jane in 1816 and the Wills children worried about the fate of their property in Sydney when George died. Sarah Howe had petitioned Governor Macquarie in 1815 to be granted the property at 96 George Street, which she and her first husband Edward Wills had originally leased for £953 and spent £4,000 on improvements. The land grant was intended as security for the Wills children. Macquarie agreed to the land grant, however, Sarah learnt a year later that the grant had been made out in George's name, not hers. Although this property had been supposedly secured by a prenuptial contract with Howe in 1812, Sarah believed it might be invalid if he died without a will. When George Howe became very ill in March 1821, he made a new will in her presence leaving everything to her.[27] This later proved to be a ruse on his part, and inheritance squabbles would later split the Wills-Howe family apart.

In the early morning of 4 April 1821 Redfern said goodbye to Sarah and their two-year-old son and boarded the *Midas* in readiness for the voyage to Van Diemen's Land. Macquarie had already embarked with Elizabeth and Lachlan Jr, his nephew Lieutenant Hector Macquarie, the topographic artist Major Taylor and an entourage of servants, baggage, horses and carriages. They sailed the next day but on leaving Port Jackson, the Pacific Ocean waves proved so mountainous the ship returned to the safety of the harbour, anchoring at noon on 6 April close to the entrance.

On Sunday, 8 April, Macquarie diarised 'Doctor Redfern having agreed to act Chaplain, we had Prayers read today to the Ship's Crew & officers; all of whom attended – and were all clean & well dressed'.[28] The next night 'nearly proved fatal' when massive waves at the harbour entrance caused the *Midas* to drag its anchor for a mile towards rocks. Macquarie worried his family was in 'eminent danger' despite assurances by Captain Beveridge that the ship was safe. But the weather got worse, and a distress signal brought rescue boats to tow the ship to a calmer location.

Redfern remained on board for the next four days to help secure the ship's anchorage, but the Macquaries and other tour members were rowed to Watson Bay to stay at the pilot's house. Macquarie recorded in his diary 'thankful to God that we had all made so miraculous an escape from a Watery Grave!'[29] On 13 April Captain Beveridge and Dr Redfern came ashore to inform Macquarie that the weather was fine enough to restart the voyage.

Within an hour the party was on board and the *Midas* set sail again for Van Diemen's Land. The weather for the next week was favourable and on 24 April the *Midas* reached Sullivans Cove at Hobart Town, where the Mulgrave Battery fired a 19-gun salute and ships anchoring in the cove repeated the salute. Macquarie and his group disembarked after a return salvo from the *Midas*. As Redfern went ashore, he recalled his visit to Hobart thirteen years earlier when John Piper had banished him to Van Diemen's Land on the *Estramina*. Then he had refused to disembark; now his status had changed significantly.

Over the next week Macquarie and his party surveyed public works, buildings, courts and convicts in and around Hobart Town. On 5 May 1821 the touring party set off to inspect Port Dalrymple (Launceston) in the north of the island. Macquarie and family were in carriages with the Lieutenant Governor William Sorell, Judge Advocate Wylde, Lieutenant Robinson, Surveyor Evans and Dr Redfern on horses. Five days later they reached Port Dalrymple. After inspecting the settlement on 15 May, Macquarie, his family and Redfern, went by barge on the Tamar River towards George Town. After nine miles carriages and horses were waiting to take the party the rest of the way. However the road proved so stony that Macquarie and family opted to continue the 'boisterous' passage down the river rather than take the coach. Redfern, with soldier Isaac Denning for protection, took the road. The barge party arrived in George Town at 8 pm where they were received with every military honour. Redfern and Denning came soon after and joined a noble dinner given by Lieutenant Colonel Cimitiere. Over the next few days, Redfern accompanied Macquarie on various inspections and dinners.[30]

On 19 May the tourists left on the return trip to Launceston. Elizabeth and son went by boat with Lieutenant Colonel Cimitiere, while Governor Macquarie rode on horses with Dr Redfern, Surveyor Evans and Dragoon Denning. The riders planned to reach the town before darkness with some minor diversions on the way. Macquarie later recalled that 'the sequel proved the fallacy of our calculations'. Two local settlers guided them through a rugged and rocky forest difficult for horses to traverse. They turned back after a guide claimed to know the bush better than the settlers, but he failed to find the main road. In heavy rain, they were led on 'such a rough, intricate, circuitous Route & so full of rocks & underwood' it took hours to find a track and, in doing so, Denning became lost. They searched until darkness without success.

When their guide left them at a track junction, Macquarie, Redfern and Evans strived to reach the main road to Launceston. But the rain, pitch-black night and rough track meant they could only walk their horses. Drenched to the skin, the three 'knew not which way to move' and wandered about in various directions for an hour. Fortunately 'Dr. Redfern's mare found the Road by his throwing the Bridle on her Neck – and allowing her to go her own way'. Once they reached the road again, they rode slowly with Evans acting as the guide. After 12 hours of riding and trekking the tired, wet and hungry men reached Launceston to be greeted by very concerned residents. The 59-year-old Macquarie wrote in his diary that he survived the ordeal 'feeling myself more fatigued and exhausted than I had ever been before in the whole course of my life'.[31] He was clearly starting to feel his age. Most likely the 46-year-old Redfern was exhausted as well, but the next day both men were fit enough to attend church service. This little misadventure reinforced the close bond between the two men.

Macquarie was particularly concerned the next day to hear that Denning had still not shown up, and he hired a tracker to search for him. To everyone's joy the lost soldier staggered into town the following morning. On 27 May the touring group set off by horse and coach for Hobart Town with planned inspections on the way, as well as naming several new townships, plains and mountains. On 6 June the touring party arrived at New Norfolk on the River Derwent northwest of Hobart Town. Here Redfern met with former Norfolk Island residents who had been relocated there. The party returned to Hobart by boat the following day.

After five weeks traversing the island, Macquarie arrived back in Hobart on 9 June where various communications were waiting. A letter from Colonial Under Secretary Goulburn informed him that Major General Thomas Brisbane would be the new Governor of

New South Wales and he would sail soon. This was welcomed by Macquarie who looked forward to returning to Scotland. On 30 June 1821 the touring group boarded the *Caroline* sailing to Sydney where they arrived on 12 July.[32]

As soon as he disembarked Redfern headed to the Antill's house to join Sarah and little 'Willey', and to hear the latest news. It was not good. George Howe had died, aged 52, on 11 May 1821 but had secretly altered his will, bequeathing nothing to his wife.[33] George had left the house, premises and land at 96 George Street, and the newspaper business, to his eldest son Robert Howe. The balance of the estate was to be sold, leased or held in trust for his children with Elizabeth Easton and Sarah's two youngest children Horatio Wills and Jane Howe. As the main beneficiary, Robert Howe now owned the land and buildings on George Street that Sarah and Edward Wills had held since 1805. These were the premises where the Wills family had always lived and it encompassed their shop, warehouse and the office of the *Gazette*. Sarah Howe was distraught at her husband's dishonesty. She challenged the will in court, testifying that prior to his death George had violent fits and was mentally deranged at the time of making the changes.[34]

This family crisis occurred while William was in Van Diemen's Land and by the time he returned, the court had declared George Howe's will and testament legal. Robert Howe requested that all debtors to the estate settle their accounts and announced the property would be auctioned. Furious pleas to Robert Howe from the five Wills children and husbands William Redfern and Henry Antill failed to gain any concessions and to protect herself Sarah Howe sold all her personal effects stored in the warehouse.[35]

The 26-year-old Robert Howe, who had worked in the printing office for years, took control of *The Sydney Gazette*. Prior to his inheritance he had been a profligate quarrelsome young man who had often been sued for libel and assault. But in 1820 he became a Wesleyan Methodist and under his editorship *The Sydney Gazette* increasingly took on morality and religious themes.[36]

Shortly after returning from the Van Diemen's Land tour, Redfern met with the committee preparing the petition for presentation to the Crown. A draft petition had been sent to rural districts and the responses were used to complete a final version, which would then be circulated for the signatures of emancipists supporting it. Much still needed to be done before October 1821 when Edward Eagar and William Redfern would depart for England on *The Duchess of York*, a ship partly owned by Eagar.[37]

Finalising travel plans was now a priority. The Redferns wanted to take James Tilley with them as a servant, but he was still a convict on a 14-year sentence. William sought to have his sentence mitigated for good behaviour and, within a week, Macquarie granted him an absolute pardon.[38] With this remittance Tilley was able to sail with the Redfern family and other servants to England.

Of critical concern to the Redferns was the proper management of the farm in their absence. This responsibility was given to Sarah's brother Thomas, who agreed to quit his bank position and manage the Redfern estate. To assist the widowed Sarah Howe, Redfern bought 270 acres of her land in Bringelly, land she had been granted in 1819. In September 1821 Redfern was granted 1180 acres of land just north of Campbellfield, a property he had been leasing since 1818.[39] Additionally Redfern purchased several neighbouring farms that enlarged the Campbellfield estate to 5100 acres on which wheat, maize and potatoes were cultivated. Fruit and vegetables were also grown on a six-acre garden and orchard. The property also held 15 horses, 790 cattle, 2656 sheep and 214 pigs. His leased farm at Bathurst grazed 815 cattle and 3190 sheep.[40] While the Redferns were in England, the management of this large estate would now be the responsibility of Thomas Wills.

William spent considerable time introducing Thomas to his farm practices and business arrangements, while Sarah and the other Wills children assisted their mother in trying to deny Robert Howe possession of their house in George Street. It was a stressful time; the first auction of the Howe estate was due on 25 September. On the day of the auction 16-year-old Edward Wills stood at the door of the house blocking Executor Joseph Underwood from entering. Underwood was outraged calling him a 'Puppy'. Edward threatened to knock him down if he said that again. 'You are a puppy!' roared Underwood and Edward promptly struck him in the face cutting his mouth. Soon after Underwood sued Edward for assault and the court ordered him to pay a fine of £5.[41]

The turmoil over George Howe's will and penurious state of his widow was probably an incentive for William to ensure that his wife had some independent financial security. On 17 October 1821 he transferred one of his £100 Bank of New South Wales shares to Sarah. The share certificate No 17, issued to William Redfern on 8 August 1818, with an endorsement to Sarah on the back, has survived and is the earliest known share certificate in Australia.[42]

On 22 October 1821, after months of preparation and debate, the petition committee, chaired by Redfern and administered by Eagar, made the final adjustments to the rights petition that had to be signed by emancipists across the colony. The document opened with a statement that the undersigned petitioners who had been transported to the colony and became free by serving out their sentence or by receiving a pardon. Emancipists and their families formed 82% of the free population (7556 men and women, 5859 children) while 18% were emigrants, excluding soldiers (1558 men and women, 878 children). As over half the colony's population were serving convicts, those becoming free annually meant a steady increase in the number of emancipists.

The document went on to say that through their hard labour and endeavour the petitioners had converted an unproductive wilderness into a thriving colony that was now an important part of the British Empire. The petitioners held the majority of investments in shipping, trade and commerce, owned three times the area of cultivable land and twice the number of sheep and cattle of other free settlers and their overall wealth was estimated nearly double of that of the emigrants. Page after page of the petition gave evidence that the colony's prosperity was mostly due to the efforts of convicts and emancipists.[43]

Governor Macquarie's humane and benevolent policies had led the petitioners to assume that the good character and rank they had gained, and the wealth they had acquired, was secured for them and their children. The recent court verdict had not only extinguished their property rights; it had unsettled the society.

> ... these decisions of the Courts of Justice in this Colony will have the effect of introducing and perpetuating party distinctions, unpleasant discussions, irritable feelings and Jealousies, heats, Animosities and diversions, between Your Majesty's free Subjects in these Territories, not only of the present Generations but for Generations to come; Will entirely take away all Encouragement,

incentive and Stimulus to good Conduct and reformation of manners, for how can these good consequences be expected where all hope of reward is withdrawn ... and the sure result of these fatal consequences will be most irretrievably to endanger, if not totally annihilate, the Agriculture and Commerce of the Colony, and so destroy possibly for ever the Labour and Fruits of Thirty Years of Laborious Industry.[44]

The petitioners called upon His Majesty to reverse the court findings and restore the emancipist's legal rights. The document was signed by Chairman William Redfern and co-signed by 1368 emancipists.[45] Governor Lachlan Macquarie fully supported the petition and provided his strongest commendations. In addition to the petition, William Redfern would convey a letter of recommendation for 'indulgent consideration and Protection' from Governor Macquarie to Lord Bathurst.

> Mr. Redfern having expressed a strong desire to be made known to your Lordship, I have yielded the more readily to his request, as I know that his character and conduct in this Colony have been very cruelly and maliciously misrepresented at Home and not unnaturally has made an unfavorable impression on your Lordship's mind against him. To remove this unfavorable impression is Mr. Redfern's most anxious wish, and I trust and hope he will be able to effect it.[46]

With this letter William Redfern hoped to restore his good name and honour in England from malicious misrepresentation he had recently received at the hand of Commissioner John Bigge.

Two days later William and Sarah said goodbye to their family and friends. On their parting, Macquarie told Redfern that he expected to sail for England within months and they would meet again in London. With that warm farewell, the Redfern family and their servants embarked the *Duchess of York*. On 25 October the ship sailed out of Port Jackson and took a northeast bearing across the South Pacific Ocean towards the island of Tahiti. At their first port of call, Papeete, the ship would take on board a cargo of coconut oil and arrowroot for later sale on the London market.

On 6 December, after 43 days at sea, the ship anchored in the harbour at Papeete. The gravely ill ruler of Tahiti, King Pomare, mistakenly feared that Edward Eagar had come to kill him because of a previous incident and forbade anyone to leave the ship. A year earlier Eagar had broken Samuel Marsden's trade monopoly by entering into an agreement with King Pomare in which his leased ship would bring a cargo of pork back to Sydney. However, the captain of Eagar's returning ship claimed the King had refused his terms, and that the pork and ship were now Pomare's property. Eagar seized the vessel in Sydney after it transpired that Samuel Marsden had bribed the captain to attempt this ruse. Eagar sued the captain in a costly but successful court case.[47]

Knowledge of William Redfern's medical expertise was already known in Tahiti. On 7 December he was requested to immediately come and treat King Pomare who suffered from 'Elephantiasis' (*lymphatic filariasis*) in his legs and arms. Redfern went to the royal residence and found a delusional man who greatly feared being attacked, asking Redfern if Eagar carried a weapon in his waistcoat. Little could be done for the King and the next day Redfern was recalled to his bedside after he had fainted. Redfern noted that 'his end was fast approaching' and shortly after the King died.

Four days later King Pomare was buried with much pomp and ceremony, attended by William and Sarah Redfern, Edward Eagar and gentlemen from the *Duchess of York*.[48] On 1 January 1822 the ship departed bearing east around Cape Horn and docked on 2 March 1822 in a hot seething Rio de Janeiro harbour at a time of political turmoil in Brazil. In a letter to D'Arcy Wentworth, Redfern told him of the Brazilians revolting against the Portuguese.[49] However, the *Duchess of York* departed unmolested and in early June 1822 arrived in London.

Exactly 21 years earlier William Redfern had left English soil on the *Canada* as a convict being transported to the penal colony in New South Wales because of a mutiny in the Royal Navy. He now returned to represent New South Wales in the presentation of an official petition to the Crown.

The reversal in Redfern's status could not have been starker.

Chapter 18

ANGEL OF DISCORD

But the Commissioner of Enquiry came amongst us as an Angel of Discord, before he had time to form any opinion he chose his party, he drew the line of demarcation, he revived every old and latent feeling of prejudice and hostility, his conduct had the effect of unduly exalting the one class and degrading the other.   Eagar to Bathurst, 1822[1]

On 7 June 1822 Edward Eagar and William Redfern went to the Colonial Office in Downing Street to present the emancipist civil rights petition to Under Secretary Robert Horton.[2] The document was to be reviewed by Lord Bathurst and discussed with legal experts before being tabled for debate in the British Parliament. If the petition was approved by Parliament, it would receive the Royal seal. Prior to these official duties, Redfern had found lodgings for his family in central London south of the Thames in the St Saviours area adjacent to the cathedral and close to the Old London Bridge.[3]

Redfern and Eagar heard that Commissioner Bigge's inquiry report had not yet been submitted to Parliament, but some leaked findings had already enraged Lachlan Macquarie's supporters in Britain. William Wentworth, now a barrister in London, was particularly agitated at the delay in publishing the full record of the inquiry interviews. On 9 March 1822 he placed an anonymous notice in *The Times* pointing out that John Bigge had been sent to New South Wales to review the administration of the colony and to report on abuses and had still not tabled these a year after his return – surely his findings could have been prepared on the return voyage! The notice reminded readers that as long as Bigge kept his report secret, he was paid an annual salary of £3000 – the delays were an unnecessary burden on the public purse.[4]

On 19 June 1822 the first of the three reports Bigge published appeared as *The Report of the Commissioner of Inquiry into the State of the Colony of New South Wales*. It was highly critical of Governor

Macquarie's policies and proposed increasing convict punishments to a degree that even the hardest criminals in Britain would fear transportation. It also recommended curtailing future convict rehabilitation efforts and the granting of emancipist rights.

Both Redfern and Eagar had expected personal condemnation in the report but were incensed at the explicitness of the published findings that were particularly damning for an official document. The 186-page report was riddled with unverified accusations by unidentified persons as well as irrational conclusions by Commissioner Bigge. Eagar's name was cited 50 times and Redfern's over 100 times.[5] Bizarrely, the report opened by praising William Redfern on improving the health of transported convicts and reducing mortality on convict ships. However, it then shifted to censuring him on almost every issue investigated by the inquiry. It strongly condemned Macquarie for appointing him as a magistrate. Indeed, Redfern's "star billing" in the report appeared to stem from his friendship to Lachlan and Elizabeth Macquarie, who had "allowed" him to enter into respectable society.

> It had been the good, or as many persons in the colony have thought, the ill fortune of Mr. Redfern, to have been distinguished by a more than ordinary share of the notice of Governor and Mrs. Macquarie. The proofs that they had received of his professional merits, and his activity and zeal in the performance of his public duties, confirmed the recommendations that they had received of him from Major General Foveaux; and they conceived that Mr. Redfern was equally fit on other grounds to be admitted to their own society, as well as to be particularly pointed out to the notice of others.[6]

It was implied that the social permissiveness of the Governor caused William Redfern to forget "where he had come from".

> Mr. Redfern's general demeanour, as from other sources of information, that his conduct in company, and even amongst those who were strangers to his situation, was both forward and obtrusive, and betrayed an entire forgetfulness in himself, of that occurrence in his life, which he will find it difficult to erase from the memory or feelings of others.[7]

After reading the draft inquiry minutes in Sydney Redfern had anticipated that Bigge's findings would be appalling but seeing the accusations printed in a public official document hurt him deeply.

Fortunately he had steeled himself for this battle on the passage to England and for months had planned to counter Bigge's insults with a fierce response.

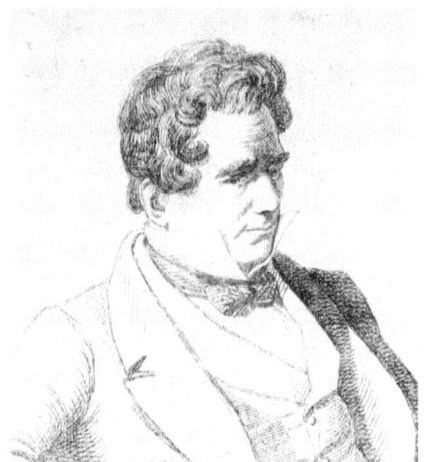 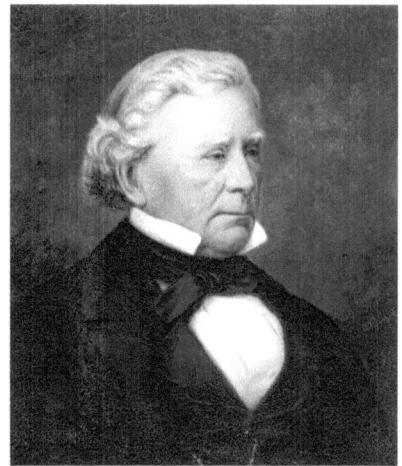

1848 and 1872 portraits of William Wentworth, son of D'Arcy Wentworth, who was a defender of Macquarie's egalitarian policies and Redfern's lawyer.

Barrister William Wentworth was also infuriated by the report. He had read Bigge's assertion that his father D'Arcy had identified him as the author of the anonymous pipe satirising Lieutenant Governor Molle. William decided to deny this – at least in public – and, declaring his reputation permanently damaged, he challenged Bigge to a duel. This caused the Colonial Under Secretary Horton to place Wentworth under police restraint, which upset him even more. Bigge offered to justify his claim about the Molle pipe in a newspaper, but Wentworth refused to accept this. Eventually the Commissioner agreed to remove the charge from the next report edition and insert an apology before it was tabled in Parliament.[8]

Revelations on the "pipe affair" were not the only matters Wentworth wanted expunged from the Bigge report. The repeated criticisms of Lachlan Macquarie and sycophantic praise of John Macarthur greatly angered him. He had been a friend of Macarthur's son, John Jr, who was a fellow barrister in London. The two fell out when William asked him for support in seeking to marry his sister Elizabeth; the same girl Redfern had treated for a walking debility years earlier. John Jr refused, and John Snr stopped the courtship in August 1818. Thereafter Wentworth vowed to 'pay him off in his own coin' and labelled John Jr a 'complete chip off the old block'.[9] One wonders what Elizabeth Macarthur's views were on the affair – by all accounts William was a personable young man who would eventually become one of Australia's richest and most powerful men. Macarthur also rejected Elizabeth's next suitor, surveyor John Oxley. She never married.

On 12 February 1822 Lachlan Macquarie and his family left Government House for the last time and were escorted by the soldiers and band of the 48th Regiment to the Sydney waterfront. The cheering crowds lining the brightly decorated and flag-festooned streets exhibited genuine regret at the governor's departure. On boarding the *Surry*, a 19-gun salute rang out in his honour and Macquarie recorded in his diary:

> The New Fort (named Fort Macquarie) and all the Rocks on Bennelong's Point, as well as Dawes Battery – and the Rocks on the Western Side of the Harbour, were covered with Men, Women, and Children, and a vast number of Boats were also sailing or rowing in the Harbour full of People, cheering us repeatedly as we passed along through them. This was to us a very grand and gratifying Sight – but at the same time a most affecting Scene, and could not be viewed by Mrs. Macquarie or myself without the deepest emotion, after a residence of upwards of Twelve Years amongst these poor attached People! [10]

The Sydney Gazette recorded the feelings of the colony 'Australia saw her Benefactor, for the last time, treading her once uncivilized and unsocial shores – and felt it too; – the parent and the child must endure the parting pang!' [11] Sailing out of Port Jackson Lachlan and Elizabeth Macquarie would have regretted leaving the many friends they had made over twelve years and who they would never see again. Undoubtedly, some tears were shed.

On 5 July 1822 the *Surry* docked in London after an uneventful voyage. Within days Lachlan Macquarie met with William Redfern, Edward Eagar, William Wentworth and General Joseph Foveaux to discuss the best way to respond to the accusations in the Bigge Report. Before this meeting Macquarie had had an encouraging interview with the Colonial Secretary Lord Bathurst, and three weeks later sent him a list of his achievements in 56 paragraphs.[12] On 5 August 1822 Lord Castlereagh, a powerful long-time friend of Macquarie, presented him to His Majesty King George IV. After these welcoming and gracious occasions, Lachlan Macquarie expected he would be received into the highest official circles. His hopes were dashed a week later when Castlereagh, who was being blackmailed over an alleged homosexual relationship, committed suicide and Macquarie lost an influential ally.

On 27 July 1822 excerpts from the Bigge Report appeared in newspapers for the first time. *The Morning Advertiser* informed readers that much of the report criticised Governor Macquarie's policies and administration. It highlighted that ex-convicts, 'many of whom are intelligent persons and men of wealth', were invited to dine at Government House and this had offended some military officers.[13] Other newspapers routinely published interesting parts of the Bigge Report. On 2 August 1822 *The Public Ledger and Daily Advertiser* went as far as to list the names and crimes of emancipists appointed by Macquarie to official posts in the colony. The list included William Redfern and Edward Eagar.[14] Two days later, the two men inserted a notice in the London newspaper *John Bull*, asking the public to withhold judgement on accusations against them until they had published their response. They also pointed out that Governor Macquarie was now in London and would use his presence 'to explain and vindicate his measures'.[15]

From his London chambers, barrister John Macarthur Jr was delighted with the publication of the Bigge findings. He believed they would help restore social order to the colony and applauded the recommendations that would assist his father's enterprises in New South Wales. He told his mother that 'Mr Redfern is wild with rage' and was preparing an answer with 'his worthy co-adjutor Mr. Eagar' – observing arrogantly, 'as if the gentry of this Country will care about the feelings or rhapsodies of two emancipated convicts'. Intriguingly, Joseph Foveaux called on John Jr to express indignation at being 'harshly treated' in the Report. Probably he also wanted to gauge the level of official support that Commissioner Bigge had in London legal circles.[16]

Two weeks after the Redfern and Eagar notice in the *John Bull*, its editor Theodore Hook published a lengthy reply. He informed his readers that he knew nothing of Mr Redfern, a delegate of the convicts in the colony, who was apparently writing a book that would 'make Ministers ashamed of themselves'. The newspaper regretted this because Governor Macquarie was closely allied to Mr

Redfern, a surgeon transported to Botany Bay for the Nore mutiny. Theodore Hook added that 'Governor Macquarie stands upon too high ground to need such an auxiliary' and was clearly 'able to fight his own battles'. The editor noted that often the commissioners sent to British colonies were 'official tinkers' who let 'personal feeling' and 'prejudice' creep into their findings. He added that a colonial governor should not 'be questioned and brow-beat by any whipper-snapper underling … send out as a sort of accredited spy'. The editor then advised that nothing should be inserted in any public report that was not 'plain truth'.[17] Redfern promptly sent a letter requesting it be inserted in the next *John Bull* edition. The editor declined, saying he understood Redfern's concerns but feared that the publication of his letter could have legal consequences.[18]

Elizabeth Macquarie's health had been poor for several years. It became worse when she reached England and was grateful to have her personal physician, Dr Redfern, close by. He became a frequent visitor to the Macquarie residence, both to treat Elizabeth and to discuss politics with Lachlan. Redfern's attention to Mrs Macquarie 'afforded some amusement in Downing Street' but neither family heeded silly gossip. When Dr Redfern advised Elizabeth to avoid London's damp weather, the Macquaries decided to spend the coming winter in France and Italy. In case Lachlan Macquarie was called before the Committee of the House of Commons during this period, he asked William Redfern to represent him in the defence of his administration.[19]

William and Sarah particularly wanted to visit members of the Redfern family whom Sarah had never met, and William had not seen for 21 years. Sarah was now three months pregnant and, while her husband was busy in responding to the Bigge Report, she met with her mother's Harding family and offered two orphaned cousins, 12-year-old Emily and 10-year-old Selina Willey, a future home. It was decided that the two girls would join them on the ship once they set sail for Australia. The Redfern's servant James Tilley had been reunited with his wife and four sons and intended to return with them to the Campbellfield estate.

The plan for Sarah and 3-year-old William to meet paternal family in England and Ireland did not eventuate. The road to Trowbridge was poor and it was probably inadvisable for the pregnant Sarah to make that coach trip. There is no record of his wife and son accompanying William when he visited his sister-in-law Ann Redfern, the widow of his brother Thomas who died in 1814, aged 51. William was indebted to Ann and Thomas for their care during his medical apprenticeship and for their generosity while he was in Coldbath Fields prison. It is also probable that they assisted him financially when he purchased land on Norfolk Island.[20] When Ann's only child, Thomas, died aged 28 a year earlier, William became her closest relative.

In late August, just prior to their European sojourn, Lachlan and Elizabeth Macquarie visited Scotland. Redfern used this break in his treatment of Elizabeth to visit his siblings in Belfast. He arrived in Dublin on 14 September 1822 and stayed at the fashionable O'Dienne's, reputably a hotel for the rich and famous.[21] From there he travelled to Belfast to visit his family. William had last seen his brother Joseph and sisters Eliza and Margaret when they were children; they were now married with families. Joseph, who had inherited the saddler business, had recently got in contact with their brother Robert in America and William would later convince Robert to migrate to Australia.[22]

After leaving Ireland William Redfern made a short stopover in London where he asked Wentworth and Eagar to charge John Bigge with violating His Majesty's instructions. Confident that that his pregnant wife was in robust health, he travelled to Edinburgh to investigate studying medicine there. He was instantly charmed by the old city and enrolled to study *Materia Medica* (pharmacology) at the University of Edinburgh for the winter semester, November to April.[23] Redfern knew he could not complete the semester, but he was eager to experience the excitement and rewards of studying the latest in medical science at this prestigious institution.

Edward Eagar proved a most effective advocate for the emancipist cause, and on 12 November he sent a 70-page rebuttal of the Bigge Report to Colonial Secretary Bathurst. In this lengthy discourse he referred to John Bigge as the 'Angel of Discord' who had, by praising one class of resident and degrading the other, divided a harmonious colony through prejudice and hostility.[24] Although Bigge hotly disputed Eagar's rebuttal, Under Secretary Horton met with Eagar and expressed some sympathy for the emancipists' cause.[25] At the same time Horton, with James Stephen and Francis Forbes, was preparing a new bill for the administration of justice in New South Wales. Francis Forbes, the former Chief Justice of Newfoundland, had just been appointed as Chief Justice in the colony to replace Judge Field. William Redfern informed D'Arcy Wentworth by letter of Forbes' appointment, writing that Forbes had interviewed him and he judged him 'the very man' for the Chief Justice post – 'a clever, humble, unafflicted and liberal man' who would 'be exceedingly popular'.[26]

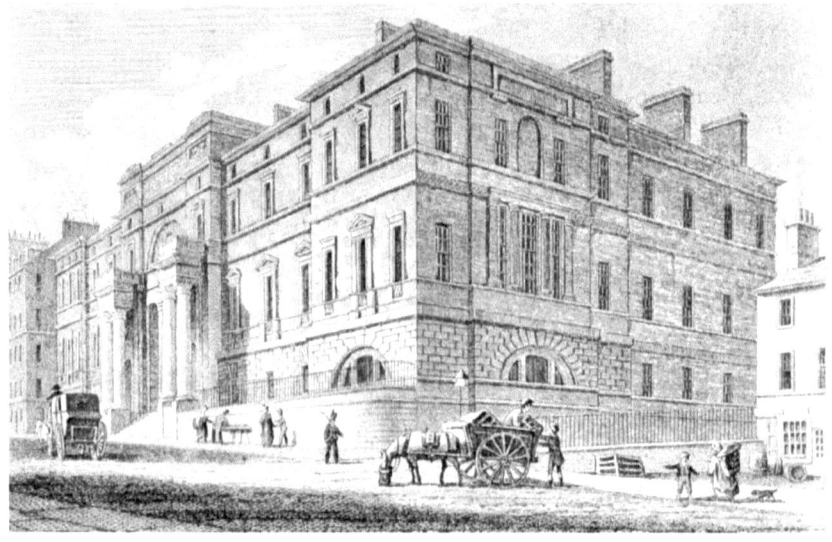

1820 engraving of University of Edinburgh where Redfern studied medicine.

In early December Redfern skipped classes at the University of Edinburgh and returned to London to be with pregnant Sarah and oversee his court action against John Bigge. On 9 December 1822 John Bigge received notice from the Clerkenwell Grand Jury that William Redfern was suing him for damages to his character and reputation arising from the report into the state of the New South Wales colony.[27] Bigge was unfazed that the indictment held him 'criminally responsible' for a report that had made false accusations against Redfern. He was only following Bathurst's instructions and therefore expected the Government Law Office to fully defend his actions.[28]

When Redfern's legal team asked Under Secretary Robert Horton to appear as their witness in the proceedings, he refused. Redfern immediately apologised and told him that he had been unaware his name had been put forward. He thanked Horton for the 'urbanity' of their last meeting in June, adding that this was in stark contrast to the manners of Bigge who had used 'his Power to nail my wing of hope, by robbing me of that which is dearer to me than life – My Good Name'. Redfern told the Under Secretary that he was about to publish a pamphlet exposing the unflattering nature of Bigge's veracity, honour and morality. He then asked Horton – clearly not as an afterthought – if he would support his request to Lord Bathurst for a half pay pension in lieu of his 18 years medical service.[29] Three weeks later Redfern met again with Horton whose conciliatory attitude gave him hope that his pension would be approved. Bathurst and Bigge eventually agreed to grant a half pay pension to Redfern provided he admitted to having used medical stores for his private practice.[30] Redfern's court action against Bigge was withdrawn after it was agreed that his name would not be slandered in the two later Bigge reports, and that earlier false accusations would be withdrawn.

William Redfern had planned to return to his medical studies in Edinburgh, but family matters intervened. His 67-year-old sister-in-law Ann Redfern was critically ill, and he went to Trowbridge with Sarah and William Jr. The imminent arrival of their second child required Sarah to be at William's side. In that village, on 7 February 1823, Sarah gave birth to a healthy boy and the proud father put a note in *The Sun* newspaper, 'Births: On Friday last, at Trowbridge, Wiltshire, the Lady of William Redfern, Esq., of a son'.[31] The boy was named Robert Joseph Foveaux Redfern after his grandfather Robert and their close friend Joseph Foveaux.

In Trowbridge, the prognosis of Ann was grim, and he could do little to help. Once Sarah and the baby were ready to travel, they returned to London and settled into a quiet area in New Kent Road Newington, south of their previous residence. Ann was left in the palliative care of locals and died on 17 May 1823.[32] In her will she bequeathed everything to William Redfern. However, her estate was £580 in debt to Rector Richardson who lent money to Thomas when he went bankrupt in 1807. After advice from Eagar, Redfern renounced all claims to the estate and its obligations.[33]

On 21 February and 13 March 1823, the long awaited second and third Reports of the Bigge Inquiry, *The Judicial Establishments* and *The State of Agriculture and Trade*, were officially released.

William Redfern was cited in the third report but not criticised. It would seem that the threat of litigation had dulled Bigge's zeal to further demean the Nore mutineer. He even rated Redfern's properties among the colony's eight top farms 'in the best state of cultivation and exhibit the greatest improvement'.

More tellingly, Bigge contradicted his first report by disputing Henry Cowper's evidence on the abysmal state of the Sydney hospital dispensary records. He now claimed they were in 'a great degree attributable to want of care in preserving them' by Cowper, and he praised the efforts of Redfern's clerk William Johnstone.[34]

> A greater degree of regularity and method appears to have taken place on the appointment of a convict clerk, named Johnstone, whom I have had occasion to mention in my former Report, and who was appointed to perform the duties of clerk at the general hospital in the month of June 1818. From the imperfect reference to the hospital books previous to this date, and from the confused manner in which the entries of discharges and deaths were noticed in them, the abstract that was made from them at my request, by Mr. Henry Cowper, is not much to be relied upon.[35]

Edward Eagar strongly criticised the second report *The Judicial Establishments*. In a letter to Bathurst in April 1823, he disputed the validity of the inquiry findings and Bigge's proposed reforms. Eagar was especially critical of objections to the colonial courts having trial by jury, a key aspect of the emancipist rights petition, and told Bathurst that emancipists insisted on its introduction.[36]

The 33-year-old William Wentworth was still unable to financially support himself as a barrister in London and had applied unsuccessfully for the position of Attorney General in New South Wales. Assisted by Redfern, he became a Fellow at Cambridge University Peterhouse College studying law for a semester.[37] While there, Wentworth entered into the Chancellor's Medal competition to write a poem on the topic for that year, 'Australasia'. He dedicated his 'crude effort' of a 443-line poem on the glories of 'new Britannia' to Lachlan Macquarie, who he labelled Australia's 'foster father' because of his liberal and humanitarian efforts.[38] Although Wentworth's poem came second in the competition, its verses would later become very popular in Australia.

Wentworth also employed his considerable energy and literary skills in revising his 1819 publication *A Statistical, Historical, and*

Political Description of the Colony. In the 1819 book he had strongly advocated an elected assembly in New South Wales, a free press, trial by jury and the settlement of Australia by free emigrants rather than convicts. In the revised edition, published in 1824 as two volumes, Wentworth expanded on these themes emphasising their importance to the future prosperity of the colony. The first volume also covered the Bigge inquiry and findings, and it is apparent that William Redfern and Edward Eagar contributed significantly to the views expressed. In fact, this book provided Redfern with a public platform to voice his criticisms of Bigge.

In London Redfern and Eagar had reluctantly come to realise the powerful influence John Bigge and the inquiry findings had on the parliament and the Tory government. Indeed legislation based on his inquiry reports was being adopted while the emancipist's petition for rights was just being tabled in the House of Commons on 12 June 1823. After many delays and scant support for the *New South Wales Jurisdiction Bill*, Scottish MP Sir James Mackintosh came to its aid on 2 July. Mackintosh had known Lachlan Macquarie in India and previously defended him against attacks in the British Parliament. Concerned that clauses on convict pardons and trial by jury may be whittled from the bill, Mackintosh re-tabled the rights petition and argued forcefully, with Eagar, Redfern and Wentworth watching from the gallery, for the inclusion of *all* the emancipist demands. His motion was defeated in a Commons dominated by Tories.[39] But Mackintosh refused to give up and eventually the inclusion of colonial pardons was agreed to, and the *Act of 1823* passed on the 7 July 1823. Mackintosh fought tenaciously for trial by jury to be routinely available in colonial courts, the debate closed when the Tory MP George Canning moved a sunset clause that allowed the legislation to be reconsidered in five years.[40]

With the passing of the *1823 Act*, pardons issued by colonial governors would have the same effect as pardons granted under the great seal, and with this statute civil rights were fully restored to emancipists. Moreover, after 35 years of autocratic colonial rule, the British had allowed the formation of the Legislative Council of New South Wales. This in turn permitted the establishment of an independent Supreme Court, a Court of Quarter Sessions and a *limited* provision for trial by jury in civil cases. The new legal system abolished the Judge Advocate Court and removed the last vestiges of military rule. Although the new Legislative Council of New South Wales was not entirely independent of Britain, it was more autonomous. Unfortunately the right of emancipists to own property was omitted from the *Act of 1823* and it would take another year of lobbying by Edward Eagar before this was allowed in the *Transportation Act of 1824*.

In late July 1823 Lachlan Macquarie and his family returned to London from their European travels, three weeks after the *Act of 1823* legislation had been passed. While in France, Macquarie had written his response to the accusations against him in the three published Reports and had sent Bathurst a lengthy discourse on 'Bigge's false, vindictive, & malicious' accounts and conclusions.[41] Although Macquarie considered the Reports to be 'of a very insidious and hostile nature', he claimed that he would have excused Bigge of 'all his invectives' had he not openly accused him of having defrauded the colony. Macquarie was confident that the 'testimony of every unprejudiced man' in the colony would consider this charge to be totally 'slanderous and unfounded'.[42]

Revitalised by a restful winter in Italy, Macquarie was ready to salvage his reputation and to secure the pension he was entitled to. He protested strongly to Bathurst but was told that the publication of his rejection of the Bigge inquiry findings would embarrass the government and might affect his pension application. Macquarie reluctantly avoided publicly defending his reputation in print, at a time when the attacks by newspapers were so scathing that he contemplated suing *The Edinburgh Review* editor for libel. Deeply hurt by the lack of official appreciation of his long governorship, he consoled himself philosophically 'that a clean conscience may defy the whole world'.[43] It was not until after his death in July 1824, that Macquarie's friends persuaded the British government to publish parts of his reply as an 1828 parliamentary paper.[44]

Once the *Act of 1823* had been passed and given the Royal Seal, William and Sarah Redfern began to plan their return to Australia. William had purchased nine merino rams and five ewes from the celebrated Essex agriculturist and Whig MP Charles Western. The merino sheep came from the famous 'Paular' flock the late King George III had imported from Spain.[45] Redfern also planned to make wine at his farm and needed to source suitable vine cuttings and a winemaker. It was decided that William would sail in

October to the Portuguese Island of Madeira off the Moroccan coast, while Sarah, the two boys and her cousins Emily and Selina, remained in London until February 1824, when they would sail to Australia and visit Madeira en route. A positive aspect of this plan was that the warm climate would benefit Redfern, who for several years had suffered from 'ill health and debility arising from his arduous services'.[46] Recently he had become exhausted from supporting the emancipist rights petition and defending his reputation against the Bigge inquiry accusations. A stress-free stay on Madeira would provide him with some much-needed rest.

Before Redfern departed for Madeira, the family visited their friends Lachlan and Elizabeth Macquarie for a last time. The former Governor presented William with a farewell gift of an 'Ivory Tooth-pick Case that had a small Magnetic Compass on top, a Mirror inside the lid and housed two Metallic Tooth-picks'.[47] The Macquaries had hoped the Redferns could visit their home on the Isle of Mull before leaving, but that was not possible.[48] The farewell would have been a sad occasion for both families. William sailed to Madeira on the *Advertiser* in October 1823 and was soon touring the island vineyards, learning viticulture and purchasing a variety of fruit trees and grape vines. He was particularly attracted to the grape variety Verdelho and would be one of the first to introduce the grape commercially into Australia.

William Wentworth's new edition of the *Statistical Account of the British Settlements in Australasia* was released in early 1824. The first 340 pages of volume 1 dealt mostly with colonial activities prior to the Bigge inquiry. In the latter pages Wentworth censures the British government for being misled by a 'booby commissioner', who was either an 'unconscious dupe, or the corrupt coadjutor of as turbulent and tyrannical a faction, as ever any community was yet cursed with'.[49] He called Bigge's reports 'nauseous trash' peppered with 'private scandal and vituperation'. Defending Macquarie's efforts for equality and reform, Wentworth claimed the Governor had been dealt a 'deadly blow' by Exclusives in the colony.[50] He also angrily criticised John Bigge and James Bowman for attempting to viciously malign William Redfern.

During Redfern's stay in Madeira, Sarah wrote two letters to Lord Bathurst in the Colonial Office on his behalf. The first on 18

October 1823 complained that her husband had not yet received an answer from the King regarding his pension.[51] In her second letter, on 13 January 1824, Sarah told Bathurst that their land in New South Wales was too small to hold the additional livestock her husband had purchased in England to improve the production of fine wool at his farm. She wrote that William was at present in Madeira 'for the benefit of his health' and to procure grape vines suitable for a vineyard. And since the civil rights uncertainties had made it almost impossible for an emancipist to purchase land, she, as a free person in the colony, was applying for land to be granted in her husband's name. Within days she received approval from Horton.[52] At the same time she also heard the sad news that her mother had died after a long illness in July 1823, aged 45.[53]

On 19 February 1824, Sarah Redfern, her two sons, cousins Emily and Selina Willey, William Wentworth, servant James Tilley and his family boarded the ship *Alfred* sailing for Madeira. Also on board was a friend of Wentworth, the London barrister Robert Wardell, his mother and his niece Jane Fisher. Wardell had been editor of the Whig newspaper *The Statesman* and had unsuccessfully applied for the position of Attorney General of New South Wales. With similar political views, the two barristers decided to continue their legal careers in Australia and to launch a new newspaper, *The Australian*. Also loaded on the *Alfred* were Redfern's merino sheep and large quantities of English grass seeds.[54]

En route to Madeira passengers on the *Alfred* complained about the dreadful cabins and poor food. Most had paid dearly for the passage and expected to be 'treated as gentlemen'. Instead, they had 'wet and comfortless' cabins, often ankle deep with water, and twice a week were served meals of salted meat and doughboys (dumplings) made with stinking water. Everything on board was filthy.[55] The *Alfred* arrived in Madeira on 2 April 1824 with William Redfern waiting on the docks with Emanuel Serown and his two children. The Serowns were a Madeira family experienced in cultivating grapes and making wine who Redfern had engaged to work at his Campbellfield farm. He had also purchased a variety of Madeira grape varieties as well as Spanish chestnut and walnut trees.[56] Although the Captain of the *Alfred* had been instructed to stay only three hours in Madeira, the passengers insisted on going ashore to purchase meat, fruit, vegetables and drinking water.

At their next port of call, St Jago in the Cape Verde Islands, the passengers bought goats to provide daily fresh milk and later asserted that without it, they would have starved on the long voyage. Passenger John Mackeness, the new Sheriff for New South Wales, would later claim that all on board suffered from bad food and cabins, and had 'literally lived worse than prisoners'!

Such complaints may have amused Redfern – he knew what it was really like to be a ship's prisoner, and this was a pleasure cruise in comparison. On the other hand, conditions aboard convict transports had improved markedly with Redfern and Fitzpatrick's reforms, while no such regulations existed yet for merchant ships. The services on private passenger ships depended entirely on the professionalism and honesty of ship owners. A year later William Wentworth and Robert Wardell sued the owner of the *Alfred* for not providing a service that was commensurate with its cost. Wentworth won £80 in damages; exactly the amount he paid for the voyage and Wardell settled his case out of court.[57]

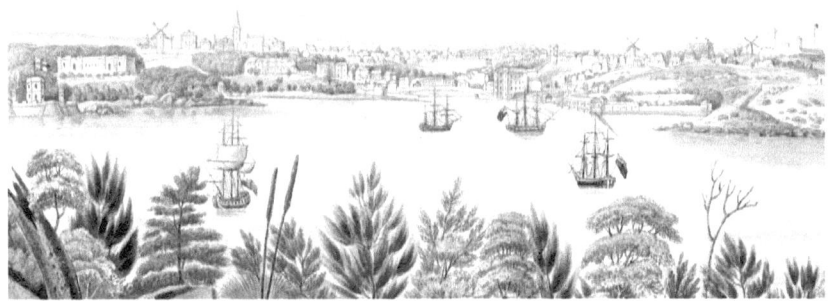

An 1825 painting of Sydney Cove viewed from the south. To the left of the cove is Bennelong Point with Fort Macquarie and Government House stables; on the right is Dawes Point.

Chapter 19

A NEW GOVERNOR

I shall not fail, on my arrival in England, to support the claims of the colonists to an extension of their civil rights. It is but justice to the free inhabitants of the colony to say, that my opinion is founded on my personal experience of their loyalty, good conduct, and private worth, during the time I have reside among them. Thomas Brisbane, 1824[1]

When the *Alfred* docked in Sydney Cove on 15 July 1824, William and Sarah would have been overjoyed at the familiar sights of the Sydney townscape. It appeared to be the same hustling bustling place they had left three years ago, but they would soon learn otherwise. Sir Thomas Brisbane had been governor of the colony for over two years and much had changed. The condemnation of Macquarie's rehabilitation efforts in the Bigge Reports had led to a harsher convict regime – much stricter punishments and the use of chain gangs had become the norm. Sydney was a penal settlement again and the sense of optimism had evaporated.

Although not appreciated by the residents of the colony at the time, Governor Brisbane privately abhorred the Bigge reforms and the harsh treatment of convicts, but his administration was obliged to follow instructions from the Colonial Office. It was also evident that Brisbane had little interest in politics or governance. He was a highly educated man who sought this governorship because it gave him an opportunity to pursue his astronomy interests and survey stars in the southern skies. Consequently his leadership style was the opposite of his predecessor. Macquarie had been a gregarious leader who sought advice from and gave opportunities to clever men of every class and profession. Brisbane made it clear from the outset that he was not inclined to socialise with colonists and, when he did, it would only be in an official capacity. By natural attrition rather than intent, emancipists in civil posts were gradually replaced and this satisfied the instructions of the Colonial Office. With their spokesmen Edward Eagar and William Redfern in

England, the emancipists kept a low profile during Brisbane's reign and reduced their campaigning for equal rights.

As a trained astronomer, Brisbane built at his own expense an observatory in Parramatta. With the help of two assistants he brought from Europe, Carl Rümker and James Dunlop, Brisbane catalogued 7000 new stars in the southern skies. This meant that he often left the leadership of the government in Sydney to others. Whereas Macquarie revelled in the minutiae of governance, Brisbane delegated most daily matters to his Colonial Secretary Frederick Goulburn or to departmental heads. The lack of strong leadership led to internal friction and excessive bureaucracy.

Brisbane's officials implemented many of the Bigge reforms and revamped the assigned convict servant system. In keeping with Macarthur's advice to Bigge, the direct payment of assigned convict servants was abolished and they were allocated according to the size of the farms and businesses. The servants were no longer given free time or any reward for extra labours. This reduced costs for masters but deprived convicts of time to grow food when off-duty and limited their ability to support a family. Convict servants were now assigned to larger estates for the entire length of their sentence, reducing administration for the government but often forcing convicts and their families to live in slave-like conditions.

The longterm servant assignments to large estates had other serious consequences for convicts. It often discouraged owners from helping valuable servants obtain a ticket of leave or a pardon. These were now only given for exceptional service and to convicts fortunate enough to have a fair and considerate master. As a further barrier to full rehabilitation, the Bigge reforms prevented ticket of leave convicts from buying property and land grants to ex-convicts were restricted to ten acres unless they already held property.[2] Such rules prejudiced under-privileged emancipists but not men like Redfern who already owned large areas of land. The new servant assignment system pleased most wealthy landholders but generated discontent and hostility in convict ranks. Governor Brisbane apparently understood the unfairness of these changes and, to his credit, avoided their rigid application where possible.

During William and Sarah's absence overseas, major changes had also been made to government institutions. In November 1822, the Sterling monetary system introduced by Macquarie was abandoned, and the Spanish Silver Dollar again became the colony's legal tender. Each silver dollar coin had a face value of 5s, but its market value in banknotes issued by the colonial bank was only 4s 2d. This 10d difference reduced government expenditure, but devalued salaries of officials by 20% and eroded the value of government payments. Farmers selling grain to government stores were short-changed and they responded by planting less wheat. The resulting shortfall in cereal production caused a flood of complaints to the Colonial Office in London. Within three years the British Parliament reversed the policy and Stirling once again became the official currency.[3]

Criticisms were voiced in Britain about the colony's administration and about Colonial Secretary Goulburn supporting only business and not the farming community. While Brisbane did not share Macquarie's zeal for social equality, he did believe in promoting meritocracy. Ironically, Macquarie's bitterest enemies, the Exclusives, initially supported Brisbane but when their demands were not prioritised, they became outspoken critics. In order to placate them, Secretary Goulburn manipulated the administration by filtering correspondence, rescinding Brisbane's explicit instructions and issuing his own official edicts. In late 1823 Brisbane became so disillusioned with continual administrative disruptions, he considered resigning. In May 1824 a frustrated Brisbane discovered that the man he had appointed to minimise his involvement in government minutia had totally usurped his authority, and he requested the Colonial Office to dismiss him.[4]

On 17 May 1824 the new Chief Justice Francis Forbes formally opened the Supreme Court. The use of trial by jury was now permitted in certain cases but was not widely supported. The Exclusives believed that it favoured the rights of commoners and therefore a dilution of their own influence. Three months later the first Legislative Council met to advise on issues presided over by the Governor. The five council members appointed by King George IV were Colonial Secretary Goulburn, Chief Justice Forbes, Lieutenant Governor William Stewart, Surveyor General John Oxley and Principal Surgeon James Bowman. The Council's role was strictly advisory; they could propose laws but only the Governor could implement them.[5] Moreover, a bill only became law if the Chief Justice certified that it was consistent with existing laws in England and the colony.

William Redfern would have been troubled by the many legal and administrative changes taking place as a result of the Bigge reforms. He understood better than most the harm it could have on convicts and emancipists and seeing their enactment would have been depressing. The optimism that convicts used to have in working off their sentence or gaining a pardon for good behaviour had largely vanished. Being an assigned servant was now more akin to slavery. Redfern realised that many of the opportunities offered to him in 1802 had disappeared; it would no longer be possible for a convict to be a surgeon, earn money and buy land. With pardons and freedom now almost out of reach for many convicts, what had Bigge and the British done to rehabilitation opportunities?

The Redfern family had quickly settled back into the pattern of farm life, as had their cousin Emily and the Portuguese Serown family. The other cousin Selina had moved in with the Antill family in Camden. In their long absence, Thomas Wills had managed the farm well despite changing government regulations and the death of his young wife and child only a year after their marriage. Emanuel Serown planted the Madeira vine cuttings on a plot 1.2 miles southeast of the Campbellfield farmhouse where Redfern built a sandstone cottage for the Serown family. This heritage-listed cottage still exists on Ben Lomond Road in Minto.[6]

The Redferns' close friend and fellow passenger on the *Alfred*, William Wentworth, had set up a lawyer's office in Macquarie Place and agreed to handle their legal and business affairs. Edward Eagar remained in London to continue his fight for emancipist rights and had asked Redfern and Wentworth to act for him in the dissolution of his partnership with Francis Ewen Forbes (not Chief Justice Francis Forbes) in the Indian and South Sea trade.[7] The firm 'Eagar & Forbes' had three partners, William Redfern, William Hutchinson and John Hosking. Francis Forbes had made some bad business decisions while Eagar was in England and the company was bankrupt. In May 1824 Hutchinson took out an injunction preventing Forbes from selling company's property.[8]

Edward Eagar intended returning to his wife Jemima and their four children in Sydney, but he never did. He later dissolved the marriage and wed a 16-year-old London girl, with whom he fathered ten children. With the closure of Eagar's firm, Wentworth and Redfern ensured his ex-wife Jemima was financially secure and had a house. In 1830, just a year after William Wentworth married Sarah Cox, he had an affair with Jemima, who bore him a son.

In August 1824 Redfern wrote to Governor Brisbane about Lord Bathurst's promise to Sarah for a land grant based on his capital. In reply, Brisbane's secretary Major John Ovens requested details of his estate. Redfern listed 1430 cattle, 4500 sheep, 22 horses, 60 pigs, 14 merino sheep, 100 bushels of wheat and agriculture implements, worth a total of £16,350, not including the value of land or buildings. The cattle were valued at £5 each, a horse £30, a pig 33s and a sheep 30s. The recently acquired merino sheep were worth £50 each. The estate employed 78 male and female servants, of which 46 were convicts.[9]

When three months passed without a response from Ovens, Redfern contacted him again. He was informed that his proposal was 'perfectly satisfactory' but, for the governor to grant him the land, matters regarding water rights on his estate needed to be resolved in order 'to remove motives of Jealousy from others'. The Governor had been informed that his farm had 'engrossed all the good water in the neighbourhood'. Since water was required for residents in nearby Campbelltown, Brisbane sought to acquire this water in exchange for more land. An astonished Redfern replied that there was 'misinformation or misconception' regarding the water on his farm. It was correct that he had 'an excellent Pond of fresh water' on his farm close to Campbelltown and on very hot days the residents were 'obliged to come considerable distances for water from that Pond'.[10] But Redfern stressed that 'it was merely a Pond, never being a running Stream'. He pointed out that it was unfair to accuse him of 'engrossing the water, calculated for the supply of the Town' because he had owned the land and 'the Pond in question' long before the town existed.

Moreover, the pond was at least one to two miles away from Campbelltown, with several farms in between and, because it was at a lower level, water could not flow to the town 'except by the intervention of Machinery'. He then claimed that nobody had ever been precluded from using the pond, and he was willing to give the town some rights to use the water but nothing 'could possibly induce me to sell my whole right to the Pond'. Redfern added that there were water sources 'much more eligible and available than the Pond in question' and suggested the Georges River might be piped to the town.¹¹ Within days the water exchange requirement was dropped, and Redfern was granted 1000 acres in Bathurst.¹²

On 16 September 1824, Chief Justice Forbes admitted William Wentworth and Robert Wardell to the bar as barristers.¹³ A month later the two launched the first edition of a new newspaper, *The Australian*, without seeking the governor's authorisation. The first editorial informed readers that 'A free Press is the most legitimate, and at the same time the most powerful weapon that can be employed to annihilate such influence, frustrate the designs of tyranny, and restrain the arm of oppression'.¹⁴ Brisbane was not concerned about the lack of governmental approval and made no attempt to block further publications. Quite the contrary; he declared that freedom of the press was essential, and that any censorship of *The Sydney Gazette* would also be discouraged.¹⁵

Not unexpectedly, Wentworth and Wardell used *The Australian* to vigorously support emancipist equal rights, the introduction of self-government, trial by jury and for emancipists to be allowed to vote and sit on court juries. The newspaper's motto was 'to convert a prison into a colony fit for a freeman'.¹⁶ William Wentworth used his editorials to attack the Exclusives and quickly became a leading political figure in the colony.

News of Lachlan Macquarie's death in London on 1 July 1824, reached William and Sarah Redfern in late October and they were deeply saddened at the loss of a close and valued friend. On 28 October 1824 *The Australian* published the notice 'The inhabitants of this colony will feel deep grief at the information contained in the following – Governor Macquarie is no more – he departed this life on the 1st inst. after a short illness'.¹⁷ The paper stated that interested parties would meet at the residence of John Campbell on 5 November to plan a funeral procession for the late Governor and secure funds for the erection of a monument in his honour. The news triggered widespread sorrow and many public tributes.

The circumstances of Lachlan Macquarie's death reached the colony somewhat later. He had travelled to London in April 1824 to defend the criticisms of his governorship and finalise details of the pension promised by Bathurst. He became extremely ill on 11 June and Elizabeth rushed from Scotland to London to be at his side. Although close to death, Lachlan insisted on informing his friends in Sydney of his final successes. On 22 June 1824 he wrote to William Wentworth telling him of his two interviews with Home Secretary Robert Peel, and that the Transportation Act had been changed to 'Restoring the emancipists to all substantial rights and privileges, not only in New South Wales, but in all His Majesty's Dominions'. This Act had now passed both Houses and been given Royal Assent.[18] Lachlan Macquarie died a week later at the age of 62. Elizabeth wrote to her friends that she believed he might have recovered if his Sydney physicians had treated him.

> I certainly think our beloved friend might have been longer spared to us, and at any rate, that his sufferings w'd have been lessened, had Drs. Wentworth and Redfern, been about him.[19]

In fact, Elizabeth was also very critical of the way the London doctors had behaved during her husband's illness.

> The Doctors behaved to me, in a manner totally different from what I had ever been used to from medical men. Their conduct to me was the reverse of what w'd have been agreeable.[20]

On 5 November 1824 friends and colleagues of the late Lachlan Macquarie met to discuss the organisation of a commemorative procession in Sydney. A mourning period of one month was decided on, and a fund set up to erect a monument in his memory. Redfern initiated the fund with a donation of £200. Despite the efforts of the committee, the funds raised were insufficient for a monument to be erected – the response of the business community was decidedly muted. On the three days prior to the funeral procession the committee requested that the church bells of St James and St Philip's churches toll at sunrise and sunset. The St James clergy refused the request because Principal Surgeon Bowman claimed it might have 'an injurious effect on the sick' in the hospital.[21] Since James Bowman was now married to John Macarthur's youngest daughter Mary, the apparent lack of sympathy for the past liberal Governor was not surprising.

Sydney commemorated Lachlan Macquarie's passing with the St Philip's bells tolling for three days at dawn and at dusk. On Sunday 14 November 1824 a procession assembled at the courthouse in Castlereagh Street and marched through streets lined with thousands of residents to the St Philip's church. The mourners were led by Reverend William Cowper followed by Major Henry Antill, John Campbell, Macquarie's former secretary and William Redfern, 'Surgeon to His late Excellency's Family'.[22] The dignified column of people included the majority of high ranking civil and military officers, followed by gentlemen, merchants and the public. Governor Brisbane was not in attendance and nor was anyone associated with John Macarthur. At St Philip's church Reverend Cowper gave a sermon and spoke glowingly of the late Governor's strength, humility and idealism. Despite opposition in the colony and from Britain, Macquarie had strived to rehabilitate prisoners and offered hope to the less fortunate.

In a real sense Lachlan Macquarie's passing marked the end of an enlightened era in colonial governance. He was not the first or the last colonial governor to face fierce political opposition from ultra-conservatives at home and abroad, but Macquarie's term ended a sequence of five progressive colonial leaders, stretching back to Arthur Phillip, who encouraged convicts to become future law-abiding citizens. Some historians have argued that the increase in convict punishments following Macquarie's tenure was a direct result of his excessive concessions to emancipists. Such arguments are specious. The dominant motive for harsher convict treatment was that Britain faced rising unemployment and petty crime, and its courts needed transportation to be a deterrent. This was an era of great wealth for the gentry in Britain, and the Tory government, who held power through rotten-borough electorates, did not want New South Wales to become a free colony; it must remain a remote prison for political dissidents and petty felons. The *sole* purpose for John Bigge going to New South Wales was to ensure that it stayed a *penal* colony. To this end Bigge ridiculed Macquarie's enlightened efforts and recommended measures that made transportation dreaded for the next two decades.

From the standpoint of establishing democracy in Australia, the colony was truly blessed when Lachlan Macquarie was appointed governor in 1809, especially as it only happened after the man chosen initially became ill at the last moment. The policies, appointments and institutions that Macquarie introduced forged the nation's democratic and egalitarian character. It seems utterly inconceivable today that a British government refused to recognise his long and distinguished leadership of the young colony, or that he had to plead for a pension! Of course, cynical observers consider that final rebuke as "another feather in his cap" – after all, the Tories saw Lachlan Macquarie as more akin to the rights activist Thomas Paine than a man who had created a prosperous democracy out of an impoverished penal colony.

In many respects it is more significant that the colony, not the colonising nation, honoured Lachlan Macquarie's fairness, energy and humanity. It was he who officially named the colony 'Australia' and is widely recognised as the nation's 'Father'. The longest-serving Governor was to be sorely missed in later years and a song celebrating those good times was often heard in colonial inns and taverns:

> Our gallant Governor has gone,
> Across the rolling sea,
> To tell the King on England's throne,
> What merry men are we.
> Macquarie was the prince of men!
> Australia's pride and joy!
> We ne'er shall see his like again.
> Here's to the old Viceroy![23]

William Wentworth continued his vigorous fight for emancipists' rights in *The Australian*. On 9 January 1825, he and Wardell lodged a request with the Supreme Court to allow emancipists to be on jury lists. Technicalities prevented them from pleading their case and it was dismissed.[24] On the 26 January, Wentworth as the President, and Redfern as his deputy, welcomed 80 men to the 37th Foundation Day dinner.[25] At this grand affair many toasts were proposed. Wentworth gave a loudly applauded speech followed by a toast to 'trial by jury'. A military band played after each of many toasts, and dinner guests sang with great enthusiasm a new song about 'the demons of discord' residing in England.[26]

The 50-year-old William Redfern seems to have lost some of his enthusiasm for political battles and he now focused more on his farm and family. He also prepared for the arrival of his brother Robert whom he had not seen for over 28 years. Robert, 56, and his son William, 16, had left Philadelphia for England where he had made a successful application to Lord Bathurst in July 1824 to become a free settler in Australia and be given a land grant.[27] On 10 March 1825 Robert and William arrived in Sydney Cove on the

Phoenix to a joyous welcome.²⁸ Within days, Robert received a 2000-acre land grant in the town of Bathurst and William made him a loan of £1000 to get started in the new country.²⁹

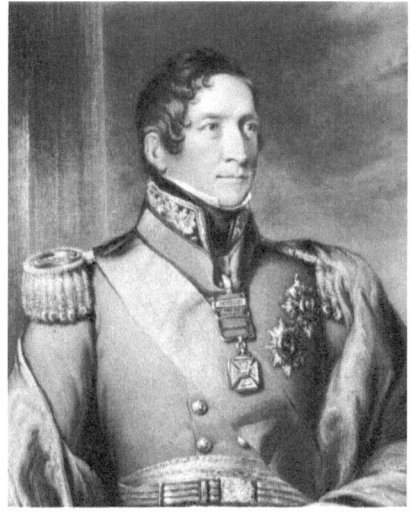 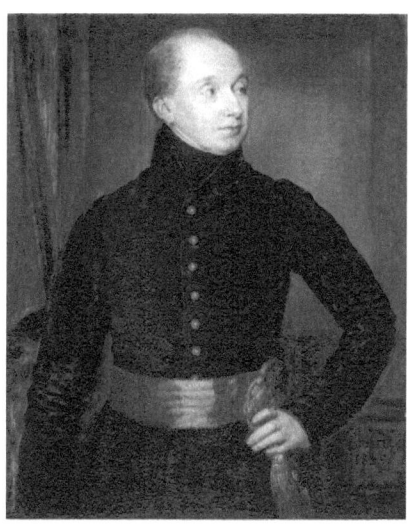

1842 portrait of Thomas Brisbane, sixth Governor of NSW (1821-25).

1825 portrait of Ralph Darling, seventh Governor of NSW (1825-31).

The announcement that General Ralph Darling would become the next governor of New South Wales was published in Britain long before Sir Thomas Brisbane received notice of his dismissal. On 28 April 1825, *The Australian* reported that the new appointment had been announced in London newspapers in December 1824, cynically observing that such an 'unceremonious dismissal' was nothing new for the British government. *The Australian* expressed disbelief that a governor 'would be treated so indecorously' as to read in the press that his 'Services [were] no longer necessary' rather than be told by official letter.³⁰ In fact, Brisbane had been notified of his replacement only days prior to *The Australian* article.

Although Governor Brisbane had sought to soften the Bigge reforms, convicts were treated much more harshly than before, and reoffenders were cruelly punished in special penal settlements in Moreton Bay and Norfolk Island. Since June 1825 Norfolk had been re-settled as a 'penitentiary island' from which there was no hope of return.³¹ Additionally, the convict transport *Phoenix* (not the *Phoenix* Robert Redfern arrived on) had been refitted as the first prison hulk in the colony.³² The hulk was moored in Hulk Bay (today Lavender Bay) and held imprisoned convicts awaiting trial or shipment to prison settlements. There is no record of what William Redfern thought of the latest purpose for Norfolk Island or the presence of a prison hulk in Sydney harbour, but he certainly would have detested both. He probably shared his criticisms with Wentworth and Wardell but wisely they did not publish them in their newspaper.

During the cold wet winter of June 1825, the 50-year-old Redfern was seriously unwell. No details of his illness are recorded but as Redfern periodically had a severe inflammation in the joints of his hands, which can be clearly seen in his handwriting, and may have suffered from arthritis. Redfern decided that 'for the benefit of his health' he would sail to England on the merchant ship *Phoenix*, the same vessel his brother had arrived on, but this time would make the journey without Sarah or the boys. On 1 July William updated his will and auctioned fifty of his milk cows that were 'well known to be some of the best Breed of Cattle in the Colony'.[33] On 7 July 1825, Redfern departed on the *Phoenix* that sailed from Sydney loaded with the largest cargo ever exported from the colony.[34] Days into the journey south to Bass Strait, the ship was badly damaged by a storm in the Pacific Ocean. High winds and massive waves washed away a longboat, the bulwarks and the cookhouse, and shredded two mainsails. Leaking heavily, Captain Francis Dixon turned back to Sydney while Redfern helped where he could with injuries and sickness on board. After 15 days at sea, the jury-rigged *Phoenix* slowly limped back into Port Jackson.[35]

To the great surprise and delight of his family and friends William Redfern had returned unexpectedly to Sydney. The shipboard traumas must have been significant because he decided not to tempt the sea gods further and cancelled his passage. *The Sydney Gazette* announced Redfern's decision on 1 September.

> Dr. Redfern, who thought of proceeding to England for the benefit of his health, and for that purpose had actually taken his passage on the Phoenix, Captain Dixon, we are pleased to learn is about abandoning his former intention in favour of future permanent residence in the Colony, and entertains the thought of shortly taking up his abode in the capital, with the view of resuming his practice, which is pretty generally remembered to have been universal. We should be sorry to offer any remark

detrimental to the interests of other Gentlemen, particularly one of peculiar eminence amongst us, but we have no hesitation in saying, that Dr. Redfern would soon have his hands full of business.[36]

The article suggests Redfern would soon resume his medical practice in Sydney, but this would take some time to eventuate.

In October 1825 Governor Brisbane prepared to return to Britain. His governorship had not been easy for the colony or himself. He was a fair person, but most in the colony found him aloof and as his administration gave limited support to struggling farmers, he had few friends in rural districts. Moreover, Brisbane was never comfortable with emancipists, and they were not sorry to see him go. However, these sentiments were about to change in a most intriguing way. Brisbane's final actions as governor gained him a level of esteem across the colony that was totally unexpected.

The surge in Brisbane's popularity started oddly; he accepted an invitation to a farewell dinner by a group of Exclusives, principally composed of John Macarthur and his friends. The news of this supposedly 'public' farewell to the governor caused indignation among prominent emancipists who were not invited. On 17 October 1825 eight gentlemen, including William Redfern, Simeon Lord, William Wentworth and Edward Hall, announced in *The Sydney Gazette* that, because the proposed farewell dinner had excluded many respectable residents, another dinner was to be held for anyone wishing to honour Governor Brisbane.[37] The next day a committee headed by William Redfern and Simeon Lord invited Brisbane to attend *their* public dinner. The Governor was puzzled why there was a need for two dinners until he was told that the Exclusives' dinner was a private affair and excluded emancipists. To avoid factionalism, Brisbane informed the Exclusives that he would gladly attend their dinner if leading emancipists in the colony were also invited.[38]

Antagonism between the elites and those they considered inferior boiled over. In the next issue of *The Australian*, Wentworth informed readers that the era when 'Nimrods of the Territory once domineered over Prisoners, Emancipists and Free alike' was about to close.[39] On 21 October 1825 a public meeting at the courthouse in Castlereagh Street was called to arrange a farewell tribute for the Governor. In a packed courtroom, Wentworth gave a passionate speech and delivered a farewell address to Governor Brisbane for debate and approval. Wentworth had also added a plea for the governor to request the British government for 'Trial by Jury' and the establishment of a House of Assembly. There were some objections, but all his proposals were eventually endorsed.[40]

The recently retired D'Arcy Wentworth was now free from the demands of public office, and he joined the colonists in this cause. A delegation of D'Arcy and William Wentworth, Thomas Raine, Daniel Cooper, William Browne, Simeon Lord, William Redfern and Edward Hall presented the governor with a written tribute. Contrary to the advice of his officials, Brisbane publicly received the delegation at Government House in the presence of the Lieutenant Governor William Stewart, Judge John Stephen and civil and military officers. The formality of the occasion gave official recognition to the emancipists' cause.[41] The Exclusives were aghast and withdrew the farewell dinner invitation to the Governor.[42] The emancipists were of course delighted that their event would now be the only dinner farewelling the governor.

Responding to the emancipists' request for support, Brisbane promised that, on arrival in England, he would help their claim for 'an extension of their civil rights'. This would be in recognition for 'their loyalty, good conduct, and private worth' during his time in the colony. He thanked the inhabitants who honoured him with their parting tribute and offered sincerest wishes for 'the continued prosperity of the country which they have adopted'.[43]

The news of his response spread like a wildfire through the colony. Sir Thomas Brisbane had managed to become a belated instant hero in a colony he had ruled for last four years. His popularity among the colony's rank and file, who included some of the richest and largest landholders in the colony, soared. The offer to support them in Britain meant that settlers finally saw Brisbane as a "good bloke", though it had taken him some time to show it.

On 4 November 1825 the men who had presented Brisbane with the farewell address were invited to dine at Government House in Parramatta.[44] At this function Redfern was advised that as a free settler "recently arrived" in Australia he was eligible to purchase Crown land in accordance with the May 1825 regulations. On 5 November he applied to Governor Brisbane for permission to purchase 5000 acres of Crown land. One of Brisbane's last official acts was to give Redfern permission to purchase a large area of Crown land in Bathurst.[45]

On 7 November 1825 the public dinner to farewell Governor Brisbane, organised by D'Arcy Wentworth and 18 stewards, was held at Nash's Inn, Parramatta.[46] It was a truly gala occasion for the 100 colonists who were able to attend – the oversubscribed event was open to all who could afford the ticket price of £1.[47] Governor Brisbane, flanked by Lieutenant Governor Stewart and most of his senior staff, arrived at the Inn with the band playing 'See the conquering Hero comes'. The hosts escorted the governor to his seat amid loud cheering and a lavish dinner followed. It was a night of high spirits and many toasts; the last toast being: 'Our Brisbane, and Freedom for ever!'[48]

The Governor then rose and gave a warm final address that was loudly applauded:

> Gentlemen: my reputation has been assailed; misrepresentations have been cast upon it; but you have cleared it (Hear, hear) and I shall now retire from this Colony under different circumstances from what I otherwise should have done (Hear, hear). You have not only given me a free clearance, but you have furnished me with a clean bill of health, such as no ship has ever quitted the Colony with before, and under similar circumstances (Hear, hear, and shouts of applause).[49]

The social and political success of the emancipists' dinner was a bitter blow for John Macarthur and the Exclusives. Sixty-one of these men voiced their disgust at this lapse in social protocol in a petition sent to Lord Bathurst. It disputed the 'wild opinions' in Brisbane's farewell address, claiming they had aroused the 'worse passions of the lower orders' and incited a 'spirit of animosity towards the upper classes' and legitimate authority. Macarthur claimed the views of 'Emancipated Convicts', aka 'the Republican Party', were not those of the respectable people in the colony.[50]

Governor Brisbane's departure from Sydney on 29 November 1825 was a quiet affair. It did not involve the colourful parades and crowds that had accompanied Macquarie's farewell, but one suspects that Brisbane would not have expected it.[51] He looked forward to returning to Britain to set up another observatory in the Scottish Highlands. His astronomical work in Australia had been highly successful and he would be made a Fellow of the Royal Society for his survey of southern skies from Parramatta.

A NEW GOVERNOR

The seventh Governor of New South Wales, Lieutenant General Ralph Darling, docked in Sydney Cove on 18 Dec 1825. The crowds attending his disembarkation gave him a muted reception. It was widely known that Darling's last post was to oversee slave plantations in Mauritius, and many considered his appointment as governor of New South Wales quite inappropriate. These concerns strengthened as Darling promptly set about rejigging the colony's administration along military lines, with strict adherence to regulation and loyalty of subordinates. Whereas Brisbane had lessened the severity of Bigge's reforms, Darling applied them in full. It was apparent that his governorship would be a stormy one.

Two days after taking office, Ralph Darling proclaimed that the Legislative Council representation would increase from five to seven men – four executive and three other members. The new members were Archdeacon Thomas Scott and John Macarthur.[52] This reversed the guarantee given by Macarthur at his 1817 court martial that he would refrain from all future political activities in the colony. Of course, there is ample evidence that Macarthur interfered in colonial politics from the day he stepped ashore in Sydney. However, his nomination to the Legislative Council gave him the opportunity to manipulate government at a much higher level and now he had *official* permission to do it. Moreover, he had two like-minded members to support him in the Council, his son-in-law Principal Surgeon James Bowman and John Bigge's brother-in-law, Archdeacon Thomas Scott.

With an ultraconservative Governor in charge and John Macarthur in the Legislative Council, the future of convicts and emancipists in the colony was about to get much grimmer.

Chapter 20

FRACTIOUS TIMES

Mr. Howe, Proprietor and Editor of the Sydney Gazette, appeared before their Worships to claim protection against Doctor Redfern.
The Sydney Gazette, 1827[1]

Buoyed by the success of Brisbane's farewell dinner, a delegation of residents advocating increased rights for emancipists sought to present a welcoming address to Governor Darling. On 2 January 1826 William Redfern, D'Arcy and William Wentworth were among fourteen colonists who met to discuss the nature of the presentation, and ten days later a draft of the address was tabled at a large public meeting chaired by William Wentworth. The draft document pointed out that expanding the Legislative Council to include members sympathetic to John Macarthur's causes was not beneficial to the colony and insisted that future Council members be elected rather than appointed. A delegation of 15 men, who included the two Wentworths, William Redfern, Edward Hall and Simeon Lord, took the address to Government House.[2]

Governor Darling thanked the men for their efforts, assuring them that he would do everything possible for the prosperity and happiness of all classes.[3] In truth, it was later divulged that he regarded the address as offensive and 'extremely injudicious'. He was already aware of the shift in political power in the colony and informed the Colonial Office Under Secretary Robert Hay that the confidence of the emancipists had by their recent actions 'gained an ascendancy'. Darling surmised that this could 'not be put down or rather kept down by the Old Settlers' who were few in number and it would 'be in vain for the old settlers who have taken the lead, to expect to retain the exclusive possession of it', as wary colonists had 'a morbid sensibility' that saw 'danger from every trifling occurrence'. Darling told Hay that he would distance himself from the emancipist faction and resist their demands.[4]

Governor Darling clearly shared Lord Bathurst's opinion of ex-convicts and believed them unworthy of consideration, let alone generous treatment. It would not be long before both convicts and emancipists experienced the diabolical consequences of Darling's application of the orders to enforce the Bigge reforms. What made matters worse, Darling treated the reforms as a discretionary weapon to be imposed lightly on those who shared his ideology and harshly on those who did not. Convicts and emancipists suffered the full severity of the new penal regulations.

But Darling was soon to realise that he did not wield the power he had in Mauritius and had misjudged the support for reform in the colony. He had not fully grasped that most residents embraced the principles of fairness and equity espoused by Macquarie and were not prepared to relinquish them for Tory inspired reforms. The resistance to the reforms was, in fact, predictable – many free and freed men saw no benefit in reversing hard-won rights gained over decades. Indeed, most wanted fewer restrictions and fairer, rather than harsher, treatment of those in servitude.

The resistance to reforms came at a time when emancipists were strongly asserting their claim to be recognised as full British citizens. Of course, John Macarthur and the Exclusives opposed such recognition, as did British Tories, and the conservative forces fought to suppress full emancipation. These diametrically opposed visions were fully appreciated by Darling, yet he placed himself firmly on the side of the elite minority. Such an alliance was not a surprise considering the rationale behind his appointment, but for him to oppose the majority aspirations of the colony supported by its wealthiest and most influential men was Sisyphean. And the governor would eventually discover this.

Darling's changes to punishments were draconian. A system of brutal chain gangs was introduced as a secondary punishment and these men built roads and bridges for the expanding colony. The gangs worked in leg-irons during the day and were shackled together at night. Darling did not hesitate sending convicts to the penal settlements of Port Macquarie, Moreton Bay or Norfolk Island where discipline was even stricter and punishments cruel. Darling believed convicts in penal settlements should expect to live permanently in irons, and this would act as a warning to any contemplating petty crimes in Britain. His experiences with slaves on Mauritius plantations seem to have guided his actions.

The Faustian benefit of this more regimented punishment system was that it provided much cheaper servant labour. In the 1820s the colony experienced an economic boom from larger farm estates and soaring profits for farm products. John Macarthur's lobbying for land development led to the formation of the Australian Agricultural Society (AAS) enabled by the 1824 Act of parliament. In late 1825 the AAS was granted one million acres of land at Port Stephens, north of Newcastle.[5] The emancipists, who were excluded from participating in the AAS, declared it a fraudulent land steal that 'must entail inevitable destruction on the industry of every loyal subject in the Colony'.[6]

With the availability of vast new tracts of land, AAS members borrowed heavily and outbid each other for the limited reserves of livestock in the colony. The rush on bank funds coincided with the re-introduction of the Sterling currency system in December 1825 and caused a foreign exchange crisis. In early 1826, reserves at the Bank of New South Wales were alarmingly low and, to make matters worse, a new bank, the *Bank of Australia*, was established on 22 February 1826 and this further reduced assets at the old bank. The new 'pure Merino Bank' was founded by Exclusives for selected clients – emancipists were excluded.[7]

The exclusiveness of the Bank of Australia led to an outcry for another bank open to anyone wanting to benefit from the boom. The lobbyists for a third colonial bank were mostly merchants and included Thomas James, Gregory Blaxland, Edward Hall, William Redfern, Samuel Terry, William Hutchinson and John Black. These men met on 27 February 1826 and proposed the creation of the *Sydney Bank* with initial capital of £100,000 in £50 shares.[8] At the meeting, William Redfern, stressed that 'every man should be ready to repel any insidious attack' on the bank assets. He urged caution in establishing a new bank and advocated for the right of all shareholders to vote on the board. He also recommended the bank's business to be conducted in Sterling currency.

> The sooner the dollars were out of the country the better, for a merchant did not know on what grounds he stood, when a cargo came from England; whereas if a sterling circulation took place, he would at once know how to act.[9]

Although the 700 £50 shares sold quickly, some investors advised that the new bank merge with the established Bank of

New South Wales. Initially the merger idea was opposed but at an 18 March meeting of Bank of New South Wales shareholders, many of whom were investors in the new bank, warned that the Sydney Bank might fail and 'almost if not entirely [be] met with annihilation'. They advised that their money would be safer in an existing bank. After a lengthy discussion, it was decided that plans for a new bank be abandoned, and the Bank of New South Wales would offer another 700 shares for public purchase.[10]

Governor Darling was asked by the Bank of New South Wales directors to approve the offer of 700 new shares at £30 each. He refused.[11] The directors responded by issuing a notice on all current shareholders requiring payment of outstanding debts on existing shares within a fortnight. On 4 May 1826 William Redfern paid £80 as the second instalment on his Bank Stock Certificates, No. 177 to 180.[12] The call on payments ensured that the Bank of New South Wales remained solvent, and on 11 May the directors applied to the governor for a loan of £20,000. They assured him this would avoid the possibility of a liquidation of bank assets and widespread bankruptcy in the colony. After examining the bank accounts, Darling approved the loan.[13] This bolstered confidence in the Bank of New South Wales and increased deposits. Within months the £20,000 was repaid in full to the government.

Since January 1826, William Redfern and his family had been in residence in 'one half of Mr. Lord's stately edifice' in Macquarie Place. The precise reason for the move from their farm to Sydney is unclear, but it was probably linked to the schooling of William Jr. Residing in Macquarie Place offered Redfern the opportunity to restart his private medical practice again, but for several months he was kept busy marketing his farm produce, overseeing his bank responsibilities and acting as executor of the estate of his friend James Meehan who had recently died aged 52. Also, much time was taken up dissolving the firm Eagar and Forbes, of which he was a partner. It took another year and several court cases to close the firm.[14]

Although Redfern did not publicise his move to Sydney, it soon became known that The Doctor was in town again and 'many poor patients' visited Macquarie Place to seek his help.[15] In May 1826, physician William Bland became seriously ill, and the closure of his busy practice affected many in Sydney. The urgent demands of

Bland's abandoned patients would have been a major reason for Redfern to re-open his medical practice. He and Bland knew each other well and both helped the Benevolent Society of New South Wales established by Macquarie in 1818 for the disadvantaged.[16] Although close colleagues they often disagreed. Bland routinely criticised Macquarie for attaching his name to public buildings and, because of some sarcastic verse lampooning the governor he spent a year in a Parramatta prison. Nevertheless, in 1822, a year after Macquarie opened the Benevolent Asylum for the aged, infirm, blind and destitute, William Bland became its pro-bono surgeon.

On 3 June 1826, Dr Redfern announced in *The Sydney Gazette* that he would provide private medical services for the next three to six months at Mrs Waple's building in Pitt Street with 'advice to the poor gratis' on Mondays and Thursday between 7 and 9 am.[17] And as Dr Bland was temporarily unable to treat the sick at the Benevolent Asylum, it is likely that Redfern did this duty as well.

Redfern became totally immersed in medicine again. One case interested him immediately; it was a Tahitian suffering from 'Elephantiasis' (*lymphatic filariasis*). Redfern first encountered the disease in 1822 when treating King Pomare on Tahiti. He found no information on the classification of this tropical disease in the four leading medical books by Sauvages, Vogel, Sagar or Cullen. This led him to write a short article for *The Sydney Gazette* about the unusual aspects of this ailment, which enlarges limbs and hardens the skin.[18] He claimed the occurrence was 'a matter of interest to every medical enquirer, who may not have had an opportunity of seeing the disease in question, in the various climates in which it occurs, and in the multifarious forms which it assumes'. Redfern took care to forewarn his Tahitian patient that other medical gentlemen might wish to come and examine him.

Dr Redfern's offer of free treatment for the poor came to the attention of staff at the Sydney hospital. On 21 June 1826, just three weeks after Redfern's practice opened, Principal Surgeon James Bowman announced that a public dispensary would be opened to provide a free medical service to the poor who were 'frequently doomed to linger on the bed of sickness'. Bowman requested that wealthier Sydney residents donate towards the new service, which would be under the patronage of Governor Darling. Dr Bowman, hospital surgeons James Mitchell and James McIntyre and military surgeons Robert Ivory and James Doyle, were to offer one hour of their services for free each week.[19] The public dispensary was not a new idea. Bowman would have known from hospital records that Redfern had proposed such a service in 1816, but it was then considered impracticable.[20]

The timing of Bowman's offer was immediately questioned in the press. A letter to *The Monitor* from 'the Scrutator' published in on 14 July wondered at the 'philanthropic feelings developed by those medical gentlemen' that led to the new service. The letter did not question the 'purity of their motives' or the sincerity of their promises, but noted that none of these medical men had ever visited the Benevolent Asylum or assisted Dr Bland's work at the asylum. The writer asked why Dr Bland was excluded from this initiative, adding, 'how prone is man to step over the praise-worthy deeds of others; climb the uneasy path of competition, and mount the eminence of self-aggrandizement!'[21]

The Australian newspaper published other criticisms. It called the sudden launch of a free dispensary a last-ditch effort by an 'expiring Faction' and said that time would reveal the hollowness of their pretensions. The editor pointed out, that while this 'Sick-List Institution' expected to cure the poor in one hour, Dr Redfern gave three hours to his poor patients. It reminded readers that Dr Bowman was unknown as a private medical practitioner in Sydney and 'never crossed the threshold of a poor man's door'. Therefore his treatment of the poor for one hour a week 'would have no great predilection'. *The Australian* asked 'Why not invite Dr. Redfern, who was in full practice, why not indeed invite all the Medical Gentlemen to join in such a praiseworthy undertaking'.[22]

The editor of *The Sydney Gazette*, Robert Howe, came to James Bowman's defence by asserting he was entitled to more credit for founding an institution of the 'purest principles of benevolence'. Howe claimed the principal surgeon had been 'roughly handled' in the other newspapers 'for lending his name to assist the poor' and the creation of the dispensary was not intended as a political manoeuvre to 'insult any gentleman or gentlemen in the Colony'. Howe observed 'the very handsome manner in which Dr. Redfern has stepped forward to contribute' to the dispensary despite the insinuations intended 'to poison his mind'.[23]

This last tribute referred to the decision by Redfern and Bland to back the public dispensary for the poor. Indeed, all members of the Redfern household enrolled as annual contributors to the dispensary fund, and William also volunteered his medical services. The annual subscription of £1 entitled a subscriber to nominate one patient for treatment at the dispensary or to be visited at home. The Redfern family payment of £9 gave nine patients free medical care for a year.[24] Dr Bland excelled in raising over half the funds collected from the general public. In January 1827 the dispensary service finally opened on Macquarie Street with Bland as a staff member. He remained in this capacity until 1845.

By early September 1826 William Redfern had become exhausted by the demands of his medical work. He terminated his private practice and the family returned to Campbellfield. The strict regime of a medical practice had made him appreciate more than ever the benefits of a farm life. Notwithstanding his passion for medicine, he had also found it difficult to practice at the same intensity as in the past and was exhausted by the late night call outs. Even so, he retained a house in Charlotte Place, and offered limited medical support to the new dispensary once it commenced operations.

On 6 September, *The Sydney Gazette* editor Robert Howe wrote that Dr Redfern expected to return to his Campbellfield farm, but it was hoped he would change his mind, as many poor patients would greatly miss his attention. Howe mischievously noted, however, that they might not miss his impolite bedside manner.

> Of Dr. Redfern's skill there can be but one opinion, since his most inveterate enemies are reluctantly obliged to do him that justice. His method, or his manner, let it be called by what term Readers please, may not be so winning or seductive as might be wished, but then his experience, his skill, and his practise, in our judgement, make ample amends for any apparent absence of overflowing politeness.[25]

Howe added he would have refrained from praising Redfern if not for the high public regard for this 'distinguished candidate for medical fame' and 'universally respected Gentleman'. Despite his esteemed status, he reminded the Doctor that in future he might be dependent on the support of his newspaper.[26]

William Redfern certainly would not have appreciated Howe's edgy public banter. This publicity would, however, be just the start of a vitriolic campaign against him by *The Sydney Gazette* editor.

The introduction of the 1827 bill in the British Parliament to replace the *Act of 1823* led to more friction with Governor Darling. Redfern and Eagar had fought hard, and successfully, to have the *Act of 1823* legitimise pardons granted in the colony, but it did not provide for trial by jury or democratic representation. These two concessions were now sought, and colonists feared the entrenched views of the governor and the Exclusives, would delay their proper consideration for another five years. The colonial Legislative Council, dominated by the Macarthur clan, opposed trial by jury. The influential settlers John Jamison, William Cox and Archibald Bell, who were ineligible to be on the Council, had recently put their weight behind the new constitutional reforms instigated by the colonists. However, in late 1826 Governor Darling had denied them permission to hold a public meeting to prepare a petition to the British Parliament and the Crown requesting these reforms.[27]

Blocking a public debate on these issues caused an avalanche of protests, and on 16 January 1827 twenty-four of the wealthiest men in the colony, both free and freed, jointly applied for a permit to discuss petitioning the King and both Houses of Parliament for three important changes: trial by jury, a House of Assembly with 100 elected members, and 'Taxation by Representation'. Among these 'men of the first rank, wealth and respectability in the Colony', whose combined wealth was £950,000, were William Redfern, D'Arcy and William Wentworth, Simeon Lord, Robert Wardell, John Jamison and Gregory Blaxland.[28]

Short of a rebellion, Governor Darling had little choice but to approve the meeting. On 26 January 1827, the 39th anniversary of Australia's foundation, colonists crowded into the courthouse on Castlereagh Street. It was the largest public meeting ever held in the colony, and free settlers, emancipists and retired members of the military and civil government debated the contents of a draft petition. At the close of the meeting William Wentworth moved that the petition be adopted, and Gregory Blaxland was appointed to take it to England. Later that day, a delegation presented the petition to Governor Darling, requesting that it be promptly forwarded to the Colonial Office.[29]

William Redfern had resumed his interest in trading commodities – something that he had started 20 years ago on Norfolk Island. He was not an adventurous trader of Simeon Lord and D'Arcy

Wentworth's ilk and only occasionally took risks, such as becoming a partner in the trading firm of Eagar & Forbes. Most of his investments were in secure stocks that he could underwrite with his large land holdings and livestock. In May 1827 Redfern stepped outside his comfort zone. To capitalise on the enormous demand for animals to stock the AAS granted land, he made the largest single sale of livestock seen in the colony. Using the agent, David Maziere, he offered five separate parcels each containing 1000 sheep, 100 cattle, 2 brood mares, 1 gelding and 4 working bullocks. The cost of each parcel was £5000, to be paid in cash or credit for up to 10 years. The total return to Redfern was £25,000 (over £2M today). Many buyers bought on credit with Redfern providing loans to those who could provide suitable collateral.[30] The editor of *The Sydney Gazette* commented on the sale:

> It will excite a little surprise in England should this incident relative to the sale of one stock-holder obtain any notice. It will not be supposed that dealings in sheep and cattle are carried on to such an extent as to twenty-five thousand pounds, at once![31]

In Ireland a few months later, the Dublin newspaper *The Morning Register* told readers of the £25,000 sale and announced that Dr Redfern, a former magistrate in New South Wales, had 'received the strongest mark of the regard and esteem of Governor Macquarie. ... He is the brother to Mr Jos. Redfern, of Belfast'.[32]

Redfern also sold wine from his vineyard. Only three men in the colony, Gregory Blaxland, John Macarthur and William Redfern had vineyards large enough to make wine, and each had brought out emigrant 'vine-dressers' from Switzerland, France and Madeira. Edward Hall, editor of *The Monitor*, informed his readers that both Blaxland and Redfern had 'gone to much greater risk than any tobacco-grower of the Chamber of Commerce, in endeavouring to produce grapes'. He proposed that in order to increase the cultivation of grape vines in Australia the prices of Cape wine, Madeira and Claret needed to increase eight-fold.[33]

During a particularly cold wet June 1827, a virulent strain of influenza reached Australia's shores. Within weeks scarcely a home in Sydney had escaped the 'epidemic visits of this species of influenza' that often created a 'house of mourning'. The disease quickly spread to outer districts with even more ferocity. When on

2 July D'Arcy Wentworth fell very ill with influenza, Dr Redfern rushed to his house at Homebush on the outskirts of Parramatta. But there was little he could do and five days later his oldest friend died, aged 65.[34] It was a devastating loss for Sarah and William. On 9 July 1827 they gathered in dismal weather at Homebush, with people from all walks of life, to pay their last respects. The mile long funeral procession of 40 carriages and 50 men on horseback led by William Redfern, accompanied the hearse and chief mourner William Wentworth on the journey to Parramatta. Following a service presided over by Reverend Samuel Marsden, D'Arcy was laid to rest in the family vault at the Parramatta St John's cemetery.[35]

Dr Wentworth's was one of the richest men in the colony, with 34,145 acres of land and an annual income from land rentals and livestock sales of over £23,000. Most of his estate was bequeathed to his children. The Homebush property was entrusted to his *de facto* wife Ann Lawes and the house on George Street was left to his companion and housekeeper, Maria Ainslie.[36] Seven months later, Ann Lawes gave birth to their eighth child.

D'Arcy Wentworth had been the president of the Bank of New South Wales board since January 1827 and his death necessitated the election of a new director and president.[37] *The Sydney Gazette* lobbied for Alexander Mackenzie, the cashier and secretary at the bank, to be elected as a new bank director. Mackenzie had been a slave dealer in the West Indies and a merchant in London before coming to Sydney in 1822.[38] Redfern distrusted him and after reading Howe's editorial decided that he would seek re-election. It turned out, the bank charter barred Mackenzie from standing and as the only candidate William Redfern became the new director and Richard Jones the new president.[39]

William Redfern re-joined the Bank of New South Wales board at a time of fierce competition from the new Bank of Australia. The rivalry forced the reorganisation of the older bank but led to bitter disputes among investors. These climaxed when the Colonial Office Secretary, Lord Bathurst, told Governor Darling that the Bank of New South Wales charter, ratified under Macquarie, was invalid and shareholders were liable for its losses.[40] The board was advised to re-establish the bank as a joint-stock company. But many shareholders opposed this change, and this prevented its reorganisation.

The banking uncertainties occurred at a time when the four Sydney newspapers, *The Australian*, *The Monitor*, *The Gleaner* and *The Sydney Gazette*, were in fierce competition for readership. The incessant analysis and denunciation of government policies were popular with readers but infuriated Governor Darling who warned the press to stop cultivating 'mutiny and insurrection' in the community. In May 1827 he imposed a government tax on every newspaper sold, followed by a series of libel suits against the editors.[41] However, the battle for newspaper readership continued unabated.

The Sydney Gazette editor, Robert Howe, who was well known for his sharp tongue, had been sued several times for libel and defamation. The new director of the Bank of New South Wales, William Redfern, became Howe's latest target. His family dispute with the Wills children, who were trying to recover their parents' George Street house from Howe, gave further impetus to his insults. The Wills siblings were also still seeking financial support for the two minors, Horatio Wills and Jane Howe, from the executors of the late George Howe's will.[42]

Robert Howe's 14-year-old stepbrother Horatio had been working at *The Sydney Gazette* for a year when the lad's guardian Thomas Wills departed for England in February 1826. Shortly after this Howe told Horatio that he could only remain at the printing office as an indentured apprentice. Without Thomas' advice, the boy was uncertain what to do and he reluctantly signed up for a seven-year indenture.[43] Learning of this, Redfern, who never indentured his medical apprentices, would certainly have strongly rebuked Howe.

Horatio Wills soon found the increased demands by George Howe intolerable. In November 1826, he was asked to account for a missing manuscript by Howe brandishing a horsewhip. When Horatio refused to enter Howe's office, the editor rushed out and began flogging him. When the 15-year-old grappled with the whip, Howe called another printer for help and the boy received a deep wound over his eye. That night Horatio and another apprentice ran away. Four days later *The Sydney Gazette* reported that the apprentice Horatio Wills was missing and information 'that will lead to his Recovery' would be rewarded. Anyone sheltering him would be prosecuted.[44] Soon after Horatio returned to the printing office.

In May 1827 Horatio's brother and guardian Thomas returned to Sydney with his new wife Marie Ann Barry. En route to England Thomas' ship had been wrecked on an island near Mauritius. He survived and during the year on the island had married Marie Ann.[45]

The Bank of New South Wales board met on 7 November 1827 to discuss the regulations for a joint-stock company and to elect new directors. Prior to this meeting *The Sydney Gazette* campaigned vigorously against William Redfern being re-elected as a director. In an editorial Howe accused Redfern of bringing criminal charges against Alexander Mackenzie to oust him from his cashier position so that his brother-in-law Thomas Wills could be appointed in his place. Howe warned Dr Redfern to stay out of bank politics and to leave Mackenzie alone. This article caused heated debates at the board meeting, but Redfern was easily re-elected as director. After charges were withdrawn against Mackenzie the cashier was also re-appointed but resigned soon after.[46]

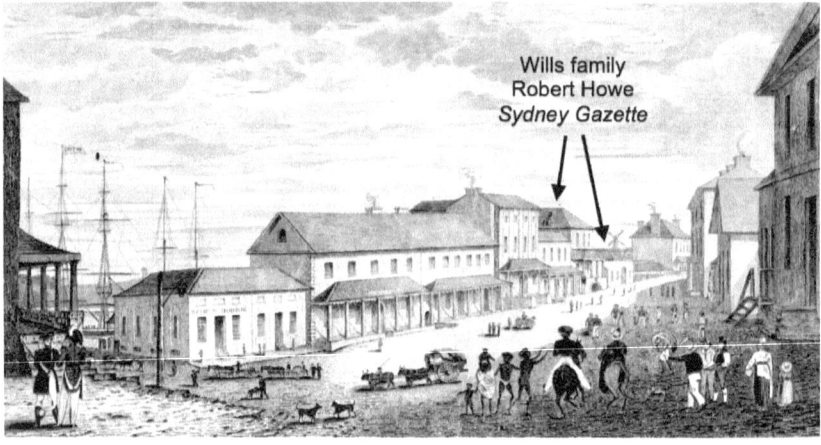

1829 engraving of Market Place on George Street. Behind the buildings is the wharf where convicts and goods were unloaded. Redfern horse-whipped Robert Howe at his house in 1827 for defamation in *The Sydney Gazette*.

Nevertheless, the relentless attack of *The Sydney Gazette* against the Bank of New South Wales and its director William Redfern continued unabated. Another bank director John Campbell was also singled out for insults, and he resigned on 20 November.[47] Days later *The Sydney Gazette* proclaimed that the old bank would fail unless certain directors were dismissed. Howe mockingly suggested emancipist Samuel Terry be appointed to the board as Redfern's accomplice.[48] Redfern was outraged at insinuations of dishonesty and promptly took his coach to physically confront the editor. Robert Howe was returning home on horseback when Redfern saw him and ordered him to stop. Howe ignored him and rode into his yard to dismount. Redfern followed and, with a horsewhip in his hand, demanded the editor explain why he 'dared to write a libel' and 'why he had mixed his name with that of Mr. Terry?' Howe responded that Terry was as good as Redfern 'as he saw no differences between Emancipists'.[49]

Incensed by Howe's arrogance Redfern struck him several times with his whip. A scuffle ensued in which Howe beat Redfern with his swordstick (small whip). The swordstick broke and Howe fled into the house pursued by an enraged Redfern. In the kitchen a servant helped Howe restrain Redfern and, hearing the ruckus, Howe's wife rushed in with a broomstick. They all began hitting the Doctor until he fell onto the stone floor, striking his head. In the adjacent office Horatio heard the shouts and rushed in to defend his brother-in-law. He pulled the servant away and Redfern retreated into the yard. Howe found another whip and chased him onto the street where passers-by witnessed a repeated flogging. With his head covered in blood, Redfern limped home, bruised but proud he had made a stand against this unhinged journalist.[50]

As soon as Howe recovered his breath and senses, he hurried to the police station and accused William Redfern of assault. Three days later Redfern, accompanied by his lawyer William Wentworth, was in court on an assault charge. To emphasise the seriousness of the charge, Howe asked for the protection of the court because a gun had recently been discharged under his window. He accused Redfern or his convict friends of threatening him and to remind him of the 'attack by an assassin some years since, a fact well known to the said Mr. Redfern'. Howe also claimed that his servant had heard Horatio Wills say that Redfern and some men intended to ambush him. Howe argued that the protection of the law was essential because the doctor was 'not of sound mind' and his life was in danger from his 'furious, ungovernable, and insane deportment' – anything was possible from 'a man of his wealth, and dangerous temperament of mind'.[51] Refuting the seriousness of the charge, Wentworth pointed out:

He really could not avoid viewing Mr. Howe's fears of being horsewhipped to death, or shot at, in the light of hypochondriacal terror; as the mere ravings of a visionary, and without any just foundation whatever. He would ask their Worships, if the Complainant might not as well claim sureties from him, Mr. W. because he dreaded chastisement for some wanton offence which possibly might now be in contemplation – in order to secure himself against the consequences?[52]

Wentworth tabled several issues of *The Sydney Gazette* containing 'malevolent insinuations' against his client that 'fully declared the nature of Mr. Howe's horror'. He claimed that there was nothing in this case that warranted a behaviour bond.

> If a person demanded sureties for another's peaceable behaviour, he himself must at least be inoffensive; he must not as in the present instance, squirt his filth in a man's face, and then demand a guarantee that he will, with the meekness of Job, suffer himself to be reviled with impunity. Mr. Howe's intention in the present application, was evidently to tie up Dr. Redfern's hands, while his quill was to be suffered to sport without control.[53]

Because Howe had sworn on oath that his life was in danger, the court bound William Redfern to keep the peace with a £100 bail and two bonds of £50 each to ensure his presence at a full hearing before the next Court of Quarter Sessions.[54] Howe fumed at the court's decision to bail Redfern, declaring that he was in danger, 'what was one hundred pounds to a man of Dr. Redfern's wealth'. The judge then informed Robert Howe that if he continued to publish offensive material about Redfern, the court would set a bail for him as well.[55]

Not unexpectedly, Horatio's assistance to Redfern during the brawl had serious consequences. Howe confronted him later at the printing office, struck him violently on the face with his clenched fist and threw a bottle at him that smashed against the wall. The next morning Horatio was told that he was fired. Howe informed Horatio's guardian Thomas Wills that the apprenticeship was cancelled but the indenture prohibiting him from working in any other printing office would remain. It is quite likely that Howe had heard that William Redfern intended setting up a rival newspaper, and under no circumstances would he allow Horatio to work for the Doctor. Two days later, a notice in *The Sydney Gazette* declared Horatio Wills to be a runaway who had neglected his work and behaved in an 'unbecoming and disrespectful Manner'. Howe warned anyone 'harbouring, encouraging, employing, or secreting the said, or any other of my Apprentices, on Pain of rigid Prosecution'.[56] Horatio now resided in the Redfern household.

Robert Howe had not finished with William Redfern yet. Howe had shares in the Bank of New South Wales, and he attended the proprietors' meeting on 12 December 1827 accusing Redfern of two improprieties. First, that he obtained loans with dubious securities, and second, that he prejudicially refused to discount Howe's bills on three occasions. He demanded an examination of the bank records and moved that Redfern be impeached for partiality and undue influence. Another director, the lawyer Robert Wardell, objected on the grounds that 'it was not fair, nor honest, to call for books, and pry into mysteries, for the purpose of finding out something to ground a charge upon'.

But Howe persisted and after the books had been examined, the board asked Redfern to explain his actions. He pointed out that his discounts were only for relatives and friends, and the records showed that 'Mr. Howe had nothing to complain of, being excluded from discounts by a law of the Board'. Redfern quipped that 'Howe had pledged himself not to issue any more of his private notes, but then who was to know if Mr. Howe would keep his promise'.[57] After Wentworth and Wardell had spoken in support of Redfern, Howe's censure motion was voted on and defeated. The board deemed that Redfern's 'conduct had been honorable and proper' while Howe's 'had been most industriously disseminated against and to the prejudice of Mr. Redfern' without foundation to 'satisfy such injurious rumours'.[58] At the adjournment of the meeting several investors offered to sell their shares, and Redfern bought them. This caused Howe to later claim in *The Sydney Gazette* that Dr Redfern now owned a quarter of the Bank of New South Wales, and it should now be considered his private bank.[59]

The never-ending libel in *The Sydney Gazette* made Redfern more determined than ever to establish his own newspaper. On 20 December 1827 the editor of *The Monitor*, Edward Hall, applauded Dr Redfern's intention to create another public journal and offered a spare printing press for his service.[60]

In the rural calm and sanctity of Campbellfield, the Redferns tried to concentrate on more sensible matters. Sarah and William needed to decide how their two boys, William and Robert, should be educated. The 8-year-old William had been taught at home, but it was time for him to attend a proper school. On 7 January 1828 William Jr began lessons at the 'Classical and Commercial School' of Jerimiah Hatch on Castlereagh Street, Sydney.[61] The Redferns expressed great hopes in the school and in Mr Hatch as a teacher.

The year 1828 opened with William Redfern on trial for assaulting Robert Howe in the Court of Quarter Sessions. On 21 January 1828 he appeared with his lawyer William Wentworth before a court and jury presided over by Judge John Stephen. The *Act of 1823* now allowed a limited number of civil trials before a jury of twelve free residents – but emancipists were ineligible. Redfern would be subjected to a judicial process that he and Edward Eagar had requested from the British Parliament and the King in 1822.

Wentworth commenced his cross-examination of Robert Howe by asking who threw the first blow in the alleged assault. Howe admitted his recollection was so vague that he could not recall this, or how his swordstick had been broken. He said that he carried it only for personal protection and had not thrown an iron pot at Redfern. Nor could he recollect putting his foot on Redfern's back when he fell over, or that his wife had hit Redfern with a broomstick. Howe did admit that if his swordstick had not broken, he almost certainly 'would have run it through his bowels'.

> He [Redfern] bled like a pig, but it was not from any blow he received; I did strike him on the head; he might have had as many as three blows on the head from the broom-stick, it was a parlour broom-stick; I consider, it was to be a creditable persecution.[62]

After questioning other witnesses, Wentworth told the jury he was extremely sorry that such an unworthy case had come before them. It was absurd in the extreme that, while Redfern sustained the most injuries and had been treated in a cowardly manner by the editor, the court was not proceeding against Howe. Wentworth admitted to the jury that 'it was a most grievous thing to be assaulted in one's own kitchen' but Redfern was not the aggressor, and he was entitled to respond to Howe's insults 'Week after week – day after day – there was another and another dish of scandal; on which the defendant was made to figure'.[63] Labelling Howe as 'a public nuisance' Wentworth asked the jury to decide who really caused the assault. After only twenty minutes the jury returned the verdict 'guilty' but recommended that the judge show 'mercy, on account of the aggravated assault!'. The courtroom burst into laughter on hearing the verdict. Redfern was fined £50, which he immediately paid by cheque, declaring the judgement a triumph and the fine was money well spent.[64]

Robert Howe was furious with the sentence and the jury, and the next *Sydney Gazette* published a two-page editorial complaining about the unfairness of the trial. It criticised barrister Wentworth who 'shot his envenomed arrows' with 'unblushing temerity' when he stated that he did not believe a word Howe said under oath. The editor accused him of misleading the court and questioned the value of trial by jury.[65] Howe's month-long rant criticised anyone associated with the bank, any friend of Redfern and every juror.

The reorganisation of the Bank of New South Wales into a joint-stock company had been stalled principally because of opposition from Howe and *The Sydney Gazette*. Appalled at the delay, twelve investors, who included William Wentworth, William Redfern, Robert Wardell and John Campbell Jr, met on 30 January 1828 to discuss forming yet another bank, to be named *The Macquarie Bank of New South Wales*. It was rumoured that these investors would sell their shares in the old bank to finance the new Macquarie Bank, each investing £2000.[66] However, this bank never got past the planning stage because its main investor, William Redfern, was to soon leave the colony.

After the assault court case, the Wills and Redfern families had hoped Howe's vindictive campaign against them would end. It did not. Howe was still after the blood of 16-year-old Horatio Wills who was residing with the Redferns. On 4 February 1828 Horatio was summoned before a magistrate on the charge of absconding from his apprenticeship contract and having, in violation of his indenture, aided Redfern in setting up a printing press.[67] The court ordered his return to his apprenticeship at *The Sydney Gazette*, whereupon his lawyer William Wentworth demanded that a summons now be issued against Howe on charges of ill treatment.

On 15 February Wentworth appealed against the court order for Horatio Wills to restart his apprenticeship and to find that Robert Howe was at fault. But, unlike Redfern's hearing before a jury, the verdict was again determined by elderly magistrates sympathetic to the age-old tradition that apprentices must be subordinate to their masters. They ruled Howe had adequately looked after Horatio, and his beating was a consequence of bad conduct. Horatio was offered the choice of resuming his apprenticeship or going to gaol.[68] The Wills and Redfern families were furious but there was little they could do, other than to carefully monitor Robert Howe's future treatment of the young lad.

Chapter 21

EDINBURGH FINALE

No words of mine can ever describe his unbounded & unlimited attention to us, Mr. Redfern had no doubt great faults, but they did not reach us. I consider him the most talented man I ever knew. The benefit he rendered his fellow Creatures you know better than I possibly can. I hope he is enjoying a degree of happiness we can have no idea of.
                    Elizabeth Macquarie to Sarah Redfern, 1833[1]

The precise reasons why William Redfern departed for England in March 1828 are unknown but the swiftness of his decision to sail would have surprised both friends and family. After all, he had just been re-elected as a director of the *Bank of New South Wales*; he was a strong advocate for establishing *The Macquarie Bank of New South Wales* and seemed committed to starting up a new newspaper. William and Sarah had long planned that their sons would be educated in Britain from the age of ten, but this had not been a matter of this urgency. William's decision to leave the colony with their eldest son immediately after Horatio Wills was found guilty of breaking his apprenticeship contract has been construed as the likely trigger for Redfern's sudden departure from the colony. The court verdict that Robert Howe could enforce his indenture on Horatio had been a setback, but it is unlikely to have caused such a major separation of the family. Whatever the reasons were, Sarah and 4-year-old Robert were to remain in the colony to manage the Campbellfield estate, assisted by her brother Thomas. Presumably it was planned that the family would meet up again later.

A number of factors may have had a bearing on Redfern going to Britain. He was dealing with several vexatious issues at the time and one or more of these could have tipped the decision. He was infuriated with Robert Howe's continual abuse of the family in *The Sydney Gazette*, and the persecution of young Horatio may have been the last straw. William may have believed that leaving the colony would stop *The Sydney Gazette* targeting his family and avoid further confrontations with Howe. Appealing as the prospect of beating Howe was, Redfern knew that assaulting him again was at best imprudent; better to avert that opportunity.

More pragmatic reasons may have led to the decision to leave. His son's new school in Sydney had attracted few students and was likely to close. William Jr was almost nine now and the Redferns might have decided to move forward their plans to educate him in Britain. Other colonists, such as D'Arcy Wentworth, had sent their boys to English boarding schools to be educated. But D'Arcy's son William had told them of his bad experiences as a 10-year-old in a cold unfriendly school. This may have convinced them that their sons needed to be accompanied overseas during their education.

Redfern may have also gone to London on a political cause. *The Colonial Advocate* claimed he was leaving 'on political business'.[2] A year earlier the colonists had sent a petition to London to amend the *Act of 1823*. Edward Eagar was still in London lobbying for an elected legislature in Australia, but the new petition had not reached London when, on 14 June 1827, Under Secretary Robert Horton sought to renew the bill in the House of Commons without amendment. Eagar was successful in delaying this for a year and a month later the petition arrived in London.[3]

At the time Howe's assault charges against Redfern were being heard in court, letters from Eagar arrived in Sydney detailing the problems encountered by the new bill in parliament. He censured his emancipist friends for 'entirely forgetting their own interests and welfare' and not pressing the British Parliament for further reforms. Eagar declared that 'New South Wales shall be condemned for years to come' and requested that an agent be appointed and funded to lobby the British. The editor of *The Monitor*, Edward Hall, agreed with Eagar, suggesting a lawyer should be sent to England. He nominated William Wentworth for the role and advocated that Edward Eagar be rewarded for his strenuous efforts in supporting colonial rights.[4]

However, Wentworth was unwilling to take up this cause as he was much too embroiled in local politics and the impeachment of Governor Darling. The deliberations of the emancipist committee steering the new petition are unknown, but with little time before the bill would be tabled, opportunities to send more support were few. It is entirely possible that they asked Redfern, who had helped Eagar and Wentworth when the Act was first passed in 1823, to be a representative and support Eagar. Such a political assignment seems, in itself, a compelling reason for Redfern to go to England. It ignores, however, the fact that he was much less interested in politics than five years earlier. As later events will suggest, William Redfern had personal motives for this trip and lobbying British parliamentarians was not one of his priorities.

In trying to understand Redfern's decision to leave his wife and youngest son in Australia and go to England, one cannot ignore medical incentives. These would have been at two levels. First, the 53-year-old was suffering from at least one major illness seriously affecting his overall health. The exact nature of his illness was never recorded but the two likely suspects are inflammation of the joints and cardiovascular disease. After the death of his friend and colleague D'Arcy Wentworth, Redfern was unlikely to have sought medical help in Sydney and probably wanted to consult physicians in England. There was also a second professional consideration. Most of his adult life William had aspired to study medicine at university, and especially at the University of Edinburgh whose lecturers were considered the most advanced in the world. The two powerful aims of rejuvenation and intellectual stimulation may have become inexorably entwined aspirations in Redfern's later years.

On 9 March 1828 William Redfern and his son William Jr departed Sydney on the fast merchant ship *Orelia* sailing directly to London. They arrived on 23 July 1828 and Redfern immediately rented a spacious residence in Grove Street in Camden Town, just a street away from Regents Park north of the Thames River.[5]

Once settled, William would have contacted Edward Eagar to discuss the progress of the bill in parliament. There had been no time to inform Eagar of his coming and Redfern's sudden presence in London would have astonished him, especially as the politics had changed radically in the months following his letters to Sydney. Disappointingly, the unchanged bill had already been rammed through parliament on 25 June 1828.[6] Eagar's lobbying efforts had been briefly curtailed when he spent several weeks in the notorious Fleet Prison for unpaid debts. He was released on 11 April 1828, a week before the bill was debated in parliament.

Governor Darling opposed further rights for the colony and advised that the Act be renewed unchanged.[7] The new Colonial Secretary George Murray and the Duke of Wellington, as Prime

Minister, had also opposed the colonists' petition for additional rights. But true to his word, the repatriated Sir Thomas Brisbane argued strongly that the colony was ready for improvement and that emancipists deserved additional rights and independence.[8]

On 18 April Sir James Mackintosh proposed amendments to the Act on behalf of the colonists that would provide for routine use of trial by jury and the establishment of a representative house of assembly in the colony. Neither amendment was accepted.[9] The new *Act of 1828* did not advance the rights of colonists, and there was nothing further to be done. The routine use of trial by jury in colonial courts was only instituted in 1832, and it was not until 1842 that a partial representative government was introduced.

William Redfern then spent weeks looking for a suitable school in London for his son. Elizabeth Macquarie, Lachlan Macquarie's widow residing in London while her son went to school there, wrote to Sarah Redfern that she had gladly met several times with William and her son. She added that she did not approve of him coming to England without Sarah but is unlikely to have broached the matter with William. In a letter to Sarah, Mrs Macquarie wrote:

> I was not well pleased to see Mr. Redfern arrive here without you, I know nothing of the motives of his journey nor shall I ever ask him any questions concerning so delicate a subject but this you may assure yourselves of, that the interest I feel in you both can only terminate with my existence.[10]

Elizabeth Macquarie noted the closeness of father and son: 'William was so shy that he would not look at me, he is a genteel smart looking child and appears to like his father very much'.[11] It would never have occurred to Redfern to tell Mrs Macquarie why Sarah was not with him – this was a family matter, and he would not have appreciated her commentary. In any case Sarah was never far from William's thoughts; husband and son had perused the best shops in London and shipped Sarah a large crate containing two bales of British linen, one cask, three cases of cutlery and four saddles.[12] He also took time to visit their mutual friend, General Joseph Foveaux, living south of Regents Park in Marylebone.

By late September 1828 Redfern had still not found a suitable school for his son and decided to move to Edinburgh. This plan was interrupted when 9-year-old William contracted measles

(*Rubeola*), a highly infectious disease endemic in England but absent in Australia until the 1850s. He became further concerned when a month later his son had 'inflammation of the Lungs', as he knew that pneumonia was a common cause of death from measles. Under his father's constant care, William Jr recovered and on 20 November wrote to his 'Dear Mama' that 'Papa bled me with leeches & blistered me twice which relieved me very much'. His letter also gives an insight into his father's health: 'Papa says that he is going to Italy, or to the south of France if he does not get better'. The affectionate letter of a homesick son urges his mother and brother Robert, who he called 'Foveaux', to join them soon.[13]

> Papa is very cross to me sometimes, but very often calls me his dear little boy, and asks me if Mama is not a very kind Mama to me. … Give my love to Foveaux and say I shall be glad to see him in London.[14]

At the close of William Jr's letter, his father added: 'The little monkey' was obliged to write 'a fresh letter' and did it in such 'a hurry it is not half so well written as the first'.[15]

The two-month convalescence of William Jr at their inner London residence allowed Redfern to leave the boy in the care of a servant and visit places of importance in the great city. Although undocumented, his would have almost certainly included visits to senior medical specialists. Redfern had always been a prolific reader and the British Library with its massive collection of medical books was only a mile away. The recently established University of London, known today as University College London, was also close by. It was the third university in England (Scotland had five) and was created through public shares as a secular alternative to Oxford and Cambridge, which offered mostly courses in classical studies at great expense and exclusiveness.

In contrast, the University of London was founded principally to serve the broader educational and technical needs of an aspiring middle class. It was modelled on the University of Edinburgh from which many founding professors came. The aim to educate a wider demographic appealed to Redfern and, since it offered a four-year course in medicine, he became a shareholder for £100.[16] It is likely Redfern attended the university's official opening on 1 October 1828 and heard the inaugural lecture by Charles Bell, Professor of

Surgery. The university buildings and museum of anatomy were open to the public and William would have relished the chance to examine their teaching facilities and discuss medicine with many of the university staff.

During his son's recovery period Redfern also renewed his acquaintance with John Hosking, an old business partner in the firm of Eagar & Forbes. Hosking had been the master of the Parramatta orphan school but after a dispute with Reverend Marsden, he and his family returned to England in 1819. Two of Hosking's sons later went back to Sydney, John Jr as a merchant in the Eagar & Forbes firm, and Peter as a surgeon. Hosking's eldest son William had been an apprentice to a builder and surveyor in Sydney, and later in London became an engineer, lecturer and a renowned architect. Redfern arranged to meet the young architect to see if he would design a mansion for the Campbellfield farm. Hosking's designs were radical for their time, and among the many papers he left for posterity was a plan dated 1830 and labelled 'a residence for W. Redfern, esq., Campbellfield'.[17] It was never built.

Dr Redfern was also concerned about the health of Sarah's brother Edward, who was studying law in London. In June 1828, a month before Redfern arrived in England, Edward was furthering his education as a Fellow at Peterhouse College in Cambridge.[18] These studies burdened him to such an extent that he showed 'symptoms of aberration of mind' and a constant fear of being persecuted. The College inquired into Edward's distress but found no basis for his concern.[19] Redfern was informed that Edward was unwell and probably visited him in Cambridge. He would have done his best to assist his agitated brother-in-law and probably paid off his debts, but little is known about his illness, other than it led Edward to take his own life two years later.

In London William Redfern and son lived extravagantly. As a wealthy man he could afford the expense, but he soon found that easy access to cash in London was limited by a highly conservative banking system. London banks and private lenders would have shown Redfern due respect but when it came to providing credit he would have been treated as a colonial of uncertain reputation. He could write cheques against funds held in Australia, but these had to be underwritten by a well-known local person and it often took twelve months for the payment of bills to be acknowledged.

The widowed Elizabeth Macquarie was a caring friend to the

Doctor and his son while they were in London. He had delivered her son Lachlan and Elizabeth made certain that she met the two regularly. She wrote to William Wentworth in Sydney that she had offered to take care of young William, but the Doctor did not want to part with his son. In the letter Elizabeth also expressed concern for Redfern's health and his finances, adding that before she 'knew how very far of his intellects have gone' she paid some of his bills. This comment is puzzling as there is no other evidence that Redfern was losing his mental abilities. It is likely that the word 'intellects' meant something different to Elizabeth and she was really questioning his "good sense", as she was certainly worried about his extravagant spending habits.

Elizabeth's letter to Wentworth was baffling in other respects. As a widow on a relatively small pension, she made Redfern a loan of £300 (£25,000 today) and had received in return his promissory note.[20] She presumably did this without realising the full extent of Redfern's wealth; he was among the richest men in Australia and repayment of the loan was never in question. Even so, she told Wentworth that in lieu of 'the many services he has rendered to us, makes me very easy in regard to the loss of this money if it should be eventually lost'.[21] Considering the enormity of this loan for a widow supporting a son on a small pension, this was an act of extreme kindness, even if Redfern had more than once saved the lives of her family. It also raises the spectre of Elizabeth seeing her friend and doctor as a man who was now unable to look after himself or his son, and this would have greatly upset her.

In early 1829 Redfern and his son were fit enough to make the move to Edinburgh. Here they rented a house in the exclusive estate of Moray Place in Edinburgh New Town.[22] In the early 1800s this area was considered to be a masterpiece of urban planning. Their house was a sumptuous Georgian four-storey terrace residence built opposite a large park bordered by a series of private gardens on the slope of the Water of Leith. The size and grandness of the house indicates that William expected Sarah and Robert to join them eventually in Edinburgh.

At his Moray Place residence William Redfern 'Esquire, former surgeon of the Sydney hospital' regularly entertained his friends and neighbours who were mostly bankers, lawyers, merchants and university professors. Each house in the terrace had stables at the rear, and this allowed William to maintain his passion for riding; he had over 60 horses on his Campbellfield estate, as well as a horse stud and racecourse with grandstand.[23] Redfern promptly bought six horses and employed a fulltime horse handler and footman. They also purchased the latest riding outfits; William acquired a pair of the finest leather riding 'Wellington Boots' made by Thomas Duncan, His Majesty's Bootmaker. From Andrew Paton's saddlery he purchased all of the gear needed to care for the horses and to harness them to a gig. Since his father Robert and brother Joseph were saddlers by trade, he only bought fittings of the highest quality. Sarah and Robert did not miss out either; William shipped them a trunk full of the latest riding apparel.[24]

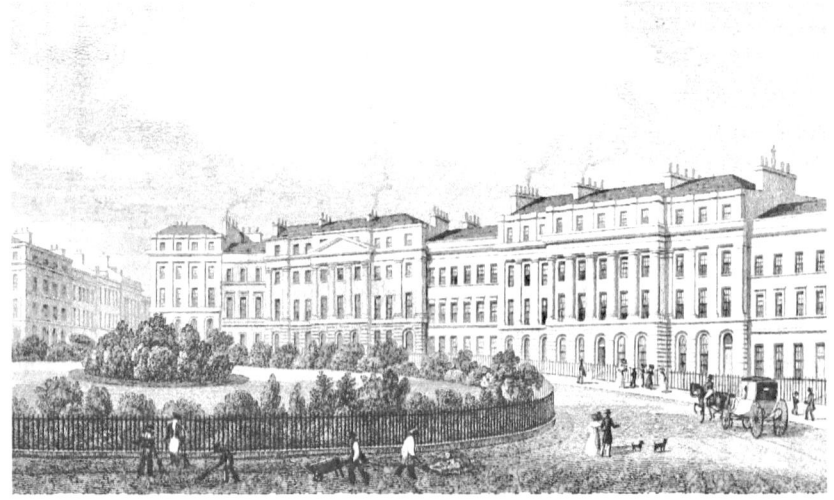

Moray Place in Edinburgh where William Redfern and his son lived in 1829.

In June 1829 William Jr began attending the fifth class at the Royal High School in Edinburgh, one of the oldest schools in Europe, which had just relocated to a grand neoclassical building on Calton Hill.[25] Just as father and son were becoming accustomed to their luxurious lifestyle, William heard from Sarah that in early January there had been a serious accident at Campbellfield when she and sister Eliza were thrown from their carriage over a fence, 'narrowly escaping death'. Eliza was unhurt but Sarah had a large splinter imbedded in her leg. Doctor Bland had come quickly from Sydney and removed the splinter, but the leg was infected.[26] Frustrated at being so far away, William fretted about Sarah's recovery, knowing that the news he received was now five months old. No antibiotics existed then, and infections were often fatal. Sarah would have also told him that the injury prevented her and Robert from travelling to Britain until the wound was fully healed.

The news that Sarah and Robert would not soon join them was distressing and disappointing after so much had been invested in creating an attractive residence for the family. Most upsetting of all, however, was that Sarah's companionship and care was greatly missed by both father and son, and they needed her to come and look after them. This would have been a difficult time for both Williams. William Jr would have missed his mother's sympathy while he was coping with a new school and a different culture. William Sr was far from healthy and felt especially vulnerable without Sarah's presence and sensibility. But the Doctor still had the resilience and determination of a man who had survived a year's solitary confinement in Coldbath Fields prison. He soldiered on and is unlikely to have shared his concerns or sympathies with his son.

Another piece of news William Redfern received in mid 1829 was far from upsetting. Robert Howe, aged 34, had drowned in January 1829 while fishing.[27] Although Horatio's apprenticeship ended with Howe's death, the 18-year-old remained a printer at *The Sydney Gazette*. Howe's widow Anne became the proprietor of the newspaper and beneficiary of much of the estate.

Not long after Redfern had learnt of Sarah's injury, Mrs Macquarie wrote to William Wentworth that she had heard from someone in Edinburgh that 'poor Mr. Redfern is going on with the most unbounded extravagance' and this worried her.[28] She expressed sympathy for Sarah because William appeared to be wasting their sons' inheritance. Elizabeth Macquarie wrote to Wentworth:

> I hope young Wills has informed you of the melancholy state to which Mr. Redfern is reduced. I find he is quite out of his mind at Edinburgh. I much fear that he will never ... [help] his Family by making away with his Property; he is surrounded by bad and low people – keeps six horses, has engaged to pay £3000 for a house, gives dinners & his kind Brother has been there from Ireland to try what could be done but returned without being able to do any good.[29]

The 'young Wills' Elizabeth refers to must have been Edward

and it appears she had no prior knowledge of the mental health issues he was personally experiencing. Elizabeth went on to say that she would not like to see Redfern 'in his present state' as 'this most unfortunate man', who had saved thousands of lives, was now 'himself reduced to the most deplorable condition'.[30] It is highly likely her claim of Redfern being 'quite out of his mind' concerned his profligacy, not his mental state. Elizabeth was a frugal Scot who abhorred any form of excess and would have been upset to hear that Redfern's health was declining; she remembered the young man who looked after them so dutifully in the colony. Elizabeth would have known that William, now aged 54, was well past the life expectancy of male Scots; at that time only 43 years.

The reliability of Elizabeth Macquarie's observations, which are among the few recorded about Redfern over this period, needs careful scrutiny. She had not seen him recently and relied entirely on the second or third hand comments from someone in Edinburgh. There is little doubt that Redfern's health was poor, but there is every indication that he remained a caring father and was relishing a life devoid of the arduous duties he had borne for the past 30 years. Elizabeth wrote that Redfern was 'engaged to pay £3000 for a house' but no records exist of him buying property in Edinburgh. It is more likely that gossip of his plans to have architect William Hosking design a house for Campbellfield that would cost £3000 (£250,000 today) was construed as the purchase of a house in Moray Place. In any case, William Redfern could afford to pay for any house in Edinburgh he wanted; in 1827 alone he had made £25,000 from a single sale of livestock.

The 'bad & low people' Elizabeth supposed Redfern was surrounded by were probably his servants and horse handlers. He would have treated these men with the same civility he showed his workers at Campbellfield. As someone who had been a convict, spent time in English prisons and assisted in the fight for emancipist equality, Redfern is likely to have mixed more easily with his staff than his neighbours. Social classes were as well defined in Scotland as in England, and fraternising with servants would have been frowned upon in Moray Place. Although Mrs Macquarie had supported her husband's promotion of emancipists in Australia, back in "the old country" she is more likely to have adhered to the established societal norms of the era.

Elizabeth Macquarie's letters to William Wentworth provide

rare information about Redfern's life in Edinburgh. However, her wording was obscure and has led to different interpretations of Redfern's behaviour and health. For this reason early historians initially saw them as intriguing gossip and personal conjecture, not reliable firsthand observations, and they avoided citing these letters as evidence of Redfern having mental problems in later life. But in 1955 Malcolm Ellis wrote that John Macarthur 'was not alone on his retreat to the world of mental malady' and listed William Redfern as another colonist who was so afflicted.[31] He renewed this claim in 1961 when he criticised the ABC television drama *The Outcasts* in which William Redfern was prominent. He wrote in *The Bulletin* that Redfern 'was actually a rather unbalanced fellow who became skilled as a medico, and who in later life went out of his mind'.[32] This led authors such as Roger Pescott and Gwyneth Dow to assert that Redfern's life in Edinburgh was one of extravagance, debt and mental deterioration.[33] All these claims appear to be based solely on Mrs Macquarie's letters. Such accusations are apocryphal. They ignore Redfern's industry and dedication to his son while in Edinburgh, as well as his interactions with his family in Sydney. There were definite indications that Redfern had reduced physical ability but there is nothing to suggest he was mentally impaired.

Another historian who referred to Elizabeth Macquarie letters was John Ritchie. He expressed strong views on Redfern in his 1969 thesis on Commissioner Bigge and supported most of Bigge's findings. Similar beliefs permeate Ritchie's 1975 book *Australia as once we were*, in which he declares 'William Redfern returned to Edinburgh and to the company of guttersnipes'.[34] In his 1986 book *Lachlan Macquarie*, Richie says of Redfern:

> the doctor's wilder extravagances plunged him into debt. Surrounded by the sweepings of Edinburgh's streets, his faculties crumbled. ... His urge to be independent in his sinning did not prevent him borrowing £300 from the late governor's widow.[35]

A general acceptance in historical circles of Redfern's mental deterioration in later years prevailed until Arthur Jones reported in 2017 that William Redfern had in 1829 enrolled to study medicine at the University of Edinburgh.[36] In the article *Surgeon William Redfern in London and Edinburgh*, Jones strongly refutes that Redfern had ever 'been out of his mind'.[37] Indeed it now seems eminently reasonable to argue that someone successfully studying medicine at university at the age of 54 may have been quixotic but it is highly unlikely he was mentally deranged.

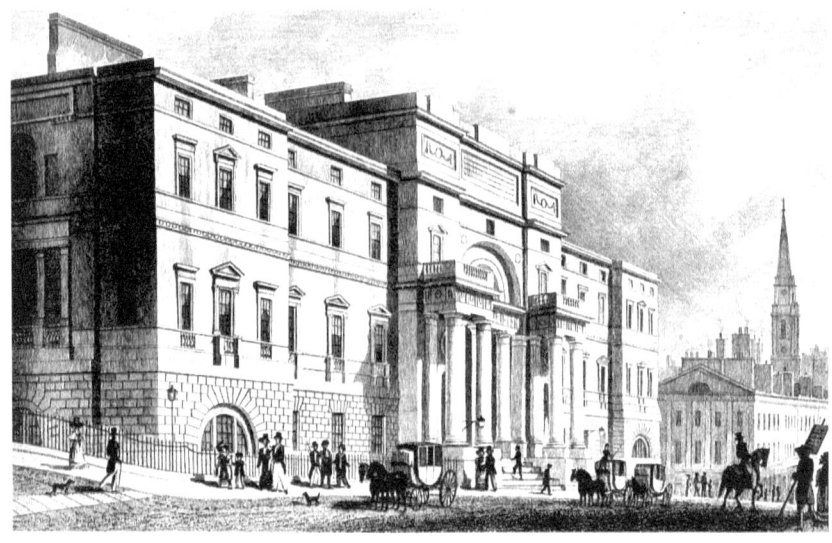

Engraving of South Bridge Street in front of the University of Edinburgh where William Redfern began his medical studies in 1829.

In October 1829, with William Jr at school, Redfern enrolled at the University of Edinburgh, an ambition he had had since the Nore mutiny robbed him of the opportunity to gain full qualifications as surgeon. He enrolled in courses for chemistry, pharmacology, midwifery, anatomy, physiology and practical anatomy; his entry record shows his country of origin as 'Londonderry Ireland'.[38] The lectures began on 4 November 1829.

Although the Edinburgh medical school had been at the fore of European medicine since the 1740s, its courses were affordable and had been used to train most surgeons in the Royal Navy. There were no entrance exams and students typically entered at the age of 15 or 16. Those enrolled for a medical diploma of the Royal College spent four years studying prescribed courses. They exited after submitting a dissertation thesis and taking a final examination in Latin. In addition to the 10 shilling entry fee to the university, students paid the lecturers directly, typically £4 6s for each course. Students were required to enter their names in the university register album during the teaching sessions and had to produce a

EDINBURGH FINALE

certificate of attendance before sitting examinations.[39]

The University buildings and medical school were located at the heart of Old Edinburgh. Lectures and demonstrations were held in the university precinct and in nearby buildings. The area known as Surgeon's Square was the focus of medical science learning. It is where several surgery lecturers lived and consulted while treating patients in the Royal Infirmary, the university's teaching hospital.

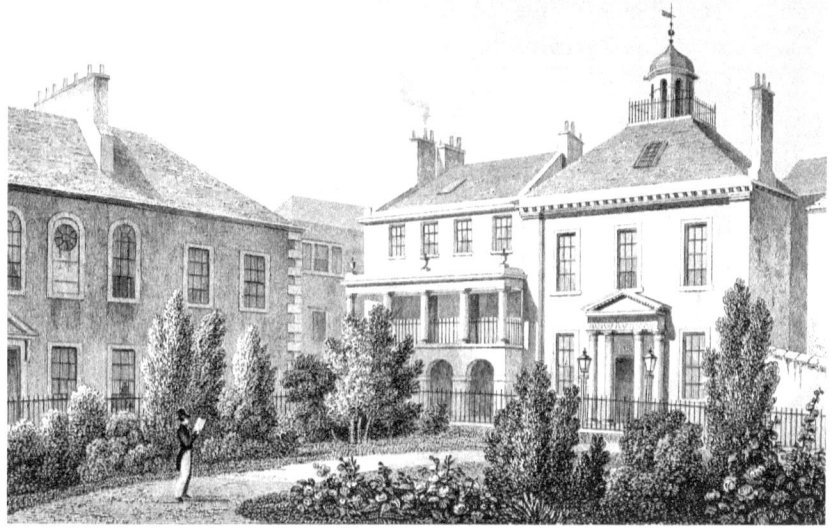

1830 engraving of Surgeon's Square at the University of Edinburgh, where William Redfern spent time as a medical student during 1829-1831.

Although the distance from Moray Place to the university was only 1.3 miles, it soon became apparent that this posed a problem with evening classes, as Redfern often arrived home late after discussions with professors. In early 1830 he moved with his son to a more convenient lodging in 18 Lothian Street, only minutes from the university district. It was an upmarket residential building providing dining room service to six unfurnished apartments. Such inner city residences were common in that era and varied from basic to swank. Moving from a luxurious house in Moray Place, Redfern would have furnished his apartment expensively. His study eventually held a library of 2000 books on medical, classical and general topics.[40] There is little doubt that both father and son would have missed ready access to horses and riding parks but may have been a pastime they pursued on weekends. In any case,

Redfern's health may have by now precluded him from such activities, and this could have been a major reason for moving to accommodation closer to his studies.

Residents at 18 Lothian Street ranged from merchants to university dons. A chemistry lecturer, John Deuchar, occupied the apartment adjacent to theirs and he offered classes in his lodgings to Ladies and Gentlemen on chemistry and experimental philosophy. Deuchar also sold medications at an adjacent shop at 20 Lothian Street. Since academics received no income during semester breaks, many lectured for a fee to the general public.[41] Only two years earlier the naturalist Charles Darwin had lodged in 11 Lothian Street while studying medicine at the university.

Few details of William Redfern's studies at the university have survived, but we can be confident he relished the experience and was fully immersed in his medical studies. As a student, he had full access to libraries, the anatomical museum and the museums of the Royal College of Surgeons. It is unknown if he joined any student societies, but it seems unlikely unless more senior lecturers were also members. Unquestionably, as an undergraduate, Redfern would have been in his element studying new medical techniques and discussing his own experiences with professors. For the other medical students, who would have been almost 40 years his junior, having a veteran physician in their midst would have been a novelty and a benefit. The skills acquired over years of medical practice meant that on occasions he would have known more than the professor did. Redfern informed his friends and family in Sydney that he was 'in the best of health' and 'studying at Edinburgh, where he intends taking out a degree'.[42]

The year 1830 was a heartbreaking one for the Redfern and Wills families. In May 1830 William heard that his brother Joseph's daughter Selina had died in Belfast aged 18 and, in late July, he was informed that his 7-year-old son Robert had died on 9 April 1830 after a short unknown illness.[43] Robert's death was a major blow to Redfern. Not only had he lost a beloved son but is likely to have felt responsible for a death that might have been avoided if he had been there. This was a massive burden that few could bear.

Robert was buried in the Sydney Devonshire Street Cemetery, today overbuilt by the Sydney Central railway station. Sarah's enormous grief is expressed on the obelisk erected on the child's grave (the boy's age was in fact seven). It read on the east side:

TO THE MEMORY
of
ROBERT FOVEAUX REDFERN
The Infant Son of
WILLIAM and SARAH REDFERN
of Campbellfield
who departed this Life April 11th 1830
Aged Six Years and three Months
Cut off at this tender age
After a short Illness
Leaving his Parents
Inconsolable for his loss

The obelisk read on the north side:

The Young as well as the Aged are Called
Be Ye ready when the Summons
Shall be sent for You
Sweet Child of Love when Death was near
A tender Mother's heart was riven
Be now her Guardian Angel here
To warn and lead her steps to heaven[44]

The emotion expressed in this inscription indicates Sarah was heart-broken by her son's death and not coping well without William and her eldest son to console her. The true extent of her anguish is unrecorded but the fact that she refused to go to Edinburgh for another three years, indicates that she was depressed and perhaps deeply resentful at her husband's absence. No letters between William and Sarah have survived from this period. Possibly Sarah held William responsible for the death; if he had been there to treat the illness, Robert may have been saved. Equally, Sarah probably felt guilty for not sailing with William and keeping his care and expertise close by. We shall never know.

With his youngest son's death, William Redfern became even more fixated on the safety of his surviving son and heir, William Jr. He resolved to protect the boy at all costs and stay in Edinburgh until he graduated. Dissatisfied with the 11-year-old's progress at the Royal High School, Redfern enrolled him in October 1830 in the third class at the Edinburgh Academy in Henderson Row New Town, an independent school for classical learning.[45] Redfern made sure the boy was accompanied to school every day and looked after by servants when he attended second year medicine classes. He had just started the 1830/31 courses in chemistry, physiology, anatomy and pharmacology.[46] The studies helped take his mind off Robert's death and Sarah's reluctance to join him.

But fate had yet another tragedy in store for the family. Edward Wills took his own life on 9 December 1830. After returning to the London courts in 1829, Edward continued to find his studies exhausting. His doctor, Peter Cosgrave, advised him to reduce his workload to avoid serious consequences. In mid 1830 Edward had severe delusions of persecution and believed that unknown enemies pursued him night and day to inflict 'desperate vengeance upon him'. Under the 'influence of mental delusion' he committed suicide. Doctor Cosgrave wrote in the coroner's report that the 25-year-old Edward was a man of 'honour and truth' who had nothing to accuse himself of, or of anything to dread. The inquest announced that the death was due to 'insanity'.[47]

A year after Robert's death, Redfern prepared a box of gifts and a letter to be sent to Sarah. The 12-year-old William Jr contributed, telling his 'Mama' that he was in the third class with 70 boys and his marks had improved since joining the Edinburgh Academy.

> I stand sixth dux in Greek & Latin, 4th in Arithmetick, 30th in Writing, & 5th in English. In all of which I was booby on the first of October 1830. You must know, Mamma, that Booby is the lowest boy in the whole class. I am sure you will regoice [*sic*] to learn that I have worked my way up so well.[48]

Young William revealed to his mother that his father's quick medical intervention had saved him from losing his sight in one eye. The injury had occurred in a ruckus with a classmate who attempted to thrust his pen into his mouth but accidentally put it in his eye. The letter describes his father's treatment:

> I have had a narrow escape from losing my eye, in consequence of a boy thrusting a pen into it. I had it leeched twice, with six leeches each time. After the inflammation went off, Papa dropt the solution of corrosive sublimate into it; & after that the wine of Opium. There is a scar right upon the pupil of the eye which Papa calls an opacity, and which he says he is afraid will never go away; and there is a mist over it & I cannot see well. It is not disfigured & nobady [*sic*] can see it without looking very close.[49]

The boy expressed a longing for his mother and hoped she was well. 'I wish you were here', he wrote and asked that she 'wear for my sake' the small gold seal he was sending her. Before closing the letter, he enclosed a lock of his hair.[50]

The need to treat his son's injured eye reaffirmed for Redfern the importance of his guardianship role while William Jr attended school in Edinburgh – there was no question of him returning to Sydney until his schooling was finished. At the end of July 1831 Redfern had completed the second year of his medical studies and the next two years involved clinical instruction in surgery and hospital work; two subjects he was particularly interested in. Redfern then made a totally unexpected decision; he discontinued his university studies. Of course, there could have been a multitude of reasons for him ceasing to attend lectures: his failing health was making it difficult to meet his own high standards of involvement in the courses; he had become less mobile and found it hard to participate in the long hospital practical sessions; he may have had a disagreement with one of the professors who were usually much younger than he was, or he may have decided that he knew more than the dons giving the next courses. Despite his decision not to re-enrol, he still could attend the surgery lectures twice a week if he wished to; these were free to surgeons and surgeon's mates of the Royal Navy, a qualification that Redfern held.

All letters coming to Edinburgh from Sydney were six months old by the time Redfern received it. He was kept abreast of management matters at Campbellfield and periodically gave advice on when to sell produce or buy more land, and their holdings flourished. By early 1833, the family's wealth had grown, and they owned over 22,000 acres of land.[51]

At Sarah's urging, the Wills' siblings made another attempt to overturn the judgement on George Howe's will. Their mother's pre-nuptial agreement with Howe protecting their inheritance had been dismissed in a lower court over a decade ago. On 25 June 1832 they challenged this finding in the Supreme Court convened by the Chief Justices Francis Forbes and James Dowling. The court ruled in favour of Sarah Howe (nee Wills and Harding), thus establishing the precedent in colonial law that a prenuptial agreement protects a wife and her children's inheritance from the 'fraudulent' action of a partner. The premises at 96 George Street now belonged to the children of Sarah Howe, not to the children of Robert Howe.[52]

William had always treasured the oval miniature portrait of Sarah framed in a gilt metal frame with a lock of her brown hair enclosed at the back. In August 1832, at the age of 57, William Redfern had his own portrait painted in miniature by the Edinburgh artist George Marshall Mather.[53] He placed the framed miniature in one of the boxes he sent to Sarah and is also likely to have included a letter asking Sarah to come to Britain, pointing out that his health was not the best, and that he and her son greatly desired to have her close by. Although no record of such plea has survived, one suspects that Redfern would have been far too proud to say just how ill he was. He desperately needed Sarah to be there but is most unlikely to have resorted to emotional blackmail.

On 31 October 1832 Redfern replied to a letter from Sarah's 21-year-old brother Horatio. The lad's wellbeing had always been a priority for William, and he was probably more of a father figure than a brother-in-law. Horatio was contemplating getting married and sought advice about his inheritance and future investment. It appears that he was considering the purchase of *The Sydney Gazette*, the newspaper he had been managing since Robert Howe's death. Redfern's letter to Horatio was wise and thoughtfully written. It also contains some personal insights into his views about life. The Doctor's last surviving letter shows no evidence that he had lost his mental faculties. Indeed, quite the opposite; it reveals an intelligent man offering carefully considered advice.

> [I] rejoice to hear that you have sown "all your wild oats" and that you are determined to become a sensible, steady, clever fellow. To become so only requires resolution. Stick close to your studies and the rest will be sure to follow. If you go on as you promise to do, you will be a credit to yourself, an honor to your relations, and a benefit to mankind. Persevere!
>
> The funds are perfectly secure. Hence you may be quite at ease on the score of the safety of your Legacy. Dread must be the Shock, that will destroy the Public debt. Its monstrous magnitude is its greatest security. There are too many interested in its preservation; to admit every trifling excitement to terminate in Revolution. All is safe. If I can guide you in any way by investing your funds in goods suitable for Colonial Market, I shall be happy to attend to your instructions. But I think, you should, previously

to taking any step in this affair, consult your brother.

The request you make in one part of your letter does credit to your heart, but I regret to say that its accomplishment is utterly impracticable; and, indeed, admitting it will, it would be unwise to attend it. The only effect it could produce would be that of honour up feelings which time has now, in some measure, tranquilized. The sufferings of some of the family have already been too severe, for me to be instrumental in their re-excitement.

I send you in Mrs. Redfern's box, Cobbetts French Grammar. I have read it as far as it is cut. It is an excellent book and if you will study it as he directs I am satisfied you cannot fail to become a good French scholar. – I regret to say that all Edinburgh cannot produce the Printers Grammar. I desired my bookseller to get it from London; but he has disappointed me. I gave an order to another, who promised to send for it, but he has not yet received it. I shall send it in the next box to Mrs. Redfern.

With every wish for your health and happiness, I remain my dear Horatio, yours ever truth.   Wm Redfern[54]

By the time Horatio received Redfern's reply, he had just started to publish a new newspaper *The Currency Lad*. In December 1832 Horatio was appointed the editor of *The Sydney Gazette*.[55]

In early 1833 Redfern's health was declining quickly, and he would have desperately hoped that his portrait and letter had convinced Sarah of the need to come to Edinburgh. This certainly seems to have been the case and on 10 March 1833 Sarah left Sydney on the fast merchant ship *Norfolk* sailing directly to London.[56]

In early July 1833 Redfern decided, and may have been advised by his personal physician, to make arrangements for approaching death. His Last Will and Testament had been drawn up in 1828 and since none of his four executors lived in Britain, he asked David Walker, an auctioneer in Lothian Street, to buy a burial plot and gravestone at the New Ground cemetery in Edinburgh in the event of his death before Sarah arrived. His greatest concern would have been for his son, and he almost certainly arranged a guardianship for the 14-year-old or enrolled him as a boarder at the Edinburgh Academy. The actual arrangements are also unrecorded. In any case, he would have kept his brother Joseph in Belfast abreast of his plans.

Despite the medical care of some of Edinburgh's best doctors, William Redfern died at 18 Lothian Street on 17 July 1833, aged

58. The cause of death is unknown.[57] On 23 July he was buried in the New Calton Burial Ground. The headstone simply reads:

WILL^M REDFERN, ESQ.
DIED 17TH JULY, 1833.

It was a lonely closure to an admirable life. William had hoped to talk to Sarah before he died and had he known that she was almost in the country, one feels certain he would have used his steely determination to hold out until she was at his bedside. Alas no such notice of Sarah's imminent arrival existed – such were the vagaries and uncertainties of 19th century communications.

The ship *Norfolk*, with Sarah on board, docked in London on 22 July.[58] She reached Edinburgh a week later to the heartbreaking news that her husband had been buried only days earlier. She had been too late to say goodbye and could only weep with her son at William's graveside.

It was not until December 1833 that the news reached the colony that Dr Redfern had died, and that his wife Sarah had arrived only days after his burial. There would have been much sadness across the settlement at the passing of the esteemed surgeon, farmer, banker and benefactor. William Wentworth in particular would have mourned the sudden loss of a friend and mentor. William Redfern had been a fatherly guardian to the Wills siblings and a dear friend of the Antill family and they would have deeply grieved at his passing. It was, in many senses, the end of an era.

Horatio Wills, the new editor of *The Sydney Gazette* and brother-in-law of The Doctor, published a short tribute.

> The long stay of the Doctor in Europe was occasioned by a paternal anxiety for his only child – a son (now in his 15th year), whose education he superintended at Edinburgh. As a professional man, the abilities of Dr. Redfern were highly respectable; as a private individual, those who were connected with him by ties of blood deeply lament a firm, liberal, and affectionate friend.[59]

Epilogue

William Redfern had made William Wentworth, Thomas Wills, Henry Antill and 'his dearly beloved wife Sarah Redfern' the executors of his will, knowing they would protect the interests of the beneficiaries and administer the estate until his only son William Lachlan Macquarie reached adulthood. In his will Redfern bequeathed the 22,500 acres of land and the houses thereon to his son William L.M. Redfern. The remaining property and most of the livestock was shared between his son and wife. Sarah also inherited the contents of the Campbellfield house and the right to use a third of the land as a *dower* for the duration of her life.

The will struck off a £1000 loan to Redfern's brother Robert. William's niece Eliza Watt was awarded £20 per year until she finished her apprenticeship and given £100 to set up her own business. Nephews Hugh and William Watt were each given £150 on reaching adulthood and his sisters Margaret Watt and Eliza McDowell given each £100.[1] The bequest made William L.M. and his mother Sarah extremely wealthy.

In accordance with the will, William L.M. remained at school in Scotland. Sarah sold most of the expensive furniture and library of books from the Lothian Street apartment for £583 (£53,860 today) and moved to Glasgow with her son to resume his schooling.[2] In Sydney, Redfern's three executors pressed debtors to the estate for payment and took court action when necessary. In March 1834 the 100 acres of land on Botany Road was subdivided into allotments of two to five acres and leased for seven years. A two-day auction at the Campbellfield estate sold the elegant furniture and other household items; Lady's dresses and wine; 400 sheep, 60 cows, 40 horses and a 'very elegant green-bodied, full-sized family carriage'.[3]

On 24 June 1834, a year after William Redfern's death, Sarah Redfern, 37, married the Glasgow merchant James Alexander, 36. After a business trip in Sydney in 1832, Glasgow-born James had returned to Britain on the same ship as Sarah. Just as her mother had, Sarah made a premarital agreement with James protecting her son's inheritance. On 9 February 1835 the couple had a daughter Sarah. In that year, William L.M., now nick-named 'Mac', began his studies at the University of Glasgow. He graduated with an Arts degree in 1837 and formed a partnership with his stepfather in the import-export trading firm *Redfern, Alexander & Co.*

In 1842 all properties of the late Dr Redfern in New South Wales were put up for sale. The firm Redfern, Alexander & Co managed the sale, and Sarah and James Alexander travelled to Australia to be present. Because of the dower clause in the will, Sarah needed her son's permission to sell the land and, while granting this, Mac also gave his mother ownership of the 30 acres of land she received as a dowry when marrying Redfern.[4] Sarah and James Alexander and their daughter Sarah arrived in Sydney in late November 1841.

In February 1842 details of the Redfern estate were announced in the press. It included 100 acres of Sydney land, 6000 acres at Campbellfield, 270 acres at Bringelly, 4700 acres on Cox's River and Lachlan River, 11,362 acres at Bathurst and other smaller plots. Also offered were 8000 sheep, a herd of cattle, milk cows, pigs, stud horses and working bullocks.[5] The 100 acres of land on Botany Road had been subdivided into 302 lots ranging in area from 400 to 4000 m^2 and was named 'Dr. Redfern's Estate'. The lots were traversed by Redfern Street and encompassed by Cleveland Street, Elizabeth Street, Phillip Street and Botany Road (Regent Street). This land is one third of today's Sydney suburb of *Redfern*. The lots sold for £22 to £155 with a 15% cash deposit and 5 to 21 year loans were offered at 10% interest. After four years, the sale of all 100 acres of land in Sydney returned £24,300 (£2.2 M today). Sale of the estate's rural land was less successful and only 1100 acres of the Campbellfield farm were sold for £8,000.[6] The unsold land was leased over the next 40 years and later valued at over £60,000.[7]

On 6 June 1842, while his mother Sarah and stepfather James were still in Sydney, William L.M. Redfern, 23, married Jane Bastable Walker, 18, in Glasgow.[8] The couple would have six children who survived to adulthood. In 1850 the Redfern and Alexander families moved to London and expanded the firm Redfern, Alexander & Co. into Australia and New Zealand. Mrs Sarah Alexander, formerly Redfern, died on 10 January 1875 at Roke Manor in Romsey Southampton, aged 78, leaving a personal wealth of £35,000 to her two children Mac and Sarah.[9] William L.M. (Mac)

EPILOGUE

Redfern died in London on 29 July 1904, aged 84, leaving an estate valued at £154,306 (£14.3 M today).[10]

Dr William Redfern had always maintained a strong relationship with his siblings Joseph, Eliza, Margaret and Robert. He had encouraged Margaret and husband Andrew Watt to educate their two oldest sons in Trowbridge Wiltshire. After finishing school in 1831, William, 18, and Hugh, 20, went to Australia and managed their uncle's farm in Bathurst. Their siblings Thomas, Ann and Elizabeth joined them later. In 1859 William Watt became the Member for Carcoar in the NSW Legislative Assembly.

Thomas Wills continued to manage the Campbellfield estate for another five years. In 1831 he helped petitioners of Campbelltown district to lobby the governor, and in 1832 was appointed the first Australian-born Justice of the Peace. In 1838 Thomas purchased land in Melbourne and a year later drove his cattle there to become a prosperous farmer, Justice of Peace, magistrate, board member of the Port Phillip Savings Bank, President of the shire and in 1843 director of the Union Bank. Thomas died in 1872 aged 72.

Horatio Wills' involvement in *The Sydney Gazette* and *The Currency Lad* newspapers ended in December 1833 when he married Elizabeth McGuire, 16, and became a farmer in the Molonglo district New South Wales. The couple had nine children, including Thomas Wills, an early renowned cricketer and the founder of Australian Rules football. In 1839 Horatio Wills and his family overlanded 5000 sheep and 500 cattle to the Port Phillip district to join his brother Thomas, where he purchased 120,000 acres land. Horatio sold the property in 1852 and moved to Melbourne, where he was elected to the Victorian Legislative Council in 1855, a position he held until 1859 when he travelled to Germany to visit his three sons at their school in Bonn. Back in Port Phillip in 1861, Horatio with his son Thomas and a party of stockmen and their families, shipped a large herd of animals to Brisbane and drove them to central Queensland to set up a station at Cullin-la-ringo near Springsure. Three weeks later, Horatio, aged 49, and 18 of his men and their families were killed when Aboriginal people attacked their camp; his son Thomas survived. The Cullin-la-ringo attack was the largest single massacre of European settlers in Australian history. The dreadful reprisals that followed resulted in the death of over 350 Aboriginal people.[11]

Henry Antill and Eliza (nee Wills) lived with their ten children on their Jarvisfield estate in Picton. After retiring from the military, Henry was made a Justice of the Peace and magistrate, and in 1829 became the Superintendent of Police for Picton. As magistrate he was meticulous and accused of showing undue sympathy towards convicts brought before him in court. Henry Antill died at Jarvisfield in 1852 aged 73 and his wife Eliza died in 1858 aged 56. In 1936 Henry's grandson Major-General John Macquarie Antill and his daughter Rose Antill-de Warren published *The Emancipist*, a historical play of three acts about Dr Redfern. The play comprises an entertaining series of clever conversations between William and Sarah Redfern, Henry Antill and Lachlan Macquarie. It relates to actual events but is certainly not an accurate historical record.[12]

In 1961 the Australian Broadcasting Corporation (ABC) produced the historical television drama *The Outcasts*, which was broadcast live on Sunday nights as twelve half-hour episodes. The central figure in *The Outcasts* was Dr William Redfern. The drama begins in 1808 when the former convict Redfern was admitted as a surgeon to the Sydney hospital and later episodes portray the struggle of emancipists for recognition in the colony. Two episodes cover the Bigge inquiry into Macquarie's administration and Bigge's dislike of Redfern. Episode 12 finishes with Redfern's going to England to plead for emancipists' causes.[13] The plot of *The Outcasts* was historically accurate and included events not widely known. Reviews and ratings were high, and the series quickly became popular viewing on Sunday night television.[14]

The journalist Malcolm Ellis, author of biographies on Lachlan Macquarie and John Macarthur, was critical of the production and its authenticity. Ellis wrote in *The Bulletin* that William Redfern was not part of Macquarie's fight for emancipists and not the humanitarian depicted. An ultra-conservative and monarchist, Ellis condemned Redfern for his involvement in the mutiny and declared he had sympathy for the officers who would not associate with the Doctor, and for the British government's opposition to his promotion. He wrote that he would not have sat at the same table as William Redfern either.[15] The ABC producer Brian Wright responded to these criticisms by defending Dr Redfern's

EPILOGUE

prominence in the drama as being true to historical records, and assured Ellis that the scriptwriter Rex Rienits had not tampered with actual events.[16]

The ABC television drama revitalised the interest of the Australian public in William Redfern's important contributions to the Sydney hospital and his efforts to improve sanitation and health aboard convict ships. In 1994 the Australasian Faculty of Public Health Medicine (AFPHM) instituted an annual *William Redfern Oration*, which commemorates Dr Redfern's pioneering work in public health and preventive medicine in Australia.

Since 1994 the William Redfern Oration has been the keynote address at the annual congress of The Royal Australasian College of Physicians (RACP). It is a tribute that would have especially pleased The Doctor.

Family of William Redfern & Sarah Wills

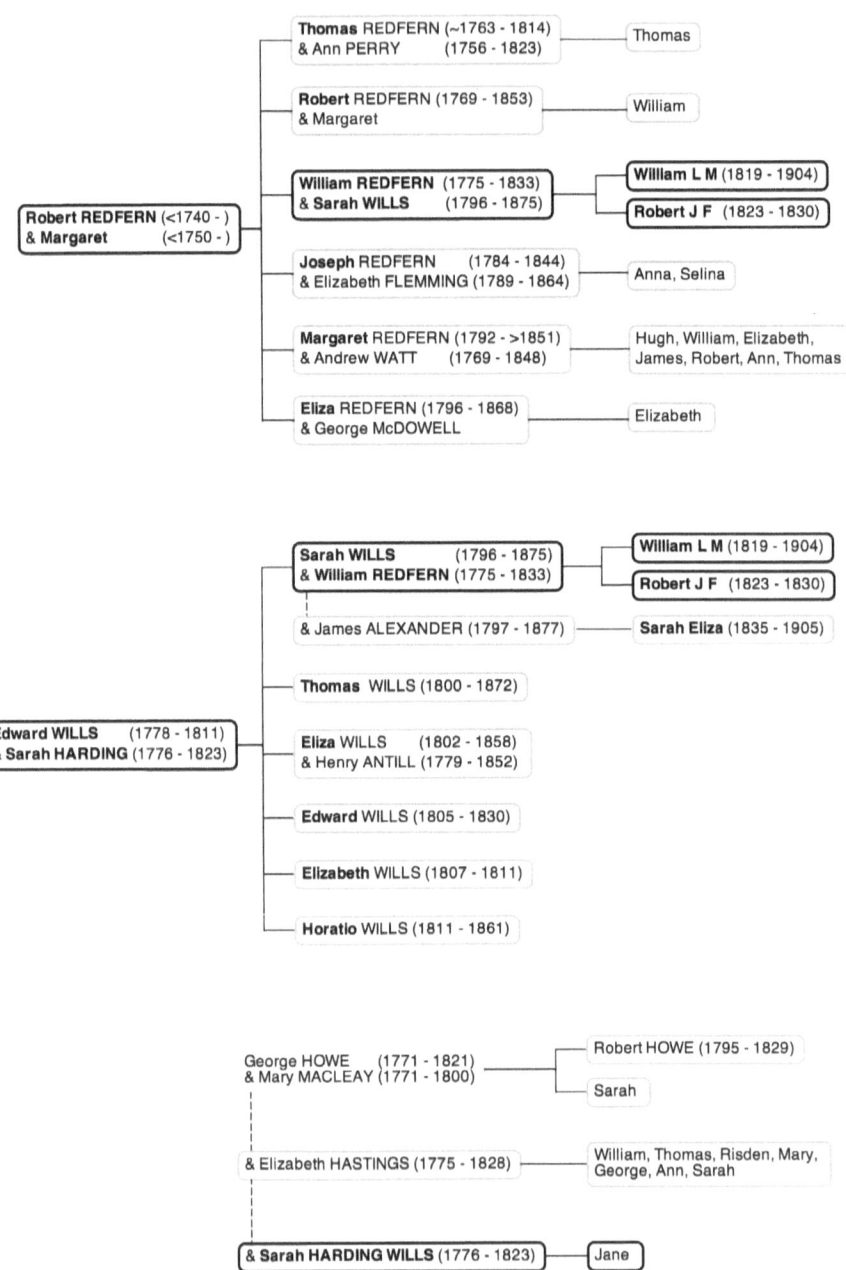

Acknowledgements

I am indebted to the Mitchell Library, the State Archives and Records of New South Wales and the National Library of Australia for access to official records, letters and dispatches cited in this book, and wish to thank the staff at the Mitchell Library Reading Room for their assistance in helping me find the more obscure records and illustrations.

I acknowledge the earlier research on William Redfern's life by Arthur Raymond Jones and his 2019 publication, *Better than Cure* – a tome that took Jones over 55 years to complete. Most original material in my biography was obtained from the digitised archives of newspapers, books and documents accessed over the Internet. In this endeavour, the web service TROVE at the National Library of Australia (NLA), and its access to the Australian Joint Copying Project, has been essential. Contemporary details of colonial life and people were extracted from newspapers, Government gazettes and publications stored electronically at the NLA library. I also wish to thank the State Library of Western Australia for electronic access to their British newspaper collection.

The NSW Land Registry Services supplied many of the historical maps and land transactions used in this book. The National Records of Scotland and The National Archives (UK) rendered documents on Redfern's trial and his family, and the National Archive of Ireland supplied details of William's brother Robert Redfern. A number of the illustrations in this book are sketches, drawings and paintings of early landscapes and portraits. These have been sourced as digital online images from the State Library of New South Wales, the Mitchell and Dixon Libraries, the National Library of Australia and the Wellcome Library London. I thank these institutions for this extremely valuable service.

I wish to thank Damian Greenish, the ggg-grandson of William Redfern, for allowing the reproduction of the miniature portraits of William and Sarah Redfern in this publication. His feedback on other aspects of this biography is also gratefully acknowledged.

I am deeply appreciative to Ruth Guss and Barbara Hall for their comments on the early draft chapters and to my husband Syd, whose efforts on many fronts has been absolutely invaluable.

BIBLIOGRAPHY

ARCHIVES AND RECORDS

AJCP	Australian Joint Copying Project
HC Deb	House of Commons Debate
HLRV	Historical Land Records Viewer, New South Wales
HRA	Historical Records Australia
HRNSW	Historical Records of New South Wales
NAI	National Archives Ireland
NLA	National Library of Australia
NRS	National Records of Scotland
PRONI	Public Record Office of Northern Ireland
SANSW	State Archives & Records of New South Wales
SLNSW	State Library of New South Wales
DX	Dixson Library
ML	Mitchell Library
TNA	The National Archives UK, Australian Joint Copying Project
WL	Wellcome Library, England

PRIMARY SOURCES

Bigge, John, *Report of the Commissioner of Inquiry into the State of the Colony of New South Wales*, House of Commons, 5 Aug 1822.

Bigge, John, *Report of the Commissioner of Inquiry on the Judicial Establishment of New South Wales and Van Diemen's Land*, House of Commons, 21 Feb 1823.

Bigge, John, *Report of the Commissioner of Inquiry into the State of Agriculture and Trade in the Colony of New South Wales*, House of Commons, 13 Mar 1823.

Bladen, F. M. (ed.), *Historical Records of New South Wales*, Vol I - VII, Government Printer, Sydney, 1892-1901.

Blane, Gilbert, *Observations on the Diseases Incident to Seamen*, London, 1785.

Burdett, Francis, *An Impartial Statement of the Inhuman Cruelties Discovered in the Coldbath-Fields Prison ... reported in the House of Commons ... the 11th July 1800*.

Cunningham, Peter, *Two Years in New South Wales*, Vol I & II, London, 1827.

Finucane, James, *Distracted Settlement: New South Wales after Bligh*, ed. Anne-Marie Whitaker, Miegunyah Press, Melbourne, 1998.

House of Commons, *Report from the Select Committee on Transportation*, 1812.

House of Commons, *Report from the Select Committee on the State of Gaols*, 1819.

Lind, James, *An Essay on the Most Effectual Means of Preserving the Health of Seamen in the Royal Navy and A Dissertation on Fevers and Infection*, London, 1774.

Lind, James, *Treatise of the Scurvy*, Edinburgh, 1753.

Macquarie, Lachlan, *Lachlan Macquarie, Governor of New South Wales, Journals of his Tours in New South Wales and Diemen's Land 1810-1822*, Trustees of the Public Library of New South Wales, Sydney, 1956.

Macquarie, Lachlan, *A Letter to the Right Honourable Viscount Sidmouth in Refutation of Statements made by the Hon. Henry Grey Bennet, MP*, London, 1821.

BIBLIOGRAPHY

Macquarie, Lachlan, *Copy of a Report by the late Major General Macquarie, on the Colony of New South Wales, to Earl Bathurst; in July 1822*, London, 1828.

Macquarie, Lachlan, *Extract of a Letter from Major General Macquarie to Earl Bathurst, in October 1823; in Answer to certain Part of the Report of Mr. Commissioner Bigge, on the State of the said Colony*, London, 1828.

Neale, William Johnson, *History of the Mutiny at Spithead and the Nore*, London, 1842.

Neild, James, *An Account of the Rise, Progress, and Present State, of the Society for the Discharge and Relief of Persons Imprisoned for Small Debts throughout England and Wales*, London, 1802.

Smellie, William, *A Treatise on the Theory and Practise of Midwifery*, London, 1766.

The Medical Calendar or Student's Guide to the Medical Schools, Maclachlan & Stewart, Edinburgh, 1828.

Thomson, Frederick, *An Essay on the Scurvy: Shewing Effectual and Practical Means for its Prevention at Sea*, London, 1790.

Trotter, Thomas, *Medicina Nautica: An Essay on the Diseases of Seamen*, Vol 1 & 2, London, 1797 & 1799.

Noah, William, *Voyage to Sydney in the Ship Hillsborough 1798-1799 and A Description of the Colony*, Library of Australian History, Sydney, 1978.

Vaux, James Hardy, *Memoirs of James Hardy Vaux*, London, 1819.

Watson, Frederick (ed.), *Historical Records of Australia*, Series I, Vol I - XIV, Series IV, Vol I, Library Committee of the Commonwealth, Government Printer, Sydney, 1914 - 1922.

Wentworth, William Charles, *Statistical, Historical, and Political Description of the Colony of New South Wales*, London, 1819.

Wentworth, William Charles, *A Statistical Account of the British Settlements in Australasia*, Vol I & II, London, 1824.

Wentworth, William Charles, *Australasia: A Poem written for the Chancellor's Medal at Cambridge*, London, 1823.

SECONDARY SOURCES

Antill, John Macquarie, Antill-De Warren, Rose, *The Emancipist: An Historical Drama in Three Acts*, Angus & Robertson, Sydney, 1936.

Atkinson, Alan, *The Europeans in Australia, Vol 1, A History*, Oxford University Press Australia, Melbourne, 1997.

Atkinson, Alan, *The Europeans in Australia, Vol 2, Democracy*, UNSW Press, Sydney, 2016.

Atkinson, Alan, *Elizabeth and John: The Macarthurs of Elizabeth Farm*, NewSouth Publishing, Sydney, 2022.

Bateson, Charles, *The Convict Ships, 1787-1868*, Brown, Son & Ferguson, Glasgow, 1959.

Baxter, Carol, *Muster and Lists, New South Wales and Norfolk Island*, Volumes: 1800-1802; 1805-1806; 1814; ABGR in association with Society of Australian Genealogists, Sydney, 1988,1989, 2006.

Baxter, Carol, *Guide to Convict Transportation Lists, Part 2: 1801-1812*, Unlock the Past, St Agnes, 2015.

Butlin, Sydney James, *Foundations of The Australian Monetary System 1788-1851*, Melbourne University Press, Carlton, 1953.

BIBLIOGRAPHY

Byrne, Paula Jane ed, *Judge Advocate Ellis Bent, Letter and Diaries 1809-1811*, Desert Pea Press, Sydney, 2012.

Clark, Manning, *A History of Australia, Vol. 1: From the Earliest Times to the Age of Macquarie*, Melbourne University Press, Carlton, 1979.

Clark, Manning, *Manning Clark's History of Australia*, abridge M. Cathcart, Melbourne University Press, Carlton, 1997.

Clune, Frank, *Bound for Botany Bay, Narrative of a Voyage in 1798 Aboard the Death Ship, Aboard the Death Ship Hillsborough*, Angus and Robertson, Sydney, 1964.

Comrie, John, *English Medicine in the Eighteenth Century*, Journal of the Royal Society of Medicine, 1935, Vol 28, pp. 1603-1610.

Connor, Michael Charles, *The Politics of Grievance: society and political controversies in New South Wales, 1819-1827*, PhD thesis, University of Tasmania, 2002.

Cummins, Cyril Joseph, *A History of Medical Administration in NSW 1788-1973*, NSW Health, Sydney, 2003.

Currey, Charles Herbert, *The Brothers Bent*, Sydney University Press, Sydney, 1968.

Dando-Collins, Stephen, *Captain Bligh's other Mutiny*, Random House, Sydney, 2007.

Dillon, Harry & Butler, Peter, *Macquarie: From colony to country*, William Heinemann, Sydney, 2010.

Dermody, Kathleen Mary, *D'Arcy Wentworth 1762-1827, A Second Chance*, PhD thesis, Australian National University, 1990.

Dugan, James, *The Great Mutiny*, Andre Deutsch, London, 1966.

Dunlop, Norman, *William Redfern, The First Australian Medical Graduate, and His Time*, Journal Royal Australian Historical Society, 14, pt 2, 1928, pp. 57-105.

Ellis, Malcolm Henry, *Lachlan Macquarie: His Life, Adventures and Times*, Angus & Robertson, Sydney, 1969.

Ellis, Malcolm Henry, *John Macarthur*, Angus & Robertson, Sydney, 1973.

Ford, Edward, *The Life and Work of William Redfern*, Annual Post-Graduate Oration, Sydney, 1953.

Gill, Conrad, *The Naval Mutinies of 1797*, University Press, Manchester, 1913.

Goddard, Jonathan Charles, *Genitourinary medicine and surgery in Nelson's navy*, Postgraduate Medical Journal, Vol 81, 2005, pp. 413-418.

Gojak, Denis, *The 1820 Influenza Outbreak in Sydney and its Impact on the Indigenous and Settler Populations*, Journal Royal Australian Historical Society, 105, pt 2, 2019, pp. 180-206.

Hall, Annegret, *In For The Long Haul, The First Fleet Voyage and Colonial Australia: The Convicts' Perspective*, ESH Publication, Nedlands, 2018.

Hall, Annegret, *Andrew Thompson, From Boy Convict to Wealthiest Settler in Colonial Australia*, ESH Publication, Nedlands, 2021.

Hill, David, *The Making of Australia*, William Heinemann, Sydney, 2015.

Hill, David, *Convict Colony: The remarkable story of the fledging settlement that survived against the odds*, Allen & Unwin, Crows Nest, 2019.

Hocking, Jenny, Donati, Laura, *Obscured but not Obscure: How History Ignored the Remarkable Story of Sarah Wills Howe*, Journal of the European Association for Studies of Australia, Vol 7, 2, 2016, pp. 58-69.

BIBLIOGRAPHY

Hughes, Robert, *The Fatal Shore, A History of the Transportation of Convicts to Australia 1787-1868*, The Folio Society, London, 1998.

Johns, Leanne, *Women in Colonial Commerce 1817-1820: The Window of understanding provided by The Bank of New South Wales Ledger and Minute Books*, thesis, Australian National University, Canberra, 2001.

Jones, Arthur Raymond, *William Redfern (1775?-1833): mutineer to colonial surgeon in New South Wales. Part I: Shock and Recovery*, Journal of Medical Biography, 7, 1999, pp. 35-41.

Jones, Arthur Raymond, *William Redfern (1775?-1833): mutineer to colonial surgeon in New South Wales. Part II: Promise and default*, Journal of Medical Biography, 7, 1999, pp. 78-85.

Jones, Arthur Raymond, *Surgeon William Redfern in London and Edinburgh 1828-1833?*, Journal Royal Australian Historical Society, 103, pt 2, 2017, pp. 201-211.

Jones, Arthur Raymond, *Better than Cure, The life and times of the ebullient and resilient William Redfern 1775-1833, Vol I, Wellbeing in the wooden world*, The Book Reality Experience, 2019.

Jones, Arthur Raymond, *Better than Cure, The life and times of the ebullient and resilient William Redfern 1775-1833, Vol II, Wellbeing in the colony*, The Book Reality Experience, 2019.

Karskens, Grace, *The Colony: A History of Early Australia*, Allen & Unwin, Crows Nest, 2010.

Karskens, Grace, *The Rocks, Life in Early Sydney*, Melbourne University Press, Carlton, 1997.

Keneally, Thomas, *Australians, Origins to Eureka*, Allen & Unwin, Crows Nest, 2009.

Kieza, Grantlee, *Macquarie*, ABC Books, Sydney, 2019.

Leroy, Paul Edwin, *The Emancipists - From Prison to Freedom: The Story of the Australian Convicts and their Descendants*, PhD thesis, Ohio State University, 1960.

Macarthur Onslow, Sibella, *Some early records of the Macarthurs of Camden*, Angus & Robertson, Sydney, 1914.

MacDonagh, Oliver, *The Inspector General, Sir Jeremiah Fitzpatrick and the Politics of Social Reform, 1783-1802*, Croom Helm, London, 1981.

Manwaring, George, Dobree, Bonamy, *The Floating Republic*, Penguin Books, London, 1937.

Nobbs, Raymond, *Norfolk Island and its first settlement 1788-1814*, Library of Australian History, Sydney, 1988.

Pfaff, Steve, Hechter, Michael, Corcoran, Katie, *The Problem of Solidarity in Insurgent Collective Action: The Nore Mutiny of 1797*, Social Science History, 40, 2016, pp. 247-270.

Pockley, Richard Vanderbyl, *Ancestor Treasure Hunt, The Edward Wills Family and Descendants in Australia*, Sydney, 1976.

Richards, David, *Transported to New South Wales: medical convicts 1788-1850*, British Medical Journal, 295, 1987, pp. 1609-1612.

Ritchie, John, *Punishment and Profit; The Reports of Commissioner Bigge on the Colonies of New South Wales and Van Diemen's Land, 1822-1823; their origins, nature and significance*, PhD thesis, Australian National University, 1969.

Ritchie, John, *Lachlan Macquarie: A Biography*, Melbourne University Press, Carlton, 1986.
Ritchie, John, *The Evidence to the Bigge Reports, New South Wales under Governor Macquarie,* Vol I & II, Heinemann, Melbourne, 1971.
Ritchie, John, *The Wentworth, Father and Son*, Melbourne University Press, Carlton, 1997.
Roe, Michael, *Trade, Life and Law at Norfolk Island 1806*-8, Tasmanian Historical Research Association, 35, No 3, 1988, pp. 93-111.
Roe, Michael, *The Slow Death of Norfolk's First Settlement*, Tasmanian Historical Research Association, 56, No 3, 2012, pp. 244-257.
Ross, John, *Attained No More: How Convicts Became Citizens*, Surry Hills, 2012.
Shann, Edward, *An Economic History of Australia*, Cambridge University Press, 1948.
Shaw, A. G. L., *Convicts & the Colonies, A Study of Penal Transportation from Great Britain & Ireland to Australia & other parts of the British Empire*, Melbourne University Press, Carlton, 1978.
Solomon, Ronald, *Barron Field and the Supreme Court of Civil Judicature: law, personality and politics in New South Wales, 1816-1824*, PhD thesis, University of New South Wales, 2013.
Starr, Fiona, *Convict artefacts from the Civil Hospital privy on Norfolk Island*, Australian Historical Archaeology, 19, 2001, pp. 39-47.
Starr, Fiona, *The Sidney Slaughter House: Convict Experience of Medical Care at the General 'Rum' Hospital, Sydney, 1816-1848*, Health and History, 19, No 2, 2017, pp. 60-89.
Tink, Andrew, *William Charles Wentworth: Australia's greatest native son*, Allen & Unwin, Crows Nest, 2012.
Walsh, Robin, *In Her Own Words: The writings of Elizabeth Macquarie*, Exisle Publishing, Wollombi, 2011.
Watson, Frederick, *The History of the Sydney Hospital from 1811 to 1911*, Government Printer, Sydney, 1911.
Whitaker, Anne-Maree, *Joseph Foveaux: A gentleman of high reputation*, Journal Royal Australian Historical Society, 83, pt 1, 1997, pp. 17-30.
Whitaker, Anne-Maree, *Swords to Ploughshares? The 1798 Irish Rebels in New South Wales*, Labour History, 75, 1998, pp. 9-21.
Whitaker, Anne-Maree, *Joseph Foveaux, Power and Patronage in Early New South Wales*, UNSW Press, Sydney, 2000.
Wills Cooke, Terry, *The Currency Lad*, 1997.

ELECTRONIC SOURCES

Ancestry	ancestry.com.au
Australian Dictionary of Biography	adb.anu.edu.au
Australian Joint Copying Project	nla.gov.au/content/australian-joint-copying-project
Biographical Database of Australia	bda-online.org.au
Findmypast	findmypast.com.au
Historical Land Record Viewer, NSW	hlrv.nswlrs.com.au
National Archives Ireland	nationalarchives.ie

BIBLIOGRAPHY

National Archives, UK	nationalarchives.gov.uk
National Library of Australia	nla.gov.au
Public Record Office of Northern Ireland	nidirect.gov.uk/campaigns/public-record-office-northern-ireland-proni
State Archives & Records NSW	records.nsw.gov.au
State Library NSW	sl.nsw.gov.au
Trove	trove.nla.gov.au

NOTES

CHAPTER 1 – Surgeon's Mate

1. Comrie, *English Medicine in the Eighteenth Century*, p. 1605.
2. There is a record of a Robert Redfern living in 1766 in Magherafelt Londonderry but without further information no connection can be made.
3. HMS *Standard* Muster, 1797, TNA: ADM 36/12239.
4. Wiltshire Record Society, by K.H. Rogers, *Early Trade Directories of Wiltshire*, Vol 47; Wiltshire Family History Society: WRO/A1/395.
5. *Northern Star*, 13 Jul 1795.
6. *The Caledonian Mercury*, 23 Nov 1833.
7. Redfern to Bigge, 26 Jun 1820, 8 Feb 1821, TNA: CO 201/124, pp. 94, 98.
8. Redfern notebook, 1796-1825, SLNSW: MAV/FM3/709.
9. Surgeons and surgeons' mates, 20 Jan 1797, TNA: ADM 104/6, p. 402.
10. HMS *Standard* Muster, 1797, TNA: ADM 36/12239.
11. Court Martial of Redfern, 23 Aug 1797, TNA: ADM 1/5486 Bk 31.
12. Goddard, *Genitourinary medicine and surgery in Nelson's navy*, p. 414.
13. Trotter, *Medicina Nautica*; Blane, *Observations on Diseases Incident to Seamen*; Thompson, *Essay on Scurvy*; Lind, *Essay on the Health of Seamen*.
14. Lind, *Treatise of Scurvy*.
15. Blane, *Observations on Diseases Incident to Seamen*, pp. 216-217.
16. Trotter, *Medicina Nautica*, pp. 221-222.

CHAPTER 2 – Mutiny at the Nore

1. Nelson to Hoste, 30 Jun 1797, Nicolas (Ed) *The Dispatches and Letters of Vice Admiral Lord Viscount Nelson*, 1845, p. 402.
2. Dugan, *The Great Mutiny*, pp. 58-59.
3. Manwaring & Bobree, *The Floating Republic*, pp. 66-67, 197.
4. Ibid.
5. Gill, *The Naval Mutinies of 1797*, pp. 6-7, 359-364.
6. Ibid.
7. Jones, *William Redfern*, Part I, pp. 35-36.
8. Gill, *The Naval Mutinies of 1797*, pp. 166-167.
9. Manwaring and Dobree, *The Floating Republic*, pp. 127-128.
10. Dando-Collins, *Captain Bligh's other Mutiny*, p. 245.
11. Gill, *The Naval Mutinies of 1797*, p. 141.
12. Manwaring and Dobree, *The Floating Republic*, pp. 144-146.
13. *The London Chronicle*, 27 May 1797.
14. Ibid.
15. Gill, *The Naval Mutinies of 1797*, pp. 351-353.
16. *The Hampshire Chronicle*, 27 May 1797.
17. Dugan, *The Great Mutiny*, pp. 187-188.
18. Dando-Collins, *Captain Bligh's other Mutiny*, p. 245.
19. Gill, *The Naval Mutinies of 1797*, pp. 167-169, 177.
20. Ibid.
21. Court Martial, 23 Aug 1797, TNA: ADM 1/5486 Bk 31, pp. 2-3.

NOTES

22 *The Evening Mail*, 31 May 1797.
23 Dugan, *The Great Mutiny*, pp. 494-495.
24 *The London Evening Post*, 1 Jun 1797.
25 Manwaring and Dobree, *The Floating Republic*, p. 72.
26 Gill, *The Naval Mutinies of 1797*, p. 275.
27 Court Martial, 24 Aug 1797, TNA: ADM 1/5486 Bk 32, pp. 68-69.
28 *Reading Mercury*, 5 Jun 1797.
29 *The Observer*, 4 Jun 1797.
30 *Northern Star*, 28 Apr 1797; Kilmainham prison, NAI: Book 1/10/1, Item 8.
31 Manwaring and Dobree, *The Floating Republic*, p. 221.
32 *The Saint James's Chronicle*, 8 Jun 1797.
33 *The General Evening Post*, 15 Jun 1797.

CHAPTER 3 – Court Martial

1 Court Martial, 24 Aug 1797, TNA: ADM 1/5486 Bk 32, pp. 34-35.
2 Pfaff et all, *Problem of Solidarity*, pp. 258-259.
3 Dugan, *The Great Mutiny*, p. 396.
4 Manwaring and Dobree, *The Floating Republic*, p. 269.
5 Gill, *The Naval Mutinies of 1797*, p. 248.
6 *The Morning Post*, 30 Jun 1797.
7 Jones, *Better than Cure*, Vol I, p. 149.
8 *The Morning Chronicle*, 30 Aug 1797.
9 Jones, *Better than Cure*, Vol I, pp. 150-152.
10 Ibid.
11 Court Martial, 24 Aug 1797, TNA: ADM 1/5486 Bk 32, pp. 61-62.
12 Ibid.
13 Court Martial, 23 Aug 1797, TNA: ADM 1/5486 Bk 31, pp. 3-7.
14 Ibid.
15 Court Martial, 24 Aug 1797, TNA: ADM 1/5486 Bk 32, pp. 68-69.
16 Ibid.
17 Court Martial, 23 Aug 1797, TNA: ADM 1/5486 Bk 31, pp. 34-42.
18 Court Martial, 24 Aug 1797, TNA: ADM 1/5486 Bk 32, pp. 48-57.
19 Bigge, *Report into the State of the Colony*, p. 84.
20 Court Martial, 24 Aug 1797, TNA: ADM 1/5486 Bk 32, pp. 30-36.
21 Ibid.
22 Ibid.
23 Court Martial, 24 Aug 1797, TNA: ADM 1/5486 Bk 32, pp. 49-50.
24 Court Martial, 24 Aug 1797, TNA: ADM 1/5486 Bk 32, p. 47.
25 Ibid.
26 Court Martial, 24 Aug 1797, TNA: ADM 1/5486 Bk 32, pp. 36-39.
27 Ibid.
28 Court Martial, 24 Aug 1797, TNA: ADM 1/5486 Bk 32, pp. 41-43.
29 Court Martial, 24 Aug 1797, TNA: ADM 1/5486 Bk 32, pp. 52-53.
30 Court Martial, 24 Aug 1797, TNA: ADM 1/5486 Bk 32, pp. 57-58.
31 Court Martial, 25 Aug 1797, TNA: ADM 1/5486 Bk 32, p. 60.
32 Court Martial, 24 Aug 1797, TNA: ADM 1/5486 Bk 32, pp. 113-114.
33 Redfern to Bigge, 5 Feb 1821, TNA: CO 201/124, p. 185.

NOTES

34 Manwaring and Dobree, *The Floating Republic*, p. 269.
35 Ford, *Life and Work of William Redfern*.
36 King's Pardon, 4 Sep 1797, TNA: HO 13/11, pp. 511-513.
37 Manwaring and Dobree, *The Floating Republic*, p. 269; King's Pardon, 4 Sep 1797, TNA: HO 13/11, pp. 511-513.
38 Manwaring and Dobree, *The Floating Republic*, p. 269.
39 Trotter, *Medicina Nautica*, Vol 2, p. 28.
40 Removal to Coldbath Fields prison, 23 Sep 1797, TNA: HO 13/11, p. 309.
41 *The Oracle*, 27 Dec 1798.
42 *The Whitehall Evening Post*, 26 Sep, 24 Oct 1797.
43 Redfern notebook, 1796-1825, SLNSW: MAV/FM3/709.
44 *The Courier*, 22 Dec 1798.
45 Redfern notebook, 1796-1825, SLNSW: MAV/FM3/709.
46 *The Oracle*, 27 Dec 1798.
47 *The Courier*, 22 Dec 1798.
48 *The London Chronicle*, 5 Jan 1799; *The True Briton*, 8 Jan 1799.
49 *The Courier*, 23 Feb 1799.
50 *The Oracle*, 7 Mar 1799.
51 Burdett, *Impartial Statement of the Inhuman Cruelties*, pp. 8-23.
52 Ibid.
53 Ibid.
54 *The Chester Courant*, 19 Aug 1800.
55 *The Star*, 1 Jan 1801.
56 Macquarie, *Letter to Sidmouth*, 1821, p. 38.
57 14 Nov 1800, TNA: HO 13/13, pp. 192-194.
58 25 Nov 1800, TNA: HO 13/13, p. 203.
59 *The General Evening Post*, 1 Jan 1801.
60 *The Oracle*, 6 Sep 1798.
61 *The Vindicator*, 13 Nov 1844.

CHAPTER 4 – Banished to NSW

1 Macquarie, *Letter to Sidmouth*, 1821, p. 38.
2 Captivity hulk, Jan 1801, TNA: HO 9/8, p. 159.
3 Fortunée and hospital hulk, 1 Apr 1801, TNA: HO 9/8, p. 32.
4 Neild, *Account of the Society for the Discharge and Relief*, pp. 312-319.
5 Bateson, *Convict Ships*, pp. 288-289.
6 Bateson, *Convict Ships*, p. 150.
7 Fitzpatrick to Rains, 13 May 1801, TNA: HO 42/62.
8 TNA: *Canada*: Wilkinson journal, May 1801, L/Mar/B/314A, pp. 5-7; *Minorca*: Leith journal, Apr-May 1801, L/Mar/B/335A, pp. 1-3; *Nile*: Sunter journal, Apr-May 1801, L/Mar/B/334A, pp. 1-5.
9 *Canada*: Wilkinson journal, 6 Jun 1801, TNA: L/Mar/B/314A, p. 9.
10 Vaux, *Memoirs*, p. 168.
11 Instructions to Surgeons, 8 Jun 1801, HRA, III, p. 98.
12 *Canada*: Wilkinson journal, 9 Jun 1801, TNA: L/Mar/B/314A, p. 9.
13 Macquarie, *Letter to Sidmouth*, 1821, p. 38.
14 Instructions, 10 Jun 1801, HRNSW, IV, pp. 399-402.

NOTES

15 Ibid.
16 *The Caledonian Mercury*, 27 Jun 1801.
17 Baxter, *Convict Transportation Lists*, pp. 15-18.
18 Instructions, 10 Jun 1801, HRNSW, IV, pp. 399-402.
19 *Canada*: Wilkinson journal, Jun 1801, TNA: L/Mar/B/314A, p. 10.
20 General Account of Persons, 2 Feb 1802, HRA, III, p. 380; Baxter, *Convict Transport List*, pp. 15-18; Bateson, *Convict Ships*, pp. 155, 288, 326; Fitzpatrick to Pelham, 21 Jun 1801, TNA: HO 11/1, HO 42/62.
21 Fitzpatrick to Pelham, 21 Jun 1801, TNA: HO 42/62.
22 Convict Indent, SLNSW: NRS 1151, [4/3999], Fiche 625.
23 *Canada*: Wilkinson journal, Jul-Aug 1801, TNA: L/Mar/B/314A, pp. 17-23.
24 *Canada*: Wilkinson journal, Aug 1801, TNA: L/Mar/B/314A, pp. 25-28.
25 Ibid.
26 *Canada*: Wilkinson journal, 28 Aug 1801, TNA: L/Mar/B/314A, pp. 40-42.
27 *Canada*: Wilkinson journal, 7 Sep 1801, TNA: L/Mar/B/314A, p. 1.
28 *Canada*: Wilkinson journal, Jul-Sep 1801, TNA: L/Mar/B/314A, p. 19.
29 *Canada*: Wilkinson journal, Aug-Sep 1801, TNA: L/Mar/B/314A, pp. 40-44.
30 *Canada*: Wilkinson journal, Oct 1801, TNA: L/Mar/B/314A, pp. 47-48.
31 *Canada*: Wilkinson journal, Dec 1801, TNA: L/Mar/B/314A, pp. 64-66.
32 Bateson, *Convict Ships*, p. 326; General return, 2 Feb 1802, HRA, III, p. 380.
33 King to King, 2 Feb 1802, HRA, III, p. 379.
34 King to Transport Commission, 2 Feb 1802, HRA, III, p. 381.

CHAPTER 5 – Norfolk Island

1   Antill, Antill-De Warren, *The Emancipist*, p. xi.
2   Redfern to Bigge, 5 Feb 1821, TNA: CO 201/124, p. 192.
3   Victualling List, 1802, TNA: CO 201/29, pp. 213-221.
4   King to King, 8 Nov 1801, HRNSW, IV, pp. 611-615.
5   P.G. King to J. King, 8 Nov 1801, HRA, III, p. 325.
6   King to Foveaux, 26 Jun 1800, HRA, II, p. 522.
7   King to Portland, 29 Apr 1800, HRA, II, p. 502.
8   Whitaker, *Joseph Foveaux*, p. 42.
9   Appointment of Foveaux by King, 26 Jun 1800, HRA, II, pp. 511-520.
10 Whitaker, *Swords to Ploughshares*, p. 9.
11 Whitaker, *Joseph Foveaux*, pp. 61-63.
12 Reg Wright, *The Fictions of 'Bucky' Jones and the Creators of Australian History*, 1998, http://www.postcolonialweb.org/australia/wright.html; Holt, Joseph, *Memoirs*, II, London, 1838; Robert Jones, *Recollections of 13 years Residence in Norfolk Island*, SLNSW: Safe 1/2d.
13 Whitaker, *Joseph Foveaux*, p. 2.
14 Victualling List, Jan 1802, TNA: CO 201/29, pp. 211-221.
15 Ibid.
16 Foveaux to King, 21 Nov 1802, SLNSW: SAFE/A 1444, pp. 42-43.
17 Ibid.
18 Richards, *Transported to NSW: medical convicts*, pp. 1609-1611.
19 State of Settlement, 27 Aug 1802, TNA: CO 201/29, p. 57.
20 Redfern to Bigge, 26 Jun 1820, TNA: CO 201/124, p. 94.

NOTES

21. State of Settlement, Aug 1802, TNA: CO 201/29, p. 56.
22. Account of Stores, 1802, TNA: CO 201/29, pp. 148, 151, 162.
23. Return of Stock, 2 Aug 1802, TNA: CO 201/29, p. 59.
24. D'Arcy Wentworth bought the land from Joseph McCaulden in 1794 and sold it again when leaving the island in 1796. Land grant and sale, 9 Jul 1802, SRNSW: NRS 898, [9/2731, p. 69], Fiche 3267; Settler's plot in cultivation, 1794, TNA: CO 700 New South Wales 12.
25. Redfern to Bigge, 5 Feb 1821, TNA: CO 201/124, p. 196.
26. Piper's Norfolk Island return, 15 May 1808, TNA: CO 201/129, p. 142.
27. Redfern to Wentworth, 16 Sep 1807, SLNSW: SAFE/A 751, pp. 201-203.
28. Government Order, 28 Jun 1802, HRNSW, IV, p. 792.
29. Government Order, 6 Jul 1802, HRNSW, IV, p. 797.
30. King to Paterson, 18 Sep 1800, HRNSW, IV, pp. 142-143.
31. King to Foveaux, Aug-Oct 1802, SLNSW: A 2015, pp. 254, 256.
32. State of Settlement, 27 Aug 1802, TNA: CO 201/29, pp. 55-57, 70.
33. Government Order, Sep-Oct 1802, HRNSW, IV, pp. 837, 853.
34. King to Portland, 21 May 1802, HRA, III, p. 490.
35. Foveaux to King, 21 Nov 1802, SLNSW: SAFE/A 1444, p. 48.
36. King to Foveaux, 25 Dec 1802, SLNSW: A 2015, p. 268.
37. Norfolk settlement report, 1802, TNA: CO 201/29, pp. 95, 253.
38. Starr, *Convict artefacts from the Civil Hospital on Norfolk Island*, pp. 39-45.
39. Jones, *Recollections of 13 years Residence in Norfolk Island*, SLNSW: Safe 1/2d, p. 16.
40. Government Order, 8 Feb 1803, HRA, IV, p. 332.
41. King to Hobart, 18, 29 Mar 1803, HRA, IV, pp. 336-338.
42. King to Foveaux, 18 Apr 1803, SLNSW: A 2015, p. 287.
43. King to Foveaux, 7 Jun 1803, SLNSW: A 2015, p. 301; *The Sydney Gazette*, 19 Jun 1803.
44. Voucher for Swine Flesh, Sep 1803, TNA: CO 201/30, pp. 108, 122-123.
45. Sick, Death & Births, May-Jun 1803, TNA: CO 201/29, p. 262.
46. Redfern on Foveaux's health, 22 Sep 1803, TNA: CO 201/30, p. 60.
47. Foveaux to King, 21 Sep 1803, SLNSW: SAFE/A 1444, pp. 63-64.
48. Victualling List, 1803, TNA: CO 201/30, p. 85.
49. King to Hobart, 1 Mar 1804, HRA, IV, pp. 454-455.
50. King to Sullivan, 7 Aug 1803, HRA, IV, pp. 366-367.
51. Government Order, 3 Jan, 8 Feb 1804 HRNSW, V, pp. 22, 300.
52. *The Sydney Gazette*, 22 Jan 1804.
53. Foveaux to King, Feb 1804, SLNSW: SAFE/A 1444, pp. 65-68.
54. Foveaux to Hobart, 1 May 1804, TNA: CO 201/30, pp. 1-4.
55. Sick, Death & Births, 17 Aug 1804, TNA: CO 201/30, p. 302.
56. Return of acres, Mar 1804, TNA: CO 201/30, pp. 56-57.
57. Voucher for Swine Flesh, May-Jun 1804, TNA: CO 201/30, pp. 233-237.
58. Redfern notebook, 1796-1825, SLNSW: MAV/FM3/709.

CHAPTER 6 – Norfolk Farmer & Trader

1. Foveaux's testimonial of Redfern, 3 Sep 1804, HRA, X, p. 275.
2. Victualing Book, Jan-Jun 1804, TNA: CO 201/30, p. 210.

NOTES

3 Dermody, *D'Arcy Wentworth*; Tink, *William Charles Wentworth*.
4 Villiers to Colonial Office, 16 Oct 1789, HO 42/15, pp. 304-305.
5 Dermody, *D'Arcy Wentworth*, pp. 31-32.
6 Cookney to Wentworth, 17 Dec 1789, SLNSW: A 715, pp. 12-12a.
7 Hobart to King, 24 Jun 1803, HRA, IV, p. 304.
8 King to Foveaux, 20 Jul 1804, HRSW, V, pp. 403-404; Foveaux to King, 10 Aug 1804, SLNSW: SAFE/A 1444, pp. 85-88.
9 Instructions to Paterson, 1 Jun 1804, HRA, V, pp. 22-24.
10 Report on Settlers on Norfolk Island, 19 Jul 1804, HRA, V, pp. 216-217.
11 King to Foveaux, 20 Jul 1804, HRNSW, V, p. 405.
12 King to Hobart, 20 Jul 1804, HRA, V, pp. 26-30.
13 King to Hobart, 19 May 1804, HRA, IV, pp. 647-648.
14 Foveaux to King, 10 Aug 1804, SLNSW: SAFE/A 1444, p. 90.
15 Piper to King, 10 Feb 1805, HRA, V, p. 327.
16 Foveaux to King, 7 Sep 1804, SLNSW: SAFE/A 1444, pp. 91-93; Foveaux to Hobart, 7 Sep 1804, TNA: CO 201/30, p. 190.
17 Foveaux's testimonial of Redfern, 3 Sep 1804, HRA, X, p. 275.
18 Class of Settlers, Mar 1805, TNA: CO 201/42, pp. 308-311.
19 Piper's Norfolk Island return, 15 May 1808, TNA: CO 201/129, p. 142.
20 Nobbs, *Norfolk Island*, p. 218.
21 Foveaux to Piper, 1 Jun 1806, SLNSW: MLMSS 681/4, p. 55.
22 Land sale, 8 Sep 1804, SRNSW: NRS 898, [9/2731, p. 69], Fiche 3267.
23 King to Piper, 6 Jan 1805, SLNSW: Safe 1/51, pp. 34-35; Number embarked, Feb 1805, TNA: CO 201/42, p. 77.
24 Inhabitants of Norfolk Island, June 1805, HRA, V, pp. 508-509.
25 Butlin, *Australian Monetary System*, pp. 26-30.
26 Butlin, *Australian Monetary System*, p. 56.
27 Voucher for Receipts, 1805, TNA: CO 201/42, pp. 168, 204.
28 Survey of salted pork, 16 Nov 1805, TNA: CO 201/42, p. 225.
29 King to Piper, 9 May 1806, HRA, V, pp. 757-758.
30 King to Marsden, 22 Feb 1806, HRA, V, p. 638.
31 Piper's Norfolk Island return, 15 May 1808, TNA: CO 201/129, p. 142.
32 Redfern to Wentworth, 16 Sep 1807, SLNSW: SAFE/A 751, pp. 201-203.
33 Wentworth to Piper, 29 Nov 1806, HRNSW, VI, p. 204.
34 Jones, *Recollections of 13 years Residence in Norfolk Island*, SLNSW: Safe 1/2d, pp. 30-32.
35 Nobbs, *Norfolk Island*, pp. 3-4, 191-209; www.wikitree.com/wiki/Piper-1325.
36 Jamison to Camden, 20 Jul 1805, HRNSW, V, pp. 667-668.
37 Bond to King, 24 Apr 1806, HRA, V, p. 712.
38 King to Camden, 15 Mar 1806, HRA, V, pp. 646-647.
39 Foveaux on Norfolk Island, Mar 1805, TNA: CO 201/42, pp. 300-307.
40 Windham to Bligh, 30 Dec 1806, HRA, VI, pp. 70-74.
41 Hall, *Andrew Thompson*, p. 143-149.
42 Roe, *Trade, Life and Law at Norfolk Island*, p. 109.
43 Piper to King, 9 Sep 1806, SANSW: NRS 898, [4/1167B, p. 107], Reel 762.
44 Regulations of Vessels, 4 Oct 1806, HRNSW, VI, pp. 193-197; Bligh to Piper, 28 Oct 1806, SLNSW: Safe 1/51, p. 53.

NOTES

45 Court Martial, 18 Jul 1807, HRNSW, VI, pp. 316-325; Bligh to Windham, 31 Oct 1807, HRA, VI, pp. 188-190.
46 Government Order, 23 Jul 1807, HRNSW, VI, p. 276; Bligh to Windham, 31 Oct 1807, HRNSW, VI, pp. 368-369.
47 *The Sydney Gazette*, 8 Mar 1807.
48 Piper to Windham, Nov 1807, TNA: CO 201/55, pp. 11-12.
49 Lord to Piper, 20 Apr 1807, SANSW: NRS 898, [ML Safe 1/51, p. 81], Reel 6040.
50 *The Sydney Gazette*, 26 Jul 1807.
51 Redfern to Wentworth, 16 Sep 1807, SLNSW: SAFE/A 751, pp. 201-203.
52 Ibid.
53 Windham to Bligh, 30 Dec 1806, HRA, VI, pp. 70-74; Bligh to Piper, 4 Sep 1807, HRA, VI, pp. 185-187.
54 Hayes to Jamison, 11 Oct 1807, TNA: C 114/37.
55 Voucher for Swine Flesh, Jan-May 1808, TNA: CO 201/55, pp. 72-75; Hayes to Jamison, 14 Feb 1808, TNA: C 114/37.
56 Nobbs, *Norfolk Island*, p. 221.
57 Settler's Address to Bligh, 1 Jan 1808, HRA, VI, pp. 373-374.
58 Macarthur's petition, 26 Jan 1808, HRA, VI, pp. 240, 723.
59 Bligh to Castlereagh, 30 Apr 1808, HRA, VI, p. 432.
60 Trial of Macarthur, 2 Feb 1808, HRNSW, VI, p. 510; Trial of Wentworth, 17 Feb 1808, HRA, VI, pp. 446-453.
61 Nobbs, *Norfolk Island*, p. 221.
62 Redfern to Wentworth, 1808, SLNSW: A 4073.
63 Ibid.
64 Piper's Norfolk Island return, 15 May 1808, TNA: CO 201/129, p. 142.
65 Nobbs, *Norfolk Island*, p. 221.

CHAPTER 7 – Medical Qualifications

1   Redfern's certificate of examination, 1 Sep 1808, HRA, VI, p. 647.
2   Johnston to Castlereagh, 11 Apr 1808, HRA, VI, p. 220; Settlers to Johnston, 11 Apr 1808, HRA, VI, pp. 572-573.
3   Settlers to Paterson, 18 Apr 1808, HRA, VI, pp. 573-574.
4   Bligh to Castlereagh, 30 Jun 1808, HRA, VI, p. 528.
5   Hall, *Andrew Thompson*, pp. 191-193.
6   Correspondence Bligh and Foveaux, 28-29 Jul 1808, HRA, VI, pp. 591-592; Foveaux to Paterson, 16 Aug 1808, HRA, VI, p. 633.
7   Macquarie to Bathurst, 28 Jun 1813, HRA, VII, pp. 786-787.
8   *The Sydney Gazette*, 31 Jul 1808.
9   Redfern's evidence, 26 Jun 1820, TNA: CO 201/124, p. 94.
10 Foveaux to Castlereagh, 4 Sep 1808, HRA, VI, p. 624.
11 Ibid.
12 Redfern's certificate of examination, 1 Sep 1808, HRA, VI, p. 647.
13 Cummins, *History of Medical Administration in NSW*, p. 157.
14 Foveaux to Castlereagh, 6 Sep 1808, HRA, VI, p. 643.
15 Government Order, 13 Sep 1808, HRNSW, VI, p. 757.
16 Redfern to Bigge, 26 Jun 1820, TNA: CO 201/124, p. 94.

NOTES

17 The street was originally named High Street; renamed in 1810 by Governor Macquarie to George Street.
18 Watson, *History of the Sydney Hospital*, p. 3.
19 Bligh to Windham, 25 Jan, 31 Oct 1807, HRA, VI, pp. 99, 169.
20 Dermody, *D'Arcy Wentworth*, pp. 220, 228.
21 Ibid.
22 Finucane, 18-21 Sep 1808, *Distracted Settlement*, pp. 65-71; Foveaux to Cooke, 21 Oct 1808, HRA, VI, p. 670.
23 Macquarie to Bigge, 6 Nov 1819, HRA, X, pp. 221-222.
24 *The Sydney Gazette*, 1 Jan 1809.
25 Foveaux to Castlereagh, 31 Dec 1808, HRA, VI, pp. 703-704.

CHAPTER 8 – Sydney Hospital Surgeon

1 Macquarie, *Letter to Sidmouth*, p. 39.
2 Finucane, 1-5 Jan 1809, *Distracted Settlement*, pp. 70-71; Foveaux to Paterson, 2 Jan 1808, HRNSW, VII, p. 5.
3 Whitaker, *Joseph Foveaux*, p. 116.
4 Finucane, 19 Jan 1809, *Distracted Settlement*, pp. 73-74.
5 Hall, *Andrew Thompson*, pp. 218-219.
6 Ibid.
7 Jones, *Better than Cure*, I, p. 21. The book was first mentioned by Edward Ford in the 1950s, but it is unknown where it is today.
8 Paterson to Bligh, 22 Feb 1809, HRNSW, VII, p. 45.
9 Government Order, 24 Feb 1809, HRNSW, VII, p. 51.
10 Finucane, 17-18 Mar 1809, *Distracted Settlement*, pp. 77-78.
11 Atkins to Johnston, 4 Mar 1809, HRA, VII, p. 63; Paterson to Johnston, 17 Mar 1809, HRA, VII, p. 64.
12 Proclamation by Bligh, 12 Mar 1809, HRA, VII, p. 73.
13 *The Sydney Gazette*, 2 Apr 1809.
14 Paterson's Proclamation against Bligh, 19 Mar 1809, HRA, VII, pp. 73-74.
15 Collins's General Order, 24 Jun 1809, HRA, VII, p. 165; Bligh to Castlereagh, 8 Jul 1809, HRA, VII, p. 161.
16 *The Sydney Gazette*, 18 Dec 1808; Government Order, 11 Feb 1809, HRNSW, VII, p. 25
17 Macquarie to Liverpool, 13 Nov 1812, HRA, VII, p. 549.
18 Redfern to Macquarie, 29 Jan 1810, SANSW: NRS 899, [4/1822 No 271, pp. 1-5], Fiche 3008.
19 Land grant, 20 May 1809, SANSW: NRS 898, [9/2731, p. 176], Fiche 3268.
20 *The Sydney Gazette*, 4, 18 Jun 1809.
21 *The Sydney Gazette*, 4 Jun 1809, 11 Jul, 17 Oct 1812, 27 Mar, 1 Jul 1813, 22 Jan, 10 Dec 1814, 15 Mar, 22 Nov 1817, 9 May, 6 Jun, 28 Aug 1818, 26 Feb 1820, 3 Feb 1821, 25 Nov 1824, 29 Apr, 2, 16 Jun, 12 Aug 1826, 4 Apr 1828.
22 *The Sydney Gazette*, 22 Oct 1809.
23 Ibid.
24 *The Sydney Gazette*, 29 Oct 1809.
25 Atkinson, *Elizabeth & John*, p. 286.
26 Miss Elizabeth Macarthur, SLNSW: A 1677/4/pp. 1101-1102.

NOTES

27 Macarthur to his wife, 3 May 1810, HRNSW, VII, p. 368.
28 Ibid.
29 Macarthur to his wife, 20 Jul 1810, HRNSW, VII, p. 397.
30 Phillips, G. and Pearn, J., *A Convict and Colonial Pharmacopoeia: Two Centuries' Changes*, History, Heritage & Health, Conference of the Australian Society of the History of Medicine, 1995, pp. 89-90.
31 Redfern notebook, 1796-1825, SLNSW: MAV/FM3/709.
32 Ibid.
33 Castlereagh to Macquarie, 14 May 1809, HRA, VII, pp. 81-82.
34 Macquarie's memoranda, 28-31 Dec 1809, SLNSW: SAFE/A 772, pp. 11-16; *The Sydney Gazette*, 7 Jan 1810.
35 Macquarie to Castlereagh, 8 Mar 1810, HRA, VII, p. 218.
36 Castlereagh to Macquarie, 14 May 1809, HRA, VII, p. 81.

CHAPTER 9 – The Rum Hospital

1 Macquarie, *Letter to Sidmouth*, 1821, pp. 38-39.
2 *The Sydney Gazette*, 7 Jan 1810.
3 Government Order, 1 Jan 1810, HRNSW, VII, pp. 253-255.
4 Foveaux to Macquarie, 10 Jan 1810, HRNSW, VII, p. 271.
5 Finucane, 24 Jan 1810, *Distracted Settlement*, p. 92.
6 Macquarie, *Letter to Sidmouth*, 1821, p. 38.
7 Proclamation, 4, 11 Jan 1810, HRA, VII, pp. 227-231.
8 Civil and Military, 3 Jan 1810, SANSW: NRS 898, [2/8332, p. 1], Fiche 3300.
9 *The Sydney Gazette*, 14 Jan 1810.
10 Macquarie's memoranda, 17-26 Jan 1810, SLNSW: SAFE/A 772, pp. 21-22.
11 *The Sydney Gazette*, 21 Jan 1810.
12 Redfern to Macquarie, 29 Jan 1810, SANSW: NRS 899, [4/1822 No 271, pp. 1-5], Fiche 3008.
13 Foveaux to Macquarie, 10 Jan 1810, HRNSW, VII, p. 271.
14 Macquarie to Castlereagh, 8 Mar 1810, HRA, VII, p. 222.
15 Campbell to Redfern, 20 Feb 1810, SANSW: NRS 935, [4/3490B, pp. 88-89], Reel 6002.
16 *The Sydney Gazette*, 24 Feb 1810.
17 Macquarie to Castlereagh, 8 Mar 1810, HRA, VII, p. 224.
18 Macquarie to Castlereagh, 30 Apr 1810, HRNSW, VII, pp. 356-357.
19 Ibid.
20 Ibid.
21 Bell evidence, Ritchie, *Evidence to the Bigge Reports*, I, pp. 89-91.
22 Ibid.
23 Arnold to his brother, 25 Feb 1810, SLNSW: A 1849/2, pp. 311-312.
24 Byrne, *Judge Advocate Ellis Bent*, p. 151; Curry, *Bent Brothers*, p. 69.
25 *The Sydney Gazette*, 24 Mar 1810.
26 Government Order, 31 Mar 1810, HRNSW, VII, p. 323.
27 Macquarie to Castlereagh, 30 Apr 1810, HRNSW, VII, pp. 356-357.
28 Johnstone evidence, 14 Dec 1819, TNA: CO 201/124, p. 76.
29 Cowper evidence, 16 Nov 1819, TNA: CO 201/124, pp. 6-10.
30 Redfern to Bigge, 19 Jul 1821, TNA: CO 201/124, p. 171.

NOTES

31. Ibid.
32. Ibid.
33. Cowper evidence, 22 Nov 1819, TNA: CO 201/124, p. 55.
34. Macquarie to Castlereagh, 12 Mar 1810, HRA, VII, p. 242.
35. Macquarie to Liverpool, 27 Oct 1810, HRA, VII, p. 343.
36. Liverpool to Macquarie, 26 Jul 1811, HRA, VII, p. 365.
37. General Statement of Inhabitants, 1 Mar 1810, TNA: CO 201/53, p. 76.
38. Macquarie to Castlereagh, 8 Mar 1810, HRA, VII, p. 223.
39. *The Sydney Gazette*, 19 May 1810; Redfern evidence, 26 Jun 1820, TNA: CO 201/124, p. 94.
40. Macquarie to Liverpool, 18 Oct 1811, HRA, VII, p. 384; Contract for hospital, 6 Nov 1810, HRA, VII, pp. 401-403.
41. Macquarie to Castlereagh, 30 Apr 1810, HRA, VII, p. 250; *The Sydney Gazette*, 3 Mar 1810.
42. Watson, *The History of the Sydney Hospital*, pp. 19-23.
43. Hospital Contract, 6 Nov 1810, HRNSW, VII, pp. 449-453.
44. *The Sydney Gazette*, 28 Apr 1810.
45. Dermody, *D'Arcy Wentworth*, p. 328.
46. SANSW: NRS 935, [4/3490C, p. 154], Reel 6002.
47. Hall, *Andrew Thompson*, pp. 258-260.
48. *The Sydney Gazette*, 3 Nov 1810.
49. Macquarie, *Journals of his tours*, pp. 1-4.
50. Ibid.
51. Macquarie, *Journals of his tours*, pp. 5-8.
52. Macquarie, *Journals of his tours*, pp. 12-14, 17.
53. Macquarie, *Journals of his tours*, pp. 20-27.
54. Macquarie, *Journals of his tours*, p. 32, 42-43.

CHAPTER 10 – Miss Sarah Wills

1. Antill, Antill-De Warren, *The Emancipist*, pp. 165-166.
2. *The Sydney Gazette*, 5 Jan 1811; Macquarie to Liverpool, 18 Oct 1811, HRA, VII, pp. 384-385.
3. Redfern to Bigge, 19 Jul 1821, TNA: CO 201/124, p. 169.
4. Hocking and Donati, *Obscured but not Obscure*, p. 61.
5. SANSW: NRS 1170, [4/4430, p. 22], Reel 774.
6. Wills Cooke, *The Currency Lad*, p. 6.
7. Officers and settlers to Johnston, 27 Jan 1808, HRA, VI, pp. 375, 732.
8. Wills Cooke, *The Currency Lad*, pp. 10-11.
9. Ibid.
10. Will of Edward Wills, 20 May 1811, SLNSW: DLWD 69.
11. Deed, 2 Mar 1811, SLNSW: SAFE A752, p. 39; William Robert received the 30-acre grant in 1794 and sold it in 1800 to John Boxley. In 1802 Thomas Laycock sold the land to Sarah Wills for £100, SLNSW: A 5407.
12. Baxter, *Muster 1805-1806*, pp. 122-123.
13. St Philip's Church Register, 4 Mar 1811, SLNSW: SAG 90.
14. *The Sydney Gazette*, 18 May 1811.
15. Jan - Dec 1811, SANSW: NRS 898, [2/8295, pp. 1-5], Reel 6024.

NOTES

16 16-19 Apr 1811, SANSW: NRS 935, [4/3490D, pp. 160-165], Reel 6002.
17 Macquarie to Bathurst, 11 Dec 1817, HRA, IX, p. 545.
18 30 Jan 1812, SANSW: NRS 935, [4/3491, pp. 172-173], Reel 6002; Wentworth & Redfern to Campbell, Feb 1812, SANSW: NRS 897, [4/1726, pp. 18-19], Reel 6043.
19 McClemens, J, Bennett, J M, *Historical Notes on the Law of Mental Illness in NSW*, Sydney Law Review, 4, 1962, pp. 59-60.
20 *The Sydney Gazette*, 28 Mar, 4 Apr 1812.
21 *The Sydney Gazette*, 1 Jun 1811.
22 Macquarie to Liverpool, 18 Oct 1811, HRA, VII, p. 388.
23 *The Sydney Gazette*, 6 Jul 1811.
24 *The Sydney Gazette*, 4 May 1811; TNA: HO 10/15.
25 Macquarie to Liverpool, 18 Oct 1811, HRA, VII, p. 388.
26 *The Sydney Gazette*, 2 Nov 1811.
27 Macquarie, *Journals of his tours*, p. 45.
28 22 May 1811, HLRV: Grant Register, Serial 7, p. 22; Parish map of Minto, HLRV: AO Map 250; Stock issued, 7 Nov 1812, HRA, VII, p. 628.
29 *The Sydney Gazette*, 1 Feb 1812.
30 Macquarie's memoranda, Apr-May 1812, SLNSW: SAFE/A 772, pp. 43-44.
31 *The Sydney Gazette*, 24 Oct 1812.
32 *The Sydney Gazette*, 11 Jul 1812.
33 *The Sydney Gazette*, 17 Oct 1812.
34 *The Sydney Gazette*, 29 Dec 1810.
35 Wills Cooke, *The Currency Lad*, pp. 12-13.
36 *The Sydney Gazette*, 10 Oct 1812, 5 Jun 1813.
37 Macquarie to Liverpool, 28 Nov 1812, HRA, VII, p. 683.
38 *The Sydney Gazette*, 2 Jan 1813.

CHAPTER 11 – Medical Pioneer

1 Redfern to Macquarie, 30 Sep 1814, HRA, VIII, p. 291.
2 *The Sydney Gazette*, 2 Jan 1813.
3 Macquarie's memoranda, 1 Jan 1813, SLNSW: SAFE/A 772, pp. 53-54.
4 *The Sydney Gazette*, 9, 16 Jan 1813.
5 *The Sydney Gazette*, 30 Jan 1813.
6 Macquarie's memoranda, 2 Feb 1813, SLNSW: SAFE/A 772, p. 55.
7 Memorial of Luttrell, 15 Nov 1812, HRA, VII, p. 556.
8 Bathurst to Macquarie, 15 Nov 1812, HRA, VII, pp. 553-555.
9 Ibid.
10 Macquarie to Bathurst 28 Jun 1813, HRA, VII, pp. 785-788.
11 Ibid.
12 Ibid.
13 House of Commons, *Select Committee on Transportation*, pp. 13-15.
14 Macquarie to Bathurst, 28 Jun 1813, HRA, VII, pp. 775-776.
15 Ibid.
16 Macquarie's memoranda, 3 Nov 1813, SLNSW: SAFE/A 772, p. 66.
17 *The Sydney Gazette*, 16 Oct 1813.
18 Macquarie's memoranda, 17 Dec 1813, SLNSW: SAFE/A 772, p. 68.

NOTES

19 Macquarie to Bathurst, 28 Apr 1814, HRA, VIII, p. 155.
20 Ford, *Life and Work of William Redfern*; Royal Australasian College of Physicians, www.racp.edu.au.
21 Macquarie to Bathurst, 28 Apr 1814, HRA, VIII, p. 140.
22 House of Commons, *Select Committee on Transportation*, p. 10.
23 No of death, 1 Jan-31 Mar 1814, SANSW: NRS 898, [2/8295], Reel 6024.
24 14 Mar 1814, SANSW: NRS 937, [4/3493, pp. 89-90], Reel 6004.
25 Redfern to Macquarie, 30 Sep 1814, HRA, VIII, pp. 275-278.
26 Ibid.
27 Macquarie's memoranda, 28 Mar 1814, SLNSW: SAFE/A 772, pp. 68-69.
28 Macquarie's memoranda, Apr 1814, SLNSW: SAFE/A 772, pp. 73-75.
29 Ibid.
30 Macquarie's memoranda, 1 May 1814, SLNSW: SAFE/A 772, pp. 75-76; St Philip's Church baptism, 1 May 1814, SLNSW: SAG 90.
31 Johnstone evidence, 14 Dec 1819, TNA: CO 201/124, p. 76.
32 Redfern to Bigge, 5 Feb 1821, TNA: CO 201/124, p. 193.
33 Redfern to Macquarie, 30 Sep 1814, HRA, VIII, pp. 275-284.
34 Ibid.
35 Macquarie to Bathurst, 24 May 1814. HRA, VIII, p. 254.
36 *The Sydney Gazette*, 21 May 1814.
37 Ibid.
38 Redfern to Macquarie, 30 Sep 1814, HRA, VIII, pp. 275-282.
39 Currey, *The Bent Brothers*, p. 100.
40 Enquiry, 30 Jul 1814, SANSW: NRS 897, [4/1731, p. 1], Reel 6044.
41 *The Sydney Gazette*, 30 Jul 1814.
42 *The Sydney Gazette*, 30 Jul 1814; NLA: MAP F 903.
43 Macquarie to Bathurst, 7 Oct 1814, HRA, VIII, p. 295.
44 Redfern to Macquarie, 30 Sep 1814, HRA, VIII, pp. 275-293.
45 Ibid.
46 Ibid.
47 *The Sydney Gazette*, 20 Aug, 3 Sep 1814.
48 Macquarie to Bathurst, 7 Oct 1814, HRA, VIII, p. 295.
49 Redfern to Macquarie, 30 Sep 1814, HRA, VIII, pp. 275-293.
50 Ibid.
51 Ibid.
52 Ibid.
53 Ibid.
54 Macquarie to Transport Board, 1 Oct 1814, HRA, VIII, pp. 274-275.
55 Bathurst to Macquarie, 3 Feb 1814, HRA, VIII, p. 130.
56 Macquarie to Bathurst, 7 Oct 1814, HRA, VIII, pp. 297-299.
57 Memorial of Medical Officers, 4 Oct 1814, HRA, VIII, pp. 324-327.
58 Baxter, *Muster 1814*; *The Sydney Gazette*, 10 Sep 1814.
59 Redfern to Bigge, 5 Feb 1821, TNA: CO 201/124, p. 194.
60 *The Sydney Gazette*, 12 Nov 1814.
61 1 Jul 1813, SANSW: NRS 897, [4/1728, p. 133], Reel 6043; *The Sydney Gazette*, 17 Jul 1813.
62 Macquarie to Bathurst, 30 Nov 1814, HRA, VIII, p. 381.
63 Bent to Macquarie, 16 Dec 1814, HRA, Series IV, I, pp. 116-117.

NOTES

CHAPTER 12 – Mountain Crossing

1. Journal of surveyor Evans, 23 May 1815, HRA, VIII, pp. 613-614.
2. Redfern to Bigge, 5 Feb 1821, TNA: CO 201/124, p. 196.
3. 15 Feb 1815, SANSW: NRS 937, [4/3493, p. 466], Reel 6004.
4. Jones, *Better than Cure*, II, p. 122.
5. Macquarie to Bathurst, 24 Mar 1815, HRA, VIII, p. 466.
6. *The Sydney Gazette*, 22 May 1813.
7. Antill journal, 1815, SLNSW: Safe 1/20a.
8. Ibid.
9. Macquarie, *Journals of his tours*, pp. 89-99.
10. Macquarie, *Journals of his tours*, pp. 89-110; Antill journal, 1815, SLNSW: Safe 1/20a.
11. Ibid.
12. Ibid.
13. *The Sydney Gazette*, 10 Feb 1816.
14. Antill journal, 1815, SLNSW: Safe 1/20a.
15. Journal of surveyor Evans, May-Jun 1815, HRA, VIII, pp. 613-614.
16. Macquarie, *Journals of his tours*, pp. 106-109.
17. Antill journal, 1815, SLNSW: Safe 1/20a.
18. Macquarie, *Journals of his tours*, pp. 108-109.
19. Macquarie to Bathurst, 24 Jun 1815, HRA, VIII, p. 564; *The Sydney Gazette*, 1 Jul 1815.
20. *The Sydney Gazette*, 10 Jun 1815.
21. Minutes of the Supreme Court, 11 May 1815, HRA, VIII, p. 515.
22. Broughton's opinion, 23 May 1815, HRA, VIII, p. 527.
23. Bent to Macquarie, 31 May 1815, HRA, VIII, p. 537.
24. Macquarie to Bent, 2 Jun 1815, HRA, VIII, p. 540.
25. Arnold journal, 18 Jun 1815, SLNSW: SAFE/C 720, p. 373.
26. Arnold to his brother, 25 Feb 1810, SLNSW: CY 339, pp. 311-312.
27. Arnold journal, 20-26 Jun 1815, SLNSW: SAFE/C 720, pp. 374-383.
28. Ibid.
29. Arnold journal, 13 Jul 1815, SLNSW: SAFE/C 720, pp. 387-393.
30. Ibid.
31. Ibid.
32. Ibid.
33. Macquarie's certificate, 30 Jun 1815, SLNSW: Safe A 752, p. 157.
34. Macquarie to Bathurst, 1 Jul 1815, HRA, VIII, p. 621.
35. Redfern to Bigge, 5 Feb 1821, TNA: CO 201/124, p. 195.
36. 21 Jul 1815, SANSW: NRS 937, [4/3494, pp. 144-145], Reel 6004.
37. *The Sydney Gazette*, 14 Oct 1815.
38. *The Sydney Gazette*, 5, 26 Aug 1815.
39. Ibid.
40. Macquarie to Bathurst, 18 Mar 1816, HRA, IX, p. 57.
41. Bathurst to Macquarie, 20 Oct 1814, HRA, VIII, p. 378; *The Sydney Gazette*, 9 Sep 1815.
42. Macquarie to Bathurst, 20 Feb 1816, HRA, IX, p. 3.
43. Macquarie to Bent, 18 Dec 1815, HRA, IX, p. 26.

NOTES

44 *The Sydney Gazette*, 11 and 18 Nov 1815.
45 Macquarie to Bent, 6 Jan 1816, HRA, IX, p. 28.

CHAPTER 13 – Bank Director

1 *The Sydney Gazette*, 8 Feb 1817.
2 13 Jan 1816, SANSW: NRS 937, [4/3494, pp. 316-317], Reel 6004.
3 Bland evidence, 23 Jan 1821, TNA: CO 201/124, p. 132.
4 *The Sydney Gazette*, 20 Jan, 3 Feb 1816.
5 Watson, *History of the Sydney Hospital*, pp. 29-34.
6 Contract for hospital, 6 Nov 1810, HRA, VII, p. 401-403; Cowper evidence, 5 Aug 1820, TNA: CO 201/124, p. 44.
7 Macquarie to York, 25 Jul 1817, HRA, IX, pp. 443-444.
8 Arnold journal, 13 Jul 1815, SLNSW: SAFE/C 720, pp. 395-397.
9 *The Sydney Gazette*, 9 Mar 1816.
10 Dermody, *D'Arcy Wentworth*, pp. 309-311.
11 *The Sydney Gazette*, 6 Apr 1816; Cowper evidence, 1819, 1820, TNA: CO 201/124, pp. 4, 44.
12 Meehan evidence, 1820, SLNSW: BT 5, pp. 2238-2239.
13 Redfern evidence, 26 Jun 1820, TNA: 201/124, pp. 93-97.
14 Redfern to Bowman, 24 Oct 1819, TNA: CO 201/124, pp. 209-210.
15 28 Sep 1816, SANSW: NRS 897, [4/1736, p. 123], Reel 6043.
16 Cowper evidence, 20 Nov 1819, TNA: CO 201/124, p. 18.
17 *The Sydney Gazette*, 28 Jun 1816.
18 Cowper evidence, 20 Nov 1819, TNA: CO 201/124, p. 54.
19 Macquarie's diary, 1-8 Sep 1816, SLNSW: SAFE/A 773, p. 44.
20 HLRV: Grant Register, 8 Sep 1816, Serial 8, p. 260; HLRV: Parish of Alexandria, AO MAP 185.
21 Macquarie to Bathurst, 24 Jun 1815, HRA, VIII, p. 554.
22 Macquarie's diary, 5 Oct 1816, SLNSW: SAFE/A 773, pp. 50-51.
23 Butlin, *Foundation of the Australian Monetary System*, pp. 110-119.
24 *The Sydney Gazette*, 30 Nov, 7 Dec 1816.
25 Wylde evidence, 1820, HRA, IV, I, p. 788.
26 Macquarie to Bathurst, 29 Mar 1817, HRA, IX, pp. 223-233.
27 Shann, *An Economic History of Australia*, p. 56.
28 Macquarie's diary, 18 Jan 1817, SLNSW: SAFE/A 773, p. 81.
29 Macquarie's memoranda, 28 Mar 1817, SLNSW: SAFE/A 772, pp. 83-84.
30 Eagar to Bathurst, 6 Nov 1822, TNA: CO 201/111, p. 257.
31 Shaw, *Convicts & Colonies*, pp. 364-365.
32 Memorial of Wentworth, 28 Mar 1817, HRA, IX, pp. 258-263.
33 Macquarie to Bathurst, 1 Apr 1817, HRA, IX, pp. 257-258.
34 Macquarie to Bathurst, 4 Apr 1817, HRA, IX, pp. 353-354.
35 *The Sydney Gazette*, 17 May 1817.
36 Macquarie to York, 25 Jul 1817, HRA, IX, pp. 446-453.
37 Macquarie to Bathurst, 13 May 1817, HRA, IX, pp. 392-393.
38 Macquarie to York, 25 Jul 1817, HRA, IX, pp. 443-444.
39 Macquarie's memoranda, 7 Aug 1817, SLNSW: SAFE/A 772, pp. 93-94.
40 Steven, Margaret, *John Macarthur*, Australian Dictionary of Biography.

NOTES

41. Macquarie's memoranda, 30 Sep 1817, SLNSW: SAFE/A 772, pp. 113-114.
42. Macarthur Onslow, *Some early records of the Macarthurs of Camden*, p. 289.
43. Macquarie to Bathurst, 18 Mar 1816, HRA, IX, p. 56-73.
44. Bathurst to Macquarie, 17 Jan 1817, HRA, IX, p. 203; Macquarie to Bathurst, 28 Nov 1817, HRA, IX, p. 495.
45. Macquarie's memoranda, 15-22 Oct 1817, SLNSW: SAFE/A 772, pp. 124-126.
46. *The Sydney Gazette*, 1 Nov 1817; Meehan evidence, 1820, SLNSW: BT 5, pp. 2238-2239; Land grant, 30 Jun 1823, SANSW: NRS 13836, [7/485], Reel 2704; HLRV: Book D No 885, Book E No 592 and 841.
47. Parrish of Minto, HLRV: AO Map 250; land grants, 20 Jun 1816, 11 Sep 1817, HLRV: Serial 8, pp. 142-143 and Serial 6, p. 132; land purchases: J. Underwood, T. Rose, J. Oadham, P. Keigham, SLNSW: A 5407.
48. Land grants and leases, 1820, TNA: CO 201/123, p. 362.
49. *The Sydney Gazette*, 9 Aug, 25 Oct 1817.
50. *The Sydney Gazette*, 30 Jan, 9 Aug 1817; 3 Jan, 27 Jun 1818; 16 Jan, 24 Apr 1819; 1 Jan 1820.
51. Macquarie to Bathurst, 1 Dec 1817, HRA, IX, pp. 495-501.

CHAPTER 14 – Calm Before the Storm

1. Macquarie to Bathurst, 15 May 1818, HRA, IX, p. 787.
2. Bigge, *State of the Colony*, pp. 88-89.
3. Ibid; Watkins to Bigge, 19 Dec 1819, TNA: CO 201/134, p. 100.
4. Macquarie's diary, 19 Jan 1818, SLNSW: SAFE/A 773, p. 136.
5. Macquarie's diary, 26 Jan 1818, SLNSW: SAFE/A 773, p. 137; Macquarie evidence, 4 Feb 1821, TNA: CO 201/142, pp. 387-388.
6. *The Sydney Gazette*, 10 Sep 1814.
7. Macquarie to Marsden 8 Jan 1818, SLNSW: A 797; *The Sydney Gazette*, 28 Mar 1818.
8. *The Sydney Gazette*, 7 Feb, 21 Mar 1818; Johns, *Women in Colonial Commerce*, pp. 111-112.
9. *The Hobart Town Gazette*, 24 Jan 1818; 26 Jun 1818, HRA, Series III, Vol 2, p. 331.
10. St Philip's Church Register, 9 Oct 1818, SLNSW: SAG 90.
11. Macquarie to Bathurst, 15 May 1818, HRA, IX, pp. 786-787.
12. Redfern to Bathurst, 24 Feb 1820, HRA, X, p. 274.
13. Cowper evidence, 16 Nov 1819, TNA: CO 201/124, p. 7.
14. Redfern to Bigge, 5 Feb 1821, TNA: CO 201/124, pp. 196-197.
15. Ibid.
16. Redfern to Bowman, 24 Oct 1819, TNA: CO 201/124, pp. 209-210.
17. Macquarie to Bathurst, 3 Apr 1817, HRA, IX, p. 330.
18. Bathurst to Sidmouth, 23 Apr 1817, HRA, X, pp. 807-808.
19. Bathurst to Bigge, 6 Jan 1819, HRA, X, pp. 4-11.
20. Ibid.
21. Ibid.
22. Tink, *William Charles Wentworth*, p. 56.
23. SLNSW: A 1272, p. 697.

NOTES

24 William Wentworth to his father, 13 Apr 1819, SLNSW: A 756, p. 139.
25 Macquarie's diary, 1 Jan 1819, SLNSW: SAFE/A 774, pp. 18-19.
26 *The Sydney Gazette*, 23 Jan 1819.
27 Macarthur Onslow, *Some early records of the Macarthurs of Camden*, p. 339.
28 Eagar to Bathurst, 6 Nov 1822, TNA: CO 201/111, p. 255; *The Sydney Gazette*, 23 Jan 1819.
29 Macquarie to Bathurst, 22 Mar 1819, HRA, X, pp. 54-65.
30 Cowper evidence, 19 Nov 1819, TNA: CO 201/124, p. 12; State of hospital, 1818-1819, TNA: CO 201/124, p. 273.
31 Macquarie to Bathurst, 24 Mar 1819, HRA, X, p. 97.
32 House of Commons, *Select Committee on Gaols*, 1819, p. 75.
33 *The Sydney Gazette*, 10 Apr 1819.
34 Wentworth to Campbell, 27 May 1819, TNA: CO 201/124, pp. 355-356.
35 Bathurst to Macquarie, 3 Jul 1818, HRA, IX, pp. 810-811; *The Sydney Gazette*, 21 Aug 1819.
36 St Philip's Church Register, 27 Jul 1819, SLNSW: SAG 90.
37 SLNSW: FM2/1897.
38 Macquarie to Bathurst, 22 Feb 1820, HRA, X, pp. 214-215.
39 Wentworth, *Statistical Account of the British Settlement*, pp. 395-396.
40 Macquarie to Bathurst, 22 Feb 1820, HRA, X, pp. 214-215.

CHAPTER 15 – The Inquisitor

1 Redfern to Bigge, 5 Feb 1821, TNA: CO 201/124, p. 184-185.
2 Bathurst to Macquarie, 30 Jan 1819, HRA, X, pp. 2-11.
3 Redfern to Bigge, 5 Feb 1821, TNA: CO 201/124, pp. 178-179.
4 Wentworth, *Statistical Account of the British Settlement*, p. 396.
5 Cowper evidence, 22 Nov 1819, TNA: CO 201/124, pp. 21-22.
6 Wentworth, *Statistical Account of the British Settlement*, pp. 396-397.
7 Redfern to Bowman, 29 Sep 1819, TNA: CO 201/124, pp. 174-175.
8 Redfern to Bigge, 5 Feb 1821, TNA: CO 201/124, pp. 178-180.
9 Ibid.
10 Johnstone evidence, 14 Dec 1819, TNA: CO 201/124, pp. 67-68.
11 Affidavit of Johnstone, 26 Jun 1820, TNA: CO 201/124, pp. 416-417.
12 Cowper evidence, 22 Nov 1819, TNA: CO 201/124, pp. 21-22.
13 Redfern evidence, 19 Jul 1820, TNA: CO 201/124, p. 172.
14 Johnstone evidence, 14 Dec 1819, TNA: CO 201/124, pp. 68-69.
15 Affidavit of Johnstone, 26 Jun 1820, TNA: CO 201/124, pp. 416-417.
16 Johnstone evidence, 14 Dec 1819, TNA: CO 201/124, pp. 68-69.
17 Macquarie's diary, 7 Oct 1819, SLNSW: SAFE/A 774/1, p. 71.
18 Redfern to Macquarie, 18 Oct 1819, HRA, X, p. 273.
19 Ibid.
20 *The Sydney Gazette*, 23 Oct 1819.
21 Redfern to Bowman, 24 Oct 1819, TNA: CO 201/124, pp. 209-211; *The Sydney Gazette*, 21 Aug 1819.
22 Redfern to Bowman, 24 Oct 1819, TNA: CO 201/124, pp. 209-211.
23 Examination of Wylde, 1820, HRA, Series IV, I, p. 789.
24 Bigge to Macquarie, 30 Oct, 1 Nov 1819, TNA: CO 201/142, pp. 22-26.

NOTES

25 Ibid.
26 Macquarie to Bigge, 6 Nov 1819, HRA, X, pp. 220-224.
27 Ibid.
28 Ibid.
29 Bigge to Macquarie, 10 Nov 1819, HRA, X, pp. 224-231.
30 Macquarie to Bigge, 12 Nov 1819, HRA, X, pp. 233-234.
31 *The Sydney Gazette*, 13 Nov 1819.
32 Macquarie to Bowman, 12 Nov 1819, TNA: CO 201/124, pp. 214-215.
33 Bigge to Bathurst, 20 Nov 1819, TNA: CO 201/142, pp. 16-19.
34 Macquarie, *Extract of a Letter to Bathurst in October 1823*, p. 25.
35 *The Monitor*, 20 Oct 1826.
36 Cowper evidence, 16, 19, 20, 22 Nov 1819, TNA: CO 201/124.
37 Johnstone evidence, 14 Dec 1819, TNA: CO 201/124, p. 76.
38 12 Oct 1819, SANSW: NRS 900, [4/1858, p. 179b], Fiche 3196; Absolute pardon, 31 Jan 1820, SANSW: NRS 1177, [4/4486], Reel 800.
39 Affidavit of Johnstone, 26 Jun 1820, TNA: CO 201/124, pp. 414-417.
40 Johnstone to Bigge, 30 Jan 1821, CO 201/124, pp. 407-411.
41 Ibid.
42 Johnstone to Bigge, 30 Jan 1821, CO 201/124, pp. 407-411.
43 Ibid.
44 Bigge, *State of the Colony*, p. 86.
45 Bigge, *State of Agriculture and Trade*, p. 105.
46 Land and stock holding, 1819, SANSW: NRS 1264, Reel 1256.
47 Bell evidence, 27 Nov 1819, Ritchie, *Evidence to the Bigge Reports*, I, pp. 88-89.
48 Redfern to Wentworth, SLNSW: FM4/9151.
49 Macquarie's diary, 27 Dec 1819, SLNSW: SAFE/ A 774/1, p. 90.

CHAPTER 16 – The Slaughter House

1 Redfern to Bigge, 5 Feb 1821, TNA: CO 201/124, p. 189.
2 Bigge to magistrates, 7 Jan 1820, TNA: CO 201/141, pp. 42-43.
3 Lowe report, 23 Jan 1820, TNA: CO 201/123, p. 192; Redfern to Bigge, 5 Feb 1821, TNA: CO 201/124, pp. 191-192.
4 Macquarie's diary, 12 Jan 1820, SLNSW: SAFE/A 774/1, p. 94.
5 Macquarie to magistrates, 15 Jan 1820, SANSW: NRS 937, [4/3501, pp. 188-191], Reel 6007.
6 Macquarie to Bathurst, 22 Feb 1820, HRA, X, pp. 237-241.
7 Macquarie to Bigge, 14 Feb 1820, HRA, X, pp. 244-245.
8 Redfern to Bigge, 5 Feb 1821, TNA: CO 201/124, p. 192.
9 Macquarie, *Letter from Macquarie to Bathurst*, p. 31.
10 Macarthur-Onslow, *Early Records of the Macarthurs of Camden*, pp. 325, 338.
11 Ibid.
12 Macquarie to Bathurst, 28 Feb 1820, HRA, X, p. 282.
13 Macquarie to Bigge, 22 Feb 1820, HRA, X, pp. 214-218.
14 Ibid.
15 Ibid.
16 Macquarie to Bathurst, 24 Feb 1820, HRA, X, pp. 272-273.
17 Macquarie to Bathurst, 22, 29 Feb 1820, HRA, X, pp. 236, 291-292.

NOTES

18 Campbell to magistrates, 20 Apr 1820, SANSW: NRS 937, [4/3502, pp. 2-5], Reel 6007; Redfern to Campbell, 24 Apr 1820, SANSW: NRS 897, [4/1744, pp. 307-310], Reel 6049.
19 Redfern to Bigge, 5 Feb 1821, TNA: CO 201/124, pp. 188-190.
20 Enquiry, 9 Jun 1820, SANSW: NRS 897, [4/1744, pp. 73-44], Reel 6049; State of hospital, May 1818-Oct 1819, TNA: CO 201/124, p. 273.
21 Cowper evidence, 1821, TNA: CO 201/124, pp. 84-85.
22 Bowman report, 23 Feb 1820, SANSW: NRS 897, [4/1744, p. 64], Reel 6049.
23 Inquest, 31 Jul 1820, SANSW: NRS 898, [4/1819, pp. 315-316], Reel 6021.
24 Enquiry, 26 Apr, 9 Jun 1820, TNA: CO 201/124, pp. 240-244.
25 Redfern to Bigge, 5 Feb 1821, TNA: CO 201/124, pp. 188-189.
26 Bigge, *State of Agriculture and Trade*, p. 111.
27 *The Monitor*, 22 Mar 1828; *The Sydney Gazette*, 28 Mar 1828.
28 Watson, *History of the Sydney Hospital*, p. 47.
29 Cummins, *History of Medical Administration in NSW*, p. 18.
30 Starr, *Sidney Slaughter House*, pp. 69-70, 85.
31 Wentworth, *Statistical Account of the British Settlements*, pp. 388-389.
32 Ellis, *Lachlan Macquarie*, p. 513.
33 Macquarie to Bathurst, 1 Sep 1820, HRA, X, p. 352.
34 Macquarie to Bathurst, 1 Sep 1820, HRA, X, pp. 351-359.
35 Eagar vs Field, 4 Apr 1820, HRA, X, pp. 358-362.
36 Redfern to Bigge, 5 Feb 1821, TNA: CO 201/124, p. 183.
37 Redfern evidence, 26 Jun 1820, TNA: CO 201/124, pp. 93-97.
38 Redfern to Bigge, 5 Feb 1821, TNA: CO 201/124, pp. 184-186.
39 Ibid.
40 Redfern to Bigge, 5 Feb 1821, TNA: CO 201/124, pp. 184-190.
41 Ibid.
42 Ibid.
43 Wentworth, *Statistical Account of the British Settlement*, pp. 398-399.
44 Redfern to Bigge, 19 Jul 1820, TNA: CO 201/124, pp. 168-172.
45 Ibid.
46 Petition of Emancipated Colonists, 22 Oct 1821, HRA, X, pp. 553-554.
47 *The Sydney Gazette*, 22 Jul 1820.
48 Land and stock at Liverpool, 1820, TNA: CO 201/123, p. 392; Land and stock at Bathurst, 9 Oct 1820, SLNSW: BT 24, p. 5196.
49 SANSW: NRS 937, [4/3501, pp. 213-214, 217], Reel 6007; NRS 937, [4/3502, pp. 60, 137-138, 292, 303, 460, 462], Reel 6007.
50 Macquarie's diary, 5 Jul 1820, SLNSW: SAFE/A 774/2, p. 139.
51 *The Sydney Gazette*, 19 Aug 1820.
52 Bigge, *State of Agriculture and Trade*, p. 81.
53 *The Sydney Gazette*, 16 Dec 1820.
54 Ibid.
55 Macquarie's diary, 1 Dec 1820, SLNSW: SAFE/A 774/2, pp. 174-177.
56 Macquarie's diary, 31 Dec 1820, SLNSW: SAFE/A 774/2, pp. 193-194.
57 Bathurst to Macquarie, 10 Jul 1820, HRA, X, pp. 310-311.

NOTES

CHAPTER 17 – Rights Activist

1. Emancipated Colonists to the King, 22 Oct 1821, HRA, X, pp. 554-556.
2. Solomon, *Barron Field and the Supreme Court*, pp. 197-198.
3. Macquarie's diary, 9 Jan 1821, SLNSW: SAFE/A 774, p. 196.
4. Redfern to Bigge, 5 Feb 1821, TNA: CO 201/124, pp. 193-194.
5. *The Sydney Gazette*, 10 Feb 1821.
6. *The Sydney Gazette*, 27 Jan 1821.
7. *The Sydney Gazette*, 27 Jan 1821; Redfern to Bigge, 5 Feb 1821, TNA: CO 201/124, p. 198.
8. *The Sydney Gazette*, 27 Jan, 3 Feb 1821.
9. Macquarie to Bigge, 4 Feb 1821, TNA: CO 201/142, pp. 382-437.
10. Ibid.
11. Ibid.
12. Ibid.
13. Redfern to Bigge, 5 Feb 1821, TNA: CO 201/124, pp. 176-198.
14. Ibid.
15. Ibid.
16. Ibid.
17. Ibid.
18. Ibid.
19. Macarthur Onslow, *Early records of the Macarthurs of Camden*, pp. 349-355.
20. Ibid.
21. Eagar to Bathurst, 12 Nov 1822, TNA: CO 201/111, pp. 246-247.
22. Redfern to Bigge, 9 Feb 1821, TNA: CO 201/124, pp. 203-204.
23. Redfern to Bigge, 8 Feb 1821, TNA: CO 201/124, pp. 98-102.
24. Ibid.
25. Macquarie's diary, 14 Feb 1821, SLNSW: A 774/2, p. 209.
26. *The Sydney Gazette*, 10 Feb 1821.
27. Pockley, *Edward Wills Family*, p. 13.
28. Macquarie, *Journals of his tours*, pp. 169-202.
29. Ibid.
30. Ibid.
31. Ibid.
32. Ibid.
33. George Howe's will, 16 May 1821, SLNSW: DLWD 69.
34. Wills Cooke, *Currency Lad*, p. 14.
35. *The Sydney Gazette*, 28 Jul 1821.
36. Byrnes, J. V, *Robert Howe*, Australian Dictionary of Biography.
37. *The Sydney Gazette*, 28 Jul 1821.
38. Petition, 20 Aug 1821, SANSW: NRS 900, [4/1863, p. 88], Fiche 3211; Pardon, 1 Sep 1821, SANSW: NRS 900, [4/1862, p. 10], Fiche 3206.
39. Land grant, 3 Sep 1821, HLRV: Serial 12, p. 257; Land purchases from S. Howe, R. Barnes, R. Knight, R. Howe, E. Myles, SLNSW: A 5407.
40. Muster, 1821, SANSW: NRS 1264, Reel 1256; NRS 1260, Reel 1252.
41. SANSW: Reel 1976, p. 286, Index 57; NRS 898, Reel 6023, X820, p. 45.
42. Freehill, Mark, *An early share certificate of the Bank of NSW*, International Bank Note Society, 1975, Vol 14, No 2, pp. 76-82; Silentworld Foundation:

NOTES

https://silentworldfoundation.org.au/collection-about/collections-ehive-objects/1211844.
43 Emancipists to King, 22 Oct 1821, HRA, X, pp. 549-555.
44 Ibid.
45 Ibid.
46 Macquarie to Bathurst, 22 Oct 1821, HRA, X, pp. 557-558.
47 Brisbane to Bathurst, 31 Aug 1822, HRA, X, p. 725.
48 NLA: Crook, Tahiti, London Missionary Society, File 58, pp. 20-23.
49 Redfern to Wentworth, 7 Mar 1822, SLNSW: SAFA/A 754/1, pp. 73-76.

CHAPTER 18 – Angel of Discord

1 Eagar to Bathurst, 6 Nov 1822, TNA: CO 201/111, p. 286.
2 Eagar to Horton, 1 Jul 1822, TNA: CO 201/111, p. 219.
3 Redfern to Bathurst, 10 Dec 1822, TNA: CO 201/111, p. 570.
4 *The Times*, 9 Mar 1822.
5 Bigge, *State of the Colony*, pp. 1-186.
6 Bigge, *State of the Colony*, p. 87.
7 Bigge, *State of the Colony*, p. 89.
8 *John Bull*, 18 Aug 1822; Bigge to Horton, 31 Jul 1822, NLA: M791, D3155, pp. 164-166.
9 Tink, *William Charles Wentworth*, p. 43.
10 Macquarie's diary, 12 Feb 1822, SLNSW: SAFE/A 775, pp. 6-8.
11 *The Sydney Gazette*, 15 Feb 1822.
12 Macquarie to Bathurst, 27 Jul 1822, HRA, X, pp. 671-701.
13 *The Morning Advertiser*, 27 Jul 1822.
14 *The Public Ledger and Daily Advertiser*, 2 Aug 1822.
15 *John Bull*, 4 Aug 1822.
16 J. Macarthur Jr to his mother, 18 Aug 1822, SLNSW: SAFE/A 2911, pp. 157-167.
17 *John Bull*, 18 Aug 1822.
18 Editor of John Bull, 25 Aug 1822, SLNSW: Ar 17.
19 J. Macarthur Jr to his mother, 18 Aug 1822, SLNSW: SAFE/A 2911, pp. 157-167.
20 Redfern to Bigge, 5 Feb 1821, TNA: CO 201/124, p. 192.
21 *The British Press*, 17 Sep 1822.
22 Mar 1821, PRONI: D3688/F/24.
23 Matriculation, 1822, SLNSW: MLMSS 7230.
24 Eagar to Bathurst, 6 Nov 1822, TNA: CO 202/111, pp. 222-290.
25 Horton, 1 Jan 1823, HRA, Series IV, Vol I, pp. 422-423.
26 Redfern to Wentworth, 3 Sep 1822, SLNSW: SAFE/A 754/1, pp. 139-141.
27 Bigge to Horton, 9 Dec 1822, TNA: M791, D3155, pp. 184-185.
28 Bigge to Horton, 12 Dec 1822, TNA: CO 201/142, pp. 243-246.
29 Redfern to Horton, 10 Dec 1822, TNA: CO 201/111, pp. 568-570.
30 Bigge on Redfern, 4 Feb 1823, SLNSW: BT 28, pp. 7038-7041.
31 *The Sun*, 10 Feb 1823.
32 Ann Redfern's burial, 17 May 1823, Wiltshire & Swindon Archives: 608/25.
33 Ann Redfern's will, 1823, Wiltshire & Swindon Archives: P1/1823/38.

NOTES

34. Bigge, *State of Agriculture and Trade*, pp. 13, 105-109.
35. Ibid.
36. Eagar to Bathurst, 3 Apr 1823, HRA, Series IV, Vol I, pp. 441-442.
37. W. Wentworth to his father, Feb 1823, SLNSW: A 756, p. 215.
38. Wentworth, *Australasia*, SLNSW: DSM/A821/W.
39. New South Wales Jurisdiction Bill, 2, 7 Jul 1823, HC Deb, Vol 9, cc 1400-1405, 1447-1452.
40. *The Times*, 7, 10 Jul 1823.
41. Macquarie's journal, 14 Jul 1823, SLNSW: SAFE/A 776/1, p. 139.
42. Macquarie, *Letter from Macquarie to Bathurst*, p. 25.
43. Ellis, *Lachlan Macquarie*, p. 514.
44. Macquarie, *Letter from Macquarie to Bathurst*.
45. Redfern to Ovens, 3 Sep 1824, SANSW: NRS 899, [4/1839A, No 808, p. 308], Fiche 3107.
46. Sarah Redfern to Bathurst, 18 Oct 1823, TNA: CO 201/47, pp. 274-275.
47. *The Monitor*, 11 Aug 1826.
48. E. Macquarie to S. Redfern, 9 Feb 1824, SLNSW: MLMSS 2381.
49. Wentworth, *Statistical Account of the British Settlements*, pp. 350, 388-389.
50. Wentworth, *Statistical Account of the British Settlements*, p. 383.
51. Sarah Redfern to Bathurst, 23 Oct 1823, TNA: CO 201/47, pp. 274-275.
52. Sarah Redfern to Bathurst, 13 Jan 1824, TNA: CO 201/157, pp. 33-34; Horton to Brisbane, 23 Jan 1824, HRA, XI, p. 202.
53. *The Sydney Gazette*, 10 Jul 1823.
54. *The Sydney Gazette*, 22 Jul 1824.
55. *The Australian*, 24 Nov 1825.
56. *The Sydney Gazette*, 22 Jul 1824.
57. *The Australian*, 24 Nov 1825.

CHAPTER 19 – A New Governor

1. *The Australian*, 26 Oct 1825.
2. Bathurst to Brisbane, 9 Sep 1822, HRA, X, pp. 784-790.
3. Butlin, *Foundation of Australian Monetary System*, pp. 151-152.
4. Brisbane to Bathurst, 1 May 1824, HRA, XI, pp. 254-258.
5. Warrant Appointing a Council, 1 Dec 1823, HRA, XI, p.p. 195-196.
6. The stone cottage is known as 'The Jug site or former Vineyards'; Heritage NSW: 5045745; wikipedia.org/wiki/Stone_Cottage,_Minto.
7. *The Sydney Gazette*, 22 Jul 1824.
8. *The Sydney Gazette*, 6 May 1824, 16 Jun 1825.
9. Redfern to Ovens, 25 Aug, 3 Sep 1824, SANSW: NRS 899, [4/1839A No 808, pp. 299-315], Fiche 3107.
10. Redfern to Brisbane, 1 Nov 1824, SANSW: NRS 899, [4/1839A No 808, pp. 291-298], Fiche 3107.
11. Ibid.
12. Land granted, 6 Nov 1824, SANSW: NRS 898, [9/2740, p. 25], Fiche 3269.
13. *The Sydney Gazette*, 16 Sep 1824.
14. *The Australian*, 14 Oct 1824.
15. Brisbane to Bathurst, 12 Jan 1825, HRA, XI, pp. 470-471.

NOTES

16. *The Australian*, 6 Jan 1825.
17. *The Australian*, 28 Oct 1824.
18. Ibid.
19. Walsh, *In Her Own Words*, pp. 168, 178.
20. Ibid.
21. *The Australian*, 18 Nov 1824.
22. *The Sydney Gazette*, 18 Nov 1824.
23. *The Colonist*, 5 Feb 1835.
24. *The Sydney Gazette*, 13 Jan 1825.
25. *The Sydney Gazette*, 27 Jan 1825.
26. *The Australian*, 3 Feb 1825.
27. Robert Redfern to Bathurst, 3 Jul 1824, TNA: CO 201/160, p. 248.
28. *The Sydney Gazette*, 10 Mar 1825.
29. Land granted, 25 Mar 1825, SANSW: NRS 898, [9/2740, p. 25], Fiche 3269; Redfern's Will, 1828, SLNSW: A 5407.
30. *The Australian*, 28 Apr 1825.
31. Bathurst to Brisbane, 22 Jul 1824, HRA, XI, pp. 321-322.
32. Brisbane to Horton, 24 Mar 1825, HRA, XI, pp. 552-553.
33. Redfern's will, SLNSW: MLMSS 2381; *The Sydney Gazette*, 7 Jul 1825.
34. *The Australian*, 14 Jul 1825.
35. *The Australian*, 28 Jul 1825.
36. *The Sydney Gazette*, 1 Sep 1825.
37. *The Sydney Gazette*, 17 Oct 1825.
38. *The Sydney Gazette*, 27 Oct 1825.
39. *The Australian*, 20 Oct 1825.
40. *The Australian*, 27 Oct 1825.
41. Scott to Bathurst, 5 Nov 1825, TNA: CO 201/168, pp. 202-203.
42. *The Australian*, 27 Oct 1825.
43. Ibid.
44. *The Colonial Times and Tasmanian Advertiser*, 2 Dec 1825.
45. 5 Nov 1825, SANSW: NRS 899, [4/1844A, No 681, p. 175], Fiche 3152; 14 Nov 1825, NRS 898, [2/1925, p. 19], Fiche 3260.
46. *The Sydney Gazette*, 3 Nov 1825.
47. *The Australian*, 6 Oct 1825.
48. *The Australian*, 10 Nov 1825.
49. *The Sydney Gazette*, 10 Nov 1825.
50. Petition to Bathurst, 30 Dec 1825, TNA: CO 201/179, pp. 220-221.
51. *The Sydney Gazette*, 1 Dec 1825.
52. Proclamation, 20 Dec 1825, HRA, XII, p. 128.

CHAPTER 20 – Fractious Times

1. *The Sydney Gazette*, 26 Nov 1827.
2. *The Sydney Gazette*, 16 Jan 1826.
3. Darling reply, 19 Jan 1826, HRA, XII, pp. 147-148.
4. Darling to Hay, 10 Dec 1825, 1 Feb 1826, TNA: CO 323/146, pp. 129-137.
5. Bathurst to Brisbane, 18 May 1825, HRA, XI, p. 591; *The Australian*, 24 Dec 1825.

NOTES

6. *The Sydney Gazette*, 22 Dec 1825.
7. *The Sydney Gazette*, 1 Mar 1826; *The Australian*, 15 Apr 1826.
8. *The Sydney Gazette*, 1 Mar 1826.
9. Ibid.
10. *The Sydney Gazette*, 22 Mar 1826.
11. *The Sydney Gazette*, 29 Apr 1826.
12. The cashier's receipt of William Redfern's payment of £80 for the second instalment on four bank shares was sold at auction in June 2022.
13. Bank of NSW, 11-12 May 1826, HRA, XII, pp. 299-306.
14. *The Sydney Gazette*, 2 Aug, 30 Dec 1826.
15. *The Sydney Gazette*, 6 Sep 1826.
16. *The Sydney Gazette*, 6 Jun 1818.
17. *The Sydney Gazette*, 3 Jun 1826; *The Monitor*, 9 Jun 1826.
18. *The Australian*, 28 Jun 1826.
19. *The Sydney Gazette*, 21 Jun 1826.
20. *The Sydney Gazette*, 12 Aug 1826.
21. *The Monitor*, 14 Jul 1826.
22. *The Australian*, 5, 9 Aug 1826.
23. *The Sydney Gazette*, 12 Aug 1826.
24. Ibid.
25. *The Sydney Gazette*, 6 Sep 1826.
26. Ibid.
27. Forbes, 15 Dec 1826, HRA, XII, p. 764; *The Australian*, 27 Jan 1827.
28. *The Sydney Gazette*, 19, 20 Jan 1827.
29. *The Sydney Gazette*, 27, 31 Jan 1827; *The Australian*, 27 Jan 1827.
30. SANSW: NRS 12992, Reel 1570; *The Colonial Times*, 22 Jun 1827.
31. *The Sydney Gazette*, 16 May 1827.
32. *The Morning Register*, 20 Oct 1827.
33. *The Australian*, 10 Mar 1827; *The Monitor*, 8 Nov 1827.
34. *The Australian*, 15 Jun 1827; *The Monitor*, 10 Jul 1827.
35. *The Australian*, 11 Jul 1827; *The Monitor*, 12 Jul 1827.
36. Dermody, *D'Arcy Wentworth*, pp. 398-399, 406-407.
37. *The Sydney Gazette*, 12 Jan 1827.
38. *Alexander Kenneth McKenzie*, Australian Dictionary of Biography.
39. *The Sydney Gazette*, 9, 18, 23 Jul 1827.
40. Bathurst to Darling, 1 Dec 1826, HRA, XII, pp. 702-703.
41. *The Monitor*, 11 May 1827; Darling to Horton, 15 Dec 1826, HRA, XII, pp. 761-763.
42. W. C. Wentworth's letters, Nov 1825, SLNSW: SAFE/A 1440, pp. 200-203.
43. *The Sydney Gazette*, 15 Feb 1828.
44. *The Sydney Gazette*, 29 Nov 1826, 15 Feb 1828.
45. Pockley, *Ancestor Treasure Hunt*, p. 24.
46. *The Sydney Gazette*, 7 Nov 1827; *The Australian*, 9 Nov 1827; *Alexander Kenneth Mckenzie*, Australian Dictionary of Biography
47. *The Sydney Gazette*, 21 Nov 1827.
48. *The Sydney Gazette*, 23 Nov 1827.
49. *The Sydney Gazette*, 26 Nov 1827; *The Monitor*, 24 Jan 1828.
50. *The Sydney Gazette*, 26 Nov 1827, 15 Feb 1828; *The Monitor*, 24 Jan 1828.

NOTES

51 *The Sydney Gazette*, 30 Nov 1827.
52 *The Monitor*, 3 Dec 1827.
53 Ibid.
54 *The Monitor*, 3 Dec 1827.
55 Ibid.
56 *The Sydney Gazette*, 29 Nov 1827, 15 Feb 1828.
57 *The Sydney Gazette*, 14 Dec 1827.
58 *The Australian*, 14 Dec 1827.
59 *The Sydney Gazette*, 17, 19 Dec 1827.
60 *The Monitor*, 20 Dec 1827.
61 *The Monitor*, 24 Dec 1827.
62 *The Australian*, 23 Jan 1828.
63 *The Australian*, 23 Jan 1828; *The Monitor*, 24 Jan 1828.
64 *The Sydney Gazette*, 23 Jan 1828; *The Australian*, 23 Jan 1828.
65 *The Sydney Gazette*, 23 Jan 1828.
66 *The Monitor*, 31 Jan 1828.
67 *The Sydney Gazette*, 4 Feb 1828.
68 *The Sydney Gazette*, 17 Feb 1828.

CHAPTER 21 – Edinburgh Finale

1 E. Macquarie to S. Redfern, 9 Sep 1833, SLNSW: MLMSS 7230.
2 *The Colonial Advocate*, 1 May 1828.
3 *The Australian*, 9 Jan 1828.
4 *The Monitor*, 14 Jan 1828.
5 *The Sydney Gazette*, 10 Mar 1828; *The Standard*, 24 Jul 1828; *The London Courier and Evening Gazette*, 26 Nov 1828.
6 *The Sydney Gazette*, 3 Jan 1829.
7 11 Apr 1828, TNA: PRIS10, Piece 056.
8 *The Sydney Monitor*, 3 Jan 1829.
9 20 Jun 1828, HC Deb: Vol 19, pp. 1456-1463; *The Sydney Monitor*, 3 Jan 1829.
10 E. Macquarie to S. Redfern, 21 Dec 1828, SLNSW: MLMSS 2381.
11 Ibid.
12 *The Sydney Gazette*, 27 Jan 1829.
13 W.L.M. Redfern to his mother, 20 Nov 1828, SLNSW: MLMSS 7230.
14 Ibid.
15 Ibid.
16 *The Times*, 21 Nov 1828.
17 Porter, Bertha, *Hosking, William, Dictionary of National Biography*, Vol 27, pp. 395-397.
18 Venn, J. A., *Alumni Cantabrigienses*, Vol 6, Part II, Cambridge, 1954, p. 511.
19 *The Times*, 14 Dec 1830.
20 E. Macquarie to W. Wentworth, undated, SLNSW: SAFE/A 757, pp. 95-97.
21 E. Macquarie to Fitzgerald, 12 Jul 1829, Walsh, *In Her Own Words*, pp. 201-202.
22 *Scottish Post Office Directories*, Edinburgh, 1829-30, p. 147.
23 Muster, Nov 1828, SANSW: NRS 1272, Reel 2555; *The Australian*, 12 Dec 1842.

NOTES

24 Redfern family papers, SLNSW: MLMSS 2381; *Sydney General Trade List*, 29 Aug 1829.
25 Edinburgh City Archive: SL 127/5/1.
26 *The Sydney Monitor*, 3 Jan 1829.
27 *The Sydney Gazette*, 31 Jan 1829.
28 E. Macquarie to W. Wentworth, 10 Jul 1829, SLNSW: SAFE/A 757, p. 29.
29 E. Macquarie to W. Wentworth, undated, SLNSW: SAFE/A 757, pp. 95-97.
30 Ibid.
31 Ellis, *John Macarthur*, p. 528.
32 *The Bulletin*, 5 Aug 1961.
33 Jones, *Surgeon William Redfern in London and Edinburgh*, p. 208.
34 Ritchie, *Punishment and Profit*; Ritchie, *Australia as once we were*, William Heinemann, 1975, p. 64.
35 Ritchie, *Lachlan Macquarie*, pp. 217-218.
36 Jones, *William Redfern, mutineer to colonial surgeon*, part II, p. 83.
37 Jones, *Surgeon William Redfern in London and Edinburgh*, pp. 201-211.
38 University of Edinburgh Matriculation Album, 1829-1830.
39 *The Medical Calendar or Students' Guide to the Medical Schools*, pp. 3-52.
40 *The Caledonian Mercury*, 21 Oct, 23 Nov 1833.
41 *Scottish Post Office Directories*, Edinburgh, 1832-33, pp. 49, 108; *The Edinburgh Evening Courant*, 16 May, 3 Sep, 29 Oct, 14 Nov 1829.
42 *The Monitor*, 5 May 1830.
43 Died 9 Apr 1830, buried 11 Apr 1830, SLNSW: SAG 90, No 512.
44 Gravestone inscription, SLNSW: B 765, p. 65. The remains and stone were removed in 1901 to La Perouse cemetery.
45 *The Edinburgh Academy Register*, Edinburgh, 1914, p. 52.
46 Jones, *Better than Cure*, Vol II, p. 400.
47 *The Times*, 9 Dec 1830.
48 W.L.M. Redfern to his mother, 11 Apr 1831, SLNSW: MLMSS 7230.
49 Ibid.
50 Ibid.
51 Calculated from known land grants and land purchases.
52 25 Jun 1832, SANSW: NRS 5869, [2/3253]; *The Sydney Gazette*, 3 Jul 1832.
53 Portraits of Sarah and William Redfern, courtesy of Damian Greenish; SLNSW: PXA 2144/Box 86, 84. Pic.Acc.2406.
54 Redfern to H. Wills, 31 Oct 1832, SLNSW: MLMSS7230.
55 *The Currency Lad*, 25 Aug 1832; *The Sydney Gazette*, 4 Jul, 18 Dec 1832.
56 *The Sydney Gazette*, 7 Mar 1833.
57 23 Jul 1833, Parish burial register, NRS: 692/2, p. 225.
58 *The Morning Advertiser*, 24 Jul 1833.
59 *The Sydney Gazette*, 26 Dec 1833.

EPILOGUE

1 Redfern estate papers, SLNSW: A 5407.
2 *The Caledonian Mercury*, 21 Oct, 23 Nov 1833; Glasgow court, 15 Nov 1834, NRS: SC36/48/24.
3 *The Sydney Gazette*, 17 Mar, 12, 16 Jun 1834.

NOTES

4 Redfern estate papers, SLNSW: A 5407.
5 *The Sydney Herald*, 3 Jan 1842; Redfern estate papers, SLNSW: A 5407; Bathurst map, 1832, NLA: MAP RaA 8 Plate 5; Redfern estate maps, SLNSW: Z/M3 812.26/1841/1 and Z/M3 812.25/1869/1.
6 *The Sydney Morning Herald*, 31 Jan, 5 Sep, 26 Dec 1842; Redfern estate papers, SLNSW: A 5407; Redfern estate Sydney, SLNSW: Z/M3 811.174/ 1842/1.
7 Report on the Redfern Estate, 1883, SLNSW: HQ 2014/1684.
8 NRS: Barony, Ref 180/255.
9 TNA: Probate 1878.
10 *The Kent & Sussex Courier*, 29 Jul 1904.
11 Sayers, C.E, *Horatio Spencer Howe Wills*, Australian Dictionary of Biography.
12 Antill, J. M., and Antill-De Warren, R., *The Emancipist*.
13 NFSA: *The Outcasts*, ABC, 1961.
14 *The Australian Women's Weekly*, 21 Jun 1961.
15 *The Bulletin*, 5 Aug 1961.
16 *The Bulletin*, 19 Aug 1961.

INDEX

Abbott, Edward, 79
ABC television
　The Outcasts series, 297, 310
Aboriginal people, 92, 175, 220, 221, 309
Abraham, Esther, 57
Act of 1823, 249, 250, 276, 284, 288
Act of 1824, 250, 271
Act of 1828, 290
Active, ship, 128
Admiral Gambier, ship, 99-101
Advertiser, ship, 251
AFPHM (Australasian Faculty of Public Health Medicine), 311
　William Redfern Oration, 141, 311
Ainslie, Maria, 68, 74, 100, 119, 278
Airds, 121, 130, 132, 159, 179, 190, 197, 200, 220, 221, 226
Albion, ship, 71, 95
Alexander, James, 307-308
Alexander, Sarah Jr, 307
Alfred, ship, 252-254, 257
Andrews, Thomas, 143
Antill, Eliza (Wills), 124, 133, 175, 183, 231, 294, 310
Antill, Henry, 109, 113, 121, 126, 130, 142, 155, 159, 161, 181, 183, 187, 200, 206, 215, 226, 230, 234, 257, 261, 307, 310
Antill, John Macquarie, 47, 123, 310
Antill-de Warren, Rose, 47, 123, 310
Aris, James, 33, 34
Arnold, Joseph, 113, 149, 161-163
Atkins, Richard, 79, 82
Australian Agricultural Society, 205, 271
Balmain, William, 50, 57, 60
Bank of Australia, 271, 278
Bank of NSW 173, 174, 182, 183, 218, 236, 271, 272, 278-280, 283, 285, 287
Banks, Joseph, 77
Barry, Marie Ann, 280
Bathurst, 157, 158, 259
Bathurst, Lord, 133, 136-140, 144, 146, 149, 150, 160, 161, 164, 166, 176-191, 196, 198, 200, 207-210, 221, 237, 239, 242, 245-252, 258, 259, 262, 267, 269, 278
Belfast, 2, 15, 66, 245, 277, 300, 305
Bell, Archibald, 113, 276
Bell, Charles, 291
Benevolent Asylum, 273, 274
Benevolent Society, 103, 175, 273
Bennet, Henry Grey, 185, 209
Bent, Ellis, 109, 114, 129, 145, 151, 152, 154, 160-164, 166, 173
Bent, Jeffery, 145, 151, 152, 154, 160-164, 166, 173, 185, 209
Bevan, David, 132
Bible Society, 103, 175
Bigge Report, 204, 212, 213, 220, 239-245, 247, 250, 251, 254-257, 263, 268, 270, 297
Bigge, John, 23, 26, 185-187, 191-194, 196-217, 221-223, 225-230, 237-251, 255, 257, 261, 268, 297, 310
Black, John, 271
Bland, William, 167, 175, 230, 272-275, 294
Blane, Gilbert, 5
Blaxcell, Garnham, 81, 119, 168
Blaxland, Gregory, 121, 155, 169, 271, 276, 277
Blaxland, John, 134
Bligh, William, 11-13, 17, 77-83, 86-90, 92-95, 97-101, 105, 107-111, 114, 115, 117, 124, 154, 177, 216
Bodie, Alexander, 128
Bohan, William, 91, 230
Bowden, Matthew, 159
Bowen, John, 61
Bowman, James, 178, 187, 190-200, 202, 206, 208-213, 216-217, 225-228, 251, 256, 260, 268, 273, 274
Brisbane, Thomas, 233, 254-256, 258-259, 261, 263, 265-269, 290
Broughton, William, 75, 81, 129, 160
Browne, William, 266
Broxbournebury, ship, 145

346

INDEX

Brumlow, William, 43
Burdett, Francis, 31-33
Burrows, John, 19, 26, 28
Campbell, John, 129, 142, 143, 156, 159, 161, 167, 174, 187, 259, 261, 280
Campbelltown, 122, 221, 258, 309
Canning, George, 249
Caroline, ship, 234
Carter, John, 114
Cartwright, Robert, 221
Castlereagh, Lord, 91, 107, 109, 112, 117, 183, 196, 242, 243
Catherine, ship, 143
Ceres, ship, 143-144
Cheeseman, Thomas, 22, 23, 25
Cimitiere, Gilbert, 232
Clark, Manning, 51
Cleaveland, Thomas, 121
Collins, David, 63, 85, 101, 111, 114, 214
Connellan, John, 74, 80
Connery, Bartholomew, 18
Cookney, Charles, 73
Cooper, Daniel, 224, 266
Cowper, Henry, 150, 153, 164, 184, 189, 194-196, 202-204, 207, 210, 217, 227, 228, 248
Cowper, William, 126, 132, 142, 150, 151, 153, 164, 175, 184, 187, 261
Cox, Sarah, 258
Cox, William, 155, 157, 159, 276
Crossley, George, 154
Crowley, Catherine, 68
Cullin-la-ringo, 309
Cummins, Cyril, 212
Darling, Ralph, 263, 268-273, 276, 278, 279, 288-289
Dart, ship, 62
Davis, Aaron, 75, 81
Davis, John, 18
Davis, Thomas, 71
Delafons, John, 20, 25
Denning, Isaac, 232-233
Despard, Edward, 30-32
Deuchar, John, 300
Diseases
    asthma, 62, 63, 71, 106, 128

cancer, 106
cold, 5, 60, 106, 220
dropsy, 128, 166
dysentery, 5, 58, 60, 61, 64, 116, 127, 128, 141, 144, 205, 210, 212
elephantiasis, 238, 273
fever, 5, 33, 41, 43, 60, 64, 128, 131, 210
haemorrhage, 128
influenza, 115, 220, 221, 277, 278
measles, 115, 290, 291
paralysis, 128
rheumatism, 5, 65, 107
scrofula, 106
scurvy, 5, 10, 41, 68, 141-144, 147
smallpox, 5, 70, 103, 104, 115, 220
tuberculosis, 80, 106
toothache, 5, 107
typhus, 5, 10, 37, 38, 116, 124, 128, 141, 145, 146
venereal, 5, 128
Dixon, Francis, 264
Dixon, John, 15
Dow, Gwyneth, 297
Dowling, James, 303
Doyle, James, 273
Druitt, George, 181, 200
Drummond, John, 78
Duchess of York, ship, 235, 237, 238
Dugan, James, 17
Duncan, Adam, 3, 4, 10, 13
Duncan, Thomas, 294
Dunlop, James, 255
Eagar, Edward, 154, 173, 174, 188, 214, 216-218, 222-224, 230, 235-240, 242, 243, 245, 247-250, 254, 257, 272-277, 284, 288, 289, 292
Eagar, Jemima, 257, 258
Earley, Henry, 43
Easton, Elizabeth, 132, 133, 234
Eddington, Margaret, 75
Edge, Mary, 83-84
Elder, James, 83-84
Elizabeth, ship, 173
Ellis, Malcolm, 213, 297, 310, 311
Erskine, James, 177, 181, 182, 187, 215

INDEX

Estramina, ship, 81, 84-86, 90, 94, 232
Evans, George, 153, 155, 157, 158, 215, 232, 233
Experiment, ship, 114
Farquhar, Walter, 177
Female School of Industry, 103
Field, Barron, 173, 177, 202, 208, 214, 217, 218, 222, 246
Finn, Bryan, 19, 26
Finucane, James, 89, 98
Fitzgerald, Hamilton, 19, 20, 24-25
Fitzpatrick, Jeremiah, 33-42, 45, 130, 253
Fitzwilliam, William Wentworth, 66, 67, 74, 94, 187
Forbes, Francis Ewen, 257, 272, 277, 292
Forbes, Francis, Chief Justice, 246, 256, 259, 303
Ford, Edward, 27
Fortune, ship, 136
Foster, Thomas, 143, 159, 171
Foveaux, Ann, 71
Foveaux, Joseph, 50-78, 80, 86-91, 94-98, 101, 102, 107-111, 114, 138, 215, 240, 242, 243, 247, 290
Francis and Eliza, ship, 165-166
Frederick, ship, 128
Freeman, Henry, 18
Frost, James, 164, 215
Fulton, Henry, 59, 87-90, 206, 222, 224
Garling, Frederick, 165, 166, 173
General Hewitt, ship, 141, 147, 148
Gilbert, John, 67, 68
Gill, John, 175
Gloves, Joseph, 19, 26
Gore, William, 119
Gorman, Thomas, 84
Goulburn, Frederick, 233, 255, 256
Gower, Erasmus, 18
Grant, John, 130, 179, 209
Griffin, Edmund, 88
Grose, Francis, 48-50, 75
Hall, Edward, 188, 202, 265, 266, 269, 271, 277, 283, 288
Harrex, James, 121
Harriet, ship, 176

Harris, John, 71, 82, 91, 100, 101, 141, 143, 167, 174, 215, 230
Harris, Samson, 18-19
Hassall, Roland, 155
Hatch, Jerimiah, 284
Hay, Robert, 269
Hayes, Michael, 74, 81
Hebe, ship, 221
Hillsborough, ship, 38, 123, 124
HMS *Bounty*, ship, 11, 77
HMS *Buffalo*, ship, 77
HMS *Dromedary*, ship, 107, 109, 111, 114, 229, 230
HMS *Glatton*, ship, 61
HMS *Hindostan*, ship, 107, 111, 113, 114, 161
HMS *Lady Nelson*, ship, 79, 81, 83, 130
HMS *Porpoise*, ship, 53, 77, 79, 81, 95, 97-101, 107, 111, 114, 138
HMS *Samarang*, ship, 134
HMS *Sirius*, ship, 48, 49
HMS *Supply*, ship, 48
Hobart, Lord, 68-70, 77
Holdsworth, William, 18, 20
Holt, Joseph, 51
Hook, Theodore, 243, 244
Hopley, William, 159, 165
Horton, Robert, 239, 241, 245-247, 252, 288
Hosking, John, 257, 292
Hosking, William, 292
Howe, George, 132, 133, 182, 231, 234, 235, 279, 303
Howe, Jane, 231, 234, 279
Howe, Richard, 8, 10
Howe, Robert, 132, 133, 234, 235, 274, 275, 279-288, 295, 304
Howe, Sarah. *See* Wills, Sarah
Hudson, Joseph, 19, 26, 28
Hughes, Richard, 141, 142
Hughes, Robert, 51
Hughes, Sarah, 75
Hunter, John, 48, 49, 78, 97
Hutchinson, William, 224, 257, 271
Indefatigable, ship, 162
Indian, ship, 125
Inett, Ann, 57

INDEX

Ingram, Archibald, 22, 25
Investigator, ship, 72
Irish Rebellion, 30, 35, 51, 53, 59
Ivory, Robert, 273
James, Thomas, 271
Jamison, John, 145, 156, 157, 159, 161, 188, 276
Jamison, Thomas, 57, 68, 71, 74, 75, 82, 86, 91-92, 94, 100, 101, 112, 145, 230
Jenkins, Robert, 134, 136, 167, 174
John Barry, ship, 192, 193, 197
John Bull, 243, 244
Johnston, George, 57, 82, 83, 87, 88, 90, 98-101, 108, 111, 114
Johnston, James, 32
Johnstone, William, 195, 196, 202-204, 248
Jones, Arthur, 297
Jones, Richard, 278
Jones, Robert, 51, 78
Jones, William, 18
Kable, Henry, 82, 214
Kelly, John, 39, 42-44
King George III, 13, 131, 250
King George IV, 243, 256
King Pomare, 237, 238, 273
King, Philip Gidley, 39, 46, 48-51, 53, 54, 57-59, 61-63, 69, 70, 72, 74, 76-78, 131, 155, 185
King, Richard, 18
Kirkwood, Robert, 4, 14, 20-24
Lady Elliot, ship, 171
Laforey, Francis, 18
Lawes, Ann, 119, 278
Lawson, William, 155, 169
Leith, John, 43
Lewin, John, 156
Lind, James, 5
Linniss, Thomas, 19, 26-28
Liverpool, 121, 132, 221
Liverpool, Earl of, 117, 133, 138, 164, 183
Lord Eldon, ship, 177, 178
Lord, Simeon, 73, 74, 78, 79, 82, 83, 86-88, 90, 96, 110, 112, 113, 115, 134, 163, 174, 188, 198, 200, 206, 207, 222, 224, 225, 265, 266, 269, 272, 276
Lowe, James, 39
Lowe, Robert, 206
Lunatic asylum, 129, 167
Luttrell, Edward, 100, 110, 136-141, 145, 149, 150, 153, 159, 165, 178, 214
Macarthur, Elizabeth, 105, 106
Macarthur, Elizabeth Jr, 105, 178, 242
Macarthur, John, 49, 50, 67, 75, 76, 78, 81-83, 87-90, 94, 97-101, 105, 106, 108, 124, 154, 177, 178, 188, 201, 202, 208, 213, 228, 229, 241, 242, 255, 260, 261, 265, 267-271, 276, 277, 297, 310
Macarthur, John Jr, 241, 243
Macarthur, Mary, 260
Mackeness, John, 253
Mackenzie, Alexander, 278, 280
Mackintosh, James, 249, 290
Mackneal, James, 119
Maclaine, John, 121, 130, 136, 142, 143, 145
Macquarie Bank of NSW, 285, 287
Macquarie, Elizabeth, 107, 113, 118, 120, 122, 130-132, 139, 155, 158, 159, 190, 221, 231, 232, 240, 242, 244, 245, 251, 259, 260, 287, 290, 292, 293, 295-297
Macquarie, Hector, 231
Macquarie, Lachlan, 95, 97, 102, 106-262, 267, 270, 273, 277, 278, 310
Macquarie, Lachlan Jr, 142, 143, 159, 175, 231
Markham, John, 18
Marsden, Anne, 105
Marsden, Samuel, 105, 115, 133, 151, 164, 175, 182, 209, 238, 278, 292
Mary and Sally, ship, 124, 133
Mather, George Marshall, 304
Matilda, ship, 177
McCann, Thomas, 42
McGuire, Elizabeth, 309
McHenry, James, 43, 47, 115
McHenry, Sarah, 43, 47, 56, 64, 71, 81, 84, 85, 92, 100, 111, 114
McHugo, Jonathan, 128, 129
McIntyre, James, 273

INDEX

McLoghlan, Arthur, 20
McNamara, Daniel, 190
Meehan, James, 121, 127, 130, 155, 158, 171, 221, 224, 272
Midas, ship, 231, 232
Mileham, James, 52-54, 75, 76, 82, 91, 100, 110, 120, 139, 149, 183, 215
Minto, 121, 179, 257
Mitchell, James, 74, 81
Mitchell, James, surgeon, 273
Molle, George, 142, 143, 161, 169, 170, 174, 176, 177, 216, 241
Moore, Thomas, 121, 206, 221
Moore, William, 154
Morisset, James, 181
Morris, John, 64
Morris, William, 20
Mountgarrett, Jacob, 61
Murphy, Jeremiah, 174
Murray, George, 289
Murray, Robert, 176
Mutiny at the Nore, 1, 7, 10-16, 27, 28, 42, 80, 95, 216
Mutiny ships
   HMS *Agamemnon*, 17
   HMS *Champion*, 17
   HMS *Comet*, 17
   HMS *Director*, 11, 15, 17, 95
   HMS *Gorgon*, 15
   HMS *Inflexible*, 17
   HMS *Isis*, ship, 17
   HMS *Lancaster*, 17
   HMS *Lion*, 17
   HMS *Marlborough*, 14
   HMS *Minotaur*, ship, 14
   HMS *Neptune*, 18, 23, 34
   HMS *Proserpine*, 17
   HMS *Pylades*, 17
   HMS *Ranger*, 17
   HMS *Sandwich*, 10, 11, 13, 18
   HMS *Standard*, 1-4, 6, 7, 12-23, 26-28, 34, 95, 138, 148, 230
   HMS *Swan*, 17
   HMS *Tysiphone*, 17
   HMS *Vestal*, 17
Nash, Samuel, 145
Native Institution, 103, 175
Neptune, ship, 67, 68

Norfolk Island, 47-85, 87, 88, 90, 95-97, 99, 101, 102, 111, 131, 179, 183, 233, 245, 263, 264, 270, 276
Norfolk, ship, 305
Northampton, ship, 160, 162
NSW Corps, 39, 41, 48-52, 57, 58, 62, 67, 70, 71, 73, 76-79, 82, 83, 87, 89, 91, 94, 95, 97, 100, 101, 107, 108, 110, 113, 115, 141
NSW Legislative Assembly, 309
NSW Legislative Council, 249, 250, 256, 268, 269, 276
O'Connell, Maurice, 109, 111
O'Connor, Bryan, 53, 54, 59, 62
Oakes, Francis, 79
Orelia, ship, 289
Orphan Institute, 103
Orphan school, 92, 131, 132, 187
Ovens, John, 258
Owen, Robert, 176, 184, 188, 195, 196, 202-204, 215
Oxley, John, 156, 159, 161, 242, 256
Paine, Thomas, 3, 262
Palmer, John, 88, 100
Parker, Richard, 11, 15, 18, 26, 162, 228
Parmeter, Thomas, 189
Parr, Thomas, 3, 13, 14, 17-22, 25-27, 148
Parramatta, 46, 71, 82, 91, 98, 100, 105, 107, 115, 119, 121, 128, 129, 132, 138, 155, 159, 178, 187, 202, 255, 266, 267, 278, 292
Parramatta hospital, 79, 86, 136, 140, 159, 165, 168
Parramatta, ship, 81
Pasley, Thomas, 18
Paterson, William, 48, 50, 70, 87, 89, 90, 94, 95, 97-104, 107-109, 115
Patton, Alexander, 66
Peel, Robert, 260
Pepys, Samuel, 8
Perceval, Spencer, 133
Pescott, Roger, 297
Philanthropic Society, 103, 175
Phillip, Arthur, 48, 75, 182, 261
Phoenix, hulk, 263
Phoenix, ship, 263, 264

INDEX

Piper, John, 70-72, 74, 75, 78, 79, 81, 83-86, 96, 131, 141, 161, 232
Pitt, ship, 50
Pitt, William, 4, 15, 31
Poldark, BBC series, 31
Power, Mary, 75, 84
Putland, John, 77, 79-81, 95
Putland, Mary, 77, 95
RACP (Royal Australasian College of Physicians), 3, 311
  William Redfern Oration, 141, 311
Raine, Thomas, 266
Ransome, Thomas, 78
Raven and *Eliza*, ship, 124
Reddall, Thomas, 221
Redfern Street, 308
Redfern Valley, 158
Redfern, Alexander & Co, 308
Redfern, Ann, sister-in-law, 245, 247
Redfern, Eliza (McDowell), sister, 2, 245, 307, 309
Redfern, Joseph, brother, 2, 35, 245, 294, 300, 305, 309
Redfern, Margaret (Watt), sister, 2, 245, 307, 309
Redfern, Margaret, mother, 2
Redfern, Robert Joseph Foveaux, 247, 284, 287, 291-295, 300- 302
Redfern, Robert, brother, 2, 15, 30, 35, 245, 262-263, 307, 309
Redfern, Robert, father, 2, 35, 247
Redfern, Sarah (Wills), 38, 123-126, 131, 132, 135, 142-144, 155, 158, 159, 168, 169, 171, 175, 181, 183, 189, 197, 221, 230, 231, 234-238, 244-247, 250-252, 254, 258, 259, 264, 278, 284, 287, 290-295, 300-308, 310
Redfern, suburb, 126, 308
Redfern, Thomas, brother, 2, 29, 35, 105, 162, 183, 245, 247
Redfern, Thomas, nephew, 105, 245

Redfern, William, Dr
  birth & education, 2, 3
  Company of Surgeons, 2-3, 229
  Hibernia, ship, 3
  surgeon's first mate, 3-8, 12-16
  mutiny trial, 17-28
  prison & hulks
    Coldbath Fields prison, 1, 29- 37, 41, 53, 74, 245, 295
    Captivity, hulk, 36
    La Fortunée, hulk, 36, 39
  transportation to NSW
    Canada, ship, 37-47, 238
    Minorca, ship, 37-47, 56, 62
    Nile, ship, 37-38, 41-44, 46
  Norfolk Island
    doctor, 52-61, 64-66, 70-73, 75, 80, 83-85
    Endeavour, ship, 84, 96
    farmer & trader, 55, 61, 64, 71-74, 78-81
    Harrington, ship, 47, 52, 72
    pardon, 59, 61
    partner. *See* McHenry, Sarah
  Sydney physician & surgeon
    convict inspection, 129, 130
    convict transportation reforms, 141-149, 228
    first medical examination, 91, 168, 230
    first medical student, 131, 151
    first quarantine camp, 146, 147
    hospital doctor, 88-96, 100, 103-107, 110-118, 123, 127-131, 136-138, 140-154, 159-166, 169-171, 175, 176, 183, 184, 187-190, 194-197
    medical board, 88, 89, 91, 138, 140, 141, 167, 230
    personal notebook, 3, 29, 30, 64, 65, 106, 107
    preventive medicine pioneer, 141
    private medical practise, 104, 114-116, 123, 143, 162, 175, 189, 190, 197, 210, 219, 265, 272-275
    prominent patients
      Bent, Ellis, 114, 162, 166
      Bligh, William, 95, 99
      Foveaux, Joseph, 62, 63, 71
      King Pomare, 238, 273
      Macarthur, Elizabeth Jr, 105, 106, 178, 241

351

INDEX

Maclaine, John, 136
Macquarie, Elizabeth, 131, 142-143, 244
Macquarie, Lachlan, 121, 171, 205, 260
Macquarie, Lachlan Jr, 178
Meehan, James, 121
Putland, John, 80, 81, 95
Redfern, Ann, 247
son William, 290-291, 302-303
Thompson, Andrew, 104, 120
Wentworth, D'Arcy, 228, 278
Wills, Edward Sn, 123, 125, 127
public dispensary, 273-275
agriculture
Bathurst, 218, 235, 259, 267, 308-309
Bringelly, 235, 308
Campbellfield, 130, 132, 150, 159, 179, 197, 218, 219, 221, 224, 235, 244, 252, 257-259, 275, 283, 287, 292, 294, 296, 303, 307-309
Sydney (Redfern), 126, 171, 307, 308
vineyard, 251, 257, 277
bank director & shares, 173, 174, 182, 183, 218, 236, 271, 272, 278-280, 283, 285
emancipist prejustice, 112, 113, 163, 181-183, 193, 194, 197-200, 208, 209, 225-230, 255
emancipist rights activist, 188, 218, 222-224, 234-237, 239, 243, 244, 249, 250, 254, 257, 265-267, 269, 276, 288, 289
magistrate, 190, 193, 198-200, 204, 206-209, 218, 221, 222, 225
marriage to Sarah Wills, 125, 126, *See* Redfern, Sarah (Wills)
personal health, 159, 160, 194, 251, 252, 264, 289, 291, 293, 295-298, 300, 303-306
philanthropy, 102, 103, 131, 132, 151, 168, 175, 187, 260, 275
travels
1810 West of Sydney, 120-122
1813 Blue Mountains, 155-159
1821 Tasmania, 230-234
1821, London, 237-253
1828, London, Edinburgh, 287-306
will, 264, 305, 307, 308

Redfern, William Lachlan Macquarie, 189, 190, 234, 244, 247, 272, 284, 287-295, 298, 299, 301, 303, 305-309
Redfern, William, nephew, 262
Reibey, Mary, 174
Reibey, Thomas, 124
Richardson, Cuthbert, 95
Rienits, Rex, 311
Riley, Alexander, 119, 139, 143, 160, 167, 168, 174, 189
Riou, Edward, 18
Ritchie, John, 297
Roberts, Thomas, 52, 53
Robinson, Henry, 232
Ross, Robert, 48
Rowley, Thomas, 50
Royal Navy, 3-10, 27
Channel Fleet, 4, 8-12, 15
North Sea Fleet, 3, 4, 10, 12-16
surgeons, 3-6, 10, 12, 14, 16, 90, 298, 303
Rümker, Carl, 255
Sael, Thomas, 18
Sarah, ship, 84
Savage, John, 70, 71, 76
Scarborough, ship, 68
Scott, Thomas, 192, 202, 207, 208, 268
Serown, Emanuel, 252, 257
Sheers, James, 131, 150, 151
Sheers, James Sr, 131
Sheers, Mary Ann, 75, 131, 141
Sherwin, Ann, 50, 57, 62, 71, 114
Sherwin, William, 50
Sidney, Algernon, 24
Sinclair, ship, 77, 88
Smellie, William, 2
Snipe, John, 10
Sorell, William, 232
Starr, Fiona, 213
Stephen, James, 245
Stephen, John, 266, 284

INDEX

Stewart, William, 256, 266, 267
Surprise, ship, 68
Surry, ship, 145-148, 242
Sydney hospital, George St, 88-94, 96, 103-106, 111-117, 123, 127-131, 140, 144, 150, 151, 153-155, 160, 161, 164, 166-168, 170, 171, 178
Sydney hospital, Macquarie St, 118, 119, 130, 151, 152, 154, 163, 166-170, 171, 175, 176, 184, 188-190, 194-197, 202-218, 225-227, 248, 260, 273, 274
Tattersall, Christopher, 197
Tawell, John, 164
Taylor, James, 231
Terry, Samuel, 134, 224, 271, 281
The Australian, 252, 259, 262, 263, 265, 274, 279
The Bulletin, 297, 310
The Caledonian Mercury, 40
The Colonial Advocate, 288
The Currency Lad, 305, 309
The Edinburgh Review, 250
The Gleaner, 279
The Hampshire Chronicle, 12
The London Chronicle, 12
The Monitor, 212, 274, 277, 279, 283, 288
The Morning Advertiser, 243
The Morning Post, 18
The Morning Register, 277
The Public Ledger and Daily Advertiser, 243
The Star, 34
The Statesman, 252
The Sun, 247
The Sydney Gazette, 61, 104, 111, 112, 119, 132, 133, 135, 151, 160, 179, 196, 200, 212, 220, 227, 230, 234, 242, 259, 264, 265, 269, 273-275, 277-280, 282, 283, 285, 287, 295, 304-306, 309
The Times, 239
The Whitehall Evening Post, 29
Thompson, Andrew, 88, 90, 96, 104, 110, 112, 113, 115, 120-122, 163, 201, 207
Thompson, William, 72

Thomson, Frederick, 99
Thomson, James, 57, 88
Three Bees, ship, 143-45, 147, 148
Throsby, Charles, 57, 58, 160
Tilley, James, 235, 244, 252
Trail, Donald, 68
Trotter, Thomas, 10, 28
Trowbridge, Wiltshire, 2, 35, 105, 106, 244, 247, 309
Underwood, James, 224
Underwood, Joseph, 235
Underwood, Michael, 105
Union, ship, 63
University of Edinburgh, 151, 245, 246, 289, 291, 297-300, 302, 303
University of London, 291
Van Diemen's Land, 45, 61, 63, 68, 74, 77, 83, 84, 87, 88, 97, 99, 101, 108, 130, 166, 183, 208, 214, 230, 231, 232, 234
Villiers, John, 67
Wakeman, William, 184
Walker, David, 305
Walker, Jane Bastable, 308
Wallace, William, 16
Wallis, John, 143
Wardell, Robert, 252, 253, 259, 262, 264, 276, 283, 285
Warlby, John, 121
Warrior, ship, 165
Watkins, William, 181
Watson, Frederick, 212
Watt, Andrew, brother-in-law, 309
Watt, Eliza, niece, 307
Watt, Hugh, nephew, 307, 309
Watt, William, nephew, 307, 309
Watts, John, 155, 175
Wellington, Duke of, 168, 289
Wentworth, D'Arcy, 55-58, 60, 61, 63, 66-75, 78-80, 82-88, 91, 94-96, 100, 102, 110, 112-115, 117-119, 121, 123, 128, 129, 131, 134, 139-141, 143, 145-147, 149-151, 153-155, 159, 162-171, 174-178, 181, 183, 184, 187-190, 194-198, 200, 202, 205-207, 210-212, 215, 217, 227, 228, 238, 241, 246, 266, 267, 269, 276-278, 288, 289

INDEX

Wentworth, D'Arcy Jr, 68
Wentworth, John, 68
Wentworth, William, 68, 119, 155, 169, 170, 187, 193, 213, 216, 217, 239, 241, 242, 245, 248, 249, 251-253, 257-260, 262, 264-266, 269, 276, 278, 281-285, 288, 293, 295, 296, 306, 307
West, Major, 165-168, 215
Western, Charles, 250
Whalan, Charles, 221
Whitaker, Anne-Maree, 51
Wilkinson, Mary, 67
Wilkinson, William, 41, 43-45
Willey, Emily, 244, 251, 252, 257
Willey, Selina, 244, 251, 252, 257
Wills, Edward, 38, 123-127, 132, 133, 231, 234
Wills, Edward Jr, 124, 235, 292, 295, 296, 302
Wills, Eliza. *See* Antill, Eliza (Wills)
Wills, Elizabeth, 124, 125
Wills, Horatio, 127, 133, 234, 279-283, 285-287, 295, 304-306, 309
Wills, Sarah. *See* Redfern, Sarah (Wills)
Wills, Sarah (Harding)/Howe, 38, 123-127, 132, 133, 178, 182, 231, 234, 235, 303, 304
Wills, Thomas, 124, 133, 182, 183, 235, 257, 279, 280, 282, 287, 307, 309
Wilson, Ralph, 62-64
Wright, Brian, 310
Wright, Reg, 51
Wylde, Thomas, 167, 173, 174, 176, 177, 198, 214, 222, 232
Yarmouth, 3, 4, 7, 10, 12, 13
Younge, Henry St. John, 140, 149, 150, 159, 166

www.ingramcontent.com/pod-product-compliance
Lightning Source LLC
Chambersburg PA
CBHW032025290426
44110CB00012B/675